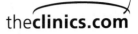

CARDIOLOGY CLINICS

Ventricular Arrhythmias

GUEST EDITOR
John M. Miller, MD

CONSULTING EDITOR
Michael H. Crawford, MD

August 2008 • Volume 26 • Number 3

SAUNDERS

An Imprint of Elsevier, Inc.
PHILADELPHIA   LONDON   TORONTO   MONTREAL   SYDNEY   TOKYO

W.B. SAUNDERS COMPANY
A Division of Elsevier Inc.

Elsevier Inc. • 1600 John F. Kennedy Blvd., Suite 1800 • Philadelphia, Pennsylvania 19103-2899

http://www.theclinics.com

CARDIOLOGY CLINICS   Volume 26, Number 3
August 2008   ISSN 0733-8651
Editor: Barbara Cohen-Kligerman   ISBN-13: 978-1-4160-6275-2
ISBN-10: 1-4160-6275-0

Cardiology Clinics (ISSN 0733-8651) is published quarterly by Elsevier Inc., 360 Park Avenue South, New York, NY 10010-1710. Months of issue are February, May, August, and November. Business and editorial Offices: 1600 John F. Kennedy Blvd., Suite 1800, Philadelphia, PA 19103-2899. Customer Service Office: 6277 Sea Harbor Drive, Orlando, FL 32887-4800. Periodicals postage paid at New York, NY, and additional mailing offices. Subscription prices are $226.00 per year for US individuals, $344.00 per year for US institutions, $113.00 per year for US students and residents, $276.00 per year for Canadian individuals, $418.00 per year for Canadian institutions, $301.00 per year for international individuals, $418.00 per year for international institutions and $150.00 per year for Canadian and foreign students/residents. To receive student/resident rate, orders must be accompanied by name of affiliated institution, data of term, and the *signature* of program/residency coordinator on institution letterhead. Orders will be billed at individual rate until proof of status is received. Foreign air speed delivery is included in all *Clinics* subscription prices. All prices are subject to change without notice. POSTMASTER: Send address changes to *Cardiology Clinics*, Elsevier Periodicals Customer Service, 6277 Sea Harbor Drive, Orlando, FL 32887-4800. **Customer Service: 1-800-654-2452 (US). From outside of the US, call 1- 407-563-6020. Fax: 1-407-363-9661. E-mail:** JournalsCustomerService-usa@elsevier.com.

Reprints. For copies of 100 or more of articles in this publication, please contact the Commercial Reprints Department, Elsevier Inc., 360 Park Avenue South, New York, NY 10010-1710. Tel.: 212-633-3812; Fax: 212-462-1935; E-mail: reprints@elsevier.com.

Cardiology Clinics is also published in Spanish by McGraw-Hill Interamericana Editores S. A., P.O. Box 5-237, 06500, Mexico D. F., Mexico; in Portuguese by Reichmann and Alfonso Editores Rio de Janeiro, Brazil; and in Greek by Dimitrios P. Lagos, 8 Pondon Street, GR115-28 Ilissia, Greece.

Cardiology Clinics is covered in *Index Medicus, Excerpta Medica, The Cumulative Index to Nursing and Allied Health Literature* (CINAHL).

Printed in the United States of America.

CONSULTING EDITOR

MICHAEL H. CRAWFORD, MD, Professor of Medicine, University of California San Francisco; Lucie Stern Chair in Cardiology, and Interim Chief of Cardiology, University of California San Francisco Medical Center, San Francisco, California

GUEST EDITOR

JOHN M. MILLER, MD, Professor of Medicine, Indiana University School of Medicine, Krannert Institute of Cardiology, Indianapolis, Indiana

CONTRIBUTORS

KELLEY P. ANDERSON, MD, FHRS, FACC, FACP, Clinical Associate Professor of Medicine, Department of Cardiology, Marshfield Clinic, University of Wisconsin Medical School, Marshfield, Wisconsin

CARLO DE ASMUNDIS, MD, Heart Rhythm Management Institute, University Hospital Brussels, Brussels, Belgium

TIM BOUSSY, MD, Heart Rhythm Management Institute, University Hospital Brussels, Brussels, Belgium

JOSEP BRUGADA, MD, PhD, Thorax Institute, Hospital Clinic University of Barcelona, Barcelona, Spain

PEDRO BRUGADA, MD, PhD, Heart Rhythm Management Institute, University Hospital Brussels, Brussels, Belgium

RAMON BRUGADA, MD, PhD, Montreal Heart Institute, Montreal Quebec, Canada

DAVID J. CALLANS, MD, Professor of Medicine, Department of Medicine, Cardiovascular Medicine Division; and Associate Director, Electrophysiology, University of Pennsylvania Health System, Hospital of the University of Pennsylvania, Philadelphia, Pennsylvania

GIAN BATTISTA CHIERCHIA, MD, Heart Rhythm Management Institute, University Hospital Brussels, Brussels, Belgium

GOPI DANDAMUDI, MD, Krannert Institute of Cardiology, Indiana University School of Medicine, Indianapolis, Indiana

MITHILESH K. DAS, MD, MRCP, FACC, Associate Professor of Medicine, Krannert Institute of Cardiology, Chief of Cardiac Arrhythmia Service, Roudebush VA Medical Center, Indiana University School of Medicine, Indianapolis, Indiana

JOHN P. DIMARCO, MD, PhD, Department of Internal Medicine, Cardiovascular Division, University of Virginia Health System, Charlottesville, Virginia

SANJAY DIXIT, MD, Assistant Professor of Medicine, Department of Medicine, Cardiovascular Medicine Division, Hospital of the University of Pennsylvania, Philadelphia, Pennsylvania

MICHAEL R. GOLD, MD, PhD, Michael E. Assey Professor of Medicine and Director, Division of Cardiology, Medical University of South Carolina, Charleston, South Carolina

STEFAN H. HOHNLOSER, MD, FHRS, FACC, FESC, Department of Medicine, Division of Cardiology, Clinical Electrophysiology Section, J.W. Goethe University, Frankfurt, Germany

HENRY H. HSIA, MD, FACC, Associate Professor of Medicine, Division of Cardiovascular Medicine, Stanford University School of Medicine, Cardiac Electrophysiology and Arrhythmia Service, Stanford University Medical Center, Stanford, California

JOSE F. HUIZAR, MD, Assistant Professor of Medicine, Virginia Commonwealth University Medical Center; Director, Arrhythmia and Device Clinic, Hunter Holmes McGuire VA Medical Center, Richmond, Virginia

KAROLY KASZALA, MD, PhD, Assistant Professor of Medicine, Virginia Commonwealth University Medical Center; Director, Cardiac Electrophysiology Laboratory, Hunter Holmes McGuire VA Medical Center, Richmond, Virginia

MATTHEW H. KLEIN, MD, Cardiology Fellow, Division of Cardiology, Medical University of South Carolina, Charleston, South Carolina

MARCIN KOWALSKI, MD, Fellow, Department of Cardiac Electrophysiology, Virginia Commonwealth University Medical Center, Richmond, Virginia

FRED KUSUMOTO, MD, Professor of Medicine, Electrophysiology and Pacing Service, Division of Cardiovascular Diseases, Department of Medicine, Mayo Clinic School of Medicine, Jacksonville Florida

SHUAIB LATIF, MD, Fellow, Department of Medicine, Cardiovascular Medicine Division, Hospital of the University of Pennsylvania, Philadelphia, Pennsylvania

RONALD LO, MD, Electrophysiology Fellow, Division of Cardiovascular Medicine, Stanford University School of Medicine, Cardiac Electrophysiology and Arrhythmia Service, Stanford University Medical Center, Stanford, California

PAMELA K. MASON, MD, Department of Internal Medicine, Cardiovascular Division, University of Virginia Health System, Charlottesville, Virginia

L. BRENT MITCHELL, MD, FRCPC, Libin Cardiovascular Institute of Alberta and Department of Cardiac Sciences, Calgary Health Region and University of Calgary, Foothills Hospital, Calgary, Alberta, Canada

GAETANO PAPARELLA, MD, Heart Rhythm Management Institute, University Hospital Brussels, Brussels, Belgium

ANDREA SARKOZY, MD, Heart Rhythm Management Institute, University Hospital Brussels, Brussels, Belgium

HILLEL STEINER, MD, Krannert Institute of Cardiology, Indiana University School of Medicine, Indianapolis, Indiana

MARK A. WOOD, MD, Professor of Medicine, Co-Director, Department of Cardiac Electrophysiology, Virginia Commonwealth University Medical Center Richmond, Virginia

CONTENTS

> Investigations of the impact of ventricular arrhythmias in populations have focused primarily on two aspects, ventricular ectopic activity and sudden cardiac death (SCD). The observation that coronary heart disease (CHD) is an important background of death due to ventricular tachyarrhythmia (VTA) remains the dominant belief today. The evidence supports the principle that reduction of deaths due to VTA is multifactorial and results from improved primary prevention, treatment of CHD complications, and secondary prevention. Recent evidence for unfavorable trends for SCD and CHD mortality raises the specter of a reversal in the gains made against fatal VTA in recent decades.

> Sudden cardiac death caused by malignant ventricular arrhythmias is the most important cause of death in the industrialized world. Most of these lethal arrhythmias occur in the setting of ischemic heart disease. A significant number of sudden deaths, especially in young individuals, are caused by inherited ventricular arrhythmic disorders, however. Genetically induced ventricular arrhythmias can be divided in two subgroups: the primary electrical disorders or channelopathies, and the secondary arrhythmogenic cardiomyopathies. This article focuses on the genetic background of these electrical disorders and the current knowledge of genotype-phenotype interactions.

> This article summarizes the current knowledge on risk stratification in patients who have structural heart disease, notably coronary artery disease and nonischemic

cardiomyopathy. Although other types of structural heart disease and inherited ion channel abnormalities are also associated with a risk of SCD, the risk stratification strategies and data in these entities are diverse and beyond the scope of this article.

Ventricular Arrhythmias in Normal Hearts

Shuaib Latif, Sanjay Dixit, and David J. Callans

Ventricular tachycardia in the structurally normal heart accounts for approximately 10% of cases. Although the overall prognosis is relatively good, with a benign course in most patients, these arrhythmias can lead to significant symptoms. Our understanding of these arrhythmias has progressed significantly, leading to effective therapies targeting their underlying mechanism. In many cases, catheter ablation is successful and the therapy of choice in patients who have sufficient symptoms. This article reviews outflow tract, idiopathic left ventricular, and automatic ventricular tachycardias.

Ventricular Arrhythmias in Heart Failure Patients

Ronald Lo and Henry H. Hsia

Ventricular arrhythmia represents a significant cause of mortality and morbidity. Its pathophysiologic mechanisms and electroanatomic substrates are slowly being elucidated. Clinical management in patients with heart failure has progressed from antiarrhythmic drugs to device therapy. Catheter ablation is an effective adjunct in the management of ventricular arrhythmia but remains a significant challenge. Advances in robotic and magnetic catheter manipulation may shorten procedural time and increase safety. Incorporation of imaging technologies such as CT, MRI, or ultrasound with electroanatomic mapping can enhance the ability to map and ablate ventricular arrhythmia. Novel imaging modalities may provide rapid characterization of the substrate for ventricular dysfunction and arrhythmia development and the capacity for serial assessment of the disease progression, improving risk stratification for ventricular dysfunction and arrhythmia development and the capacity for serial assessment of the disease progression, improving risk stratification.

Role of Drug Therapy for Sustained Ventricular Tachyarrhythmias

L. Brent Mitchell

Antiarrhythmic drug therapy, broadly defined, is the mainstay of treatment and prevention of ventricular tachycardia (VT)/ventricular fibrillation (VF), which can lead to sudden death. This article evaluates the evidence for and appropriate use of class I antiarrhythmic drugs, class III antiarrhythmic drugs, beta-blockers, nondihydropyridine calcium-channel blockers, statins, angiotensin enzyme inhibitors, angiotensin receptor blockers, aldosterone blockers, and digoxin for antiarrhythmic benefits in patients who have a propensity for VT/VF and therefore are at risk of sudden death.

Use of Traditional and Biventricular Implantable Cardiac Devices for Primary and Secondary Prevention of Sudden Death

Matthew H. Klein and Michael R. Gold

Sudden cardiac death is the leading cause of cardiac mortality, particularly among high-risk populations with known left ventricular systolic dysfunction. Multiple randomized clinical trials demonstrated a significant mortality benefit of the implantable cardioverter defibrillator (ICD) compared with antiarrhythmic drug therapy or standard medical care. Initial ICD trials showed a mortality improvement for patients who previously had experienced aborted sudden cardiac death or sustained ventricular tachycardia (secondary prevention). Primary prevention trials in selected high-risk patients who had both ischemic and nonischemic cardiomyopathy also demonstrated a mortality benefit associated with ICD treatment. More recently, cardiac resynchronization therapy with or without defibrillator capability has been shown to reduce morbidity and mortality among advanced heart failure patients with a prolonged QRS duration.

Unresolved Issues in Implantable Cardioverter-Defibrillator Therapy 433
Pamela K. Mason and John P. DiMarco

Over the last 15 years, a series of well-designed randomized clinical trials has clearly demonstrated that implantable cardioverter-defibrillator (ICD) therapy reduces mortality in select high-risk populations. Despite the widespread acceptance of ICD therapy, many questions related to its optimal use remain. This article discusses several key issues now confronting clinicians.

Problems with Implantable Cardiac Device Therapy 441
Marcin Kowalski, Jose F. Huizar, Karoly Kaszala, and Mark A. Wood

Implantable cardioverter-defibrillators (ICDs) improve survival in patients who have left ventricular dysfunction; however, they are associated with numerous problems at implant and during follow-up. The diagnosis and management of these problems is usually straightforward, but more difficult problems may include the management of patients who have elevated energy requirements to terminate ventricular fibrillation or of those who have postoperative device infections. Long-term issues in ICD patients include the occurrence of inappropriate or frequent appropriate shocks. ICD generators and leads are more prone to failures than are pacing systems alone; management of patients potentially dependent on "recalled" devices to deliver life-saving therapy is a particularly complex issue. The purpose of this article is to review the diagnosis and management of these more troublesome ICD problems.

Role of Ablation Therapy in Ventricular Arrhythmias 459
Mithilesh K. Das, Gopi Dandamudi, and Hillel Steiner

Catheter ablation is an effective therapy for symptomatic ventricular arrhythmia (VA) in patients with and without structural heart disease. It is the treatment of choice to cure or reduce recurrent VA in patients who have an implantable cardioverter defibrillator and can be a life-saving procedure in patients who have electrical storm. Catheter ablation for VAs remains a challenging procedure and requires a precise understanding of cardiac electrophysiology, the arrhythmia mechanisms, and mapping techniques. Various mapping techniques such as pace mapping, activation mapping, entrainment mapping, and substrate mapping are used. These techniques complement each other in localizing the critical isthmus of a reentrant VT or the source of origin of a focal VT. Most VAs can be ablated endocardially. Epicardial ablation is needed for VAs with an epicardial circuit or a focal source.

A Comprehensive Approach to Management of Ventricular Arrhythmias 481
Fred Kusumoto

This review presents five cases that highlight the complexity of taking care of patients with ventricular arrhythmias. Three of the cases discuss management of patients with nonsustained ventricular tachycardia in the setting of structural heart disease: dilated cardiomyopathy, hypertrophic cardiomyopathy, and after myocardial infarction. A fourth case asks whether data from implantable cardioverter defibrillator (ICD) trials can be extrapolated to older patients, and the fifth case discusses management of recurrent ventricular arrhythmias in a patient with an ICD.

Index 497

FORTHCOMING ISSUES

RECENT ISSUES

VISIT OUR WEB SITE

The Clinics are now available online!
Access your subscription at www.theclinics.com

ELSEVIER
SAUNDERS

Cardiol Clin 26 (2008) ix

CARDIOLOGY
CLINICS

Foreword

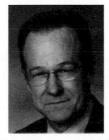

Michael H. Crawford, MD
Consulting Editor

The management of sudden cardiac death (SCD) has moved from acute treatment and secondary prevention to primary prevention. My first encounter with SCD was in the coronary care unit (CCU), which was devoted to the treatment of ventricular arrhythmias, usually from acute myocardial infarction (MI). With reperfusion therapy the CCU has become an anachronism because very few acute MIs have ventricular arrhythmias of any consequence. Next, SCD prevention focused on patients who had an event but survived because of CPR or an automatic external defibrillator. These patients usually had coronary artery disease and required revascularization. As more patients have been revascularized, the focus on SCD has changed to primary prevention. This focus has targeted conditions in which SCD is more common, such as heart failure attributable to left ventricular systolic dysfunction, and genetic conditions, such as the Brugada syndrome.

I was delighted when Dr. Miller again agreed to guest edit an issue on this topic, because he did an outstanding job editing the May 2000 issue.

As a testament to the remarkable changes in this field in the last 8 years, only one topic from the 2000 issue is included in the current issue, namely, the role of drug therapy for sustained ventricular arrhythmias, which is again ably discussed by Dr. Mitchell. All the other topics are new and cover a remarkable spectrum from the genetic basis of ventricular arrhythmias to practical approaches to ventricular arrhythmia management. Dr. Miller has assembled an outstanding group of authors and selected extremely relevant topics. I know you are going to enjoy this timely issue.

Michael H. Crawford, MD
Division of Cardiology
Department of Medicine
University of California, San Francisco Medical
Center
505 Parnassus Avenue, Box 0124
San Francisco, CA 94143-0124, USA

E-mail address: crawfordm@medicine.ucsf.edu

CARDIOLOGY CLINICS

Cardiol Clin 26 (2008) xi–xii

Preface

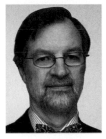

John M. Miller, MD
Guest Editor

Sudden cardiac death because of ventricular arrhythmias (ventricular tachycardia or fibrillation) continues to be a major public health problem in industrialized societies. In the 8 years since publication of the last issue of *Cardiology Clinics* devoted to ventricular arrhythmias, substantial progress has been made in our understanding of the basic pathophysiologic mechanisms of these arrhythmias, as well as their diagnosis and management. In the last several years, identifying and treating individuals who have suffered and survived an episode of ventricular tachycardia (VT) or ventricular fibrillation (VF)—also known as secondary prevention—has become well established, and increasing attention has been turned to primary prevention: that is, identifying and prophylactically treating individuals to prevent sudden death before an episode of VT or VF occurs. This issue explores the current status of this rapidly moving field, including new insights into genetic bases of certain forms of ventricular arrhythmias, changes in the epidemiology of ventricular arrhythmias, application of new as well as old diagnostic tests to identify patients at risk, and results of clinical trials upon which current therapy is based. With advances in the treatment of heart failure, VT and VF have increased in prevalence as causes of death, posing challenges in identification and prophylactic treatment of patients at risk.

Just two decades ago, antiarrhythmic drugs were standard therapy for malignant ventricular arrhythmias, although implantable cardioverter-defibrillators (ICDs) were rapidly developing. Now that ICD technology has largely matured, it has become the default therapy in most cases, but not without problems. Several articles deal with current indications for and application of ICD and cardiac resynchronization therapy, as well as unresolved questions and new problems caused by ICD therapy. Catheter ablation is assuming an increasingly important role in therapy, not only in individuals who have no discernible structural heart disease, but even in those with rapid ventricular arrhythmias previously not considered treatable with ablation. Although antiarrhythmic drug therapy maintains a role in the treatment of ventricular arrhythmias, it has diminished significantly in importance, while other, nonantiarrhythmic medications such as statins and inhibitors of the renin-angiotensin-aldosterone system, are receiving increasing attention for their potential role in preventing ventricular arrhythmias. Several articles deal with these aspects as well. Finally, the last article includes a series of diverse cases illustrating the practical application of many of the current principles of diagnosis and therapy.

As new knowledge is acquired in this field, new questions always arise. This is a very exciting time to be involved in this discipline, with rapid changes leading to improved patient outcomes. With a greater focus on working backwards on the timeline of arrhythmias—better understanding of and rectifying risk factors, as well as greater public awareness and primary care physician identification of patients at risk for VT and VF episodes—we can hope to see even more dramatic decreases in the tremendous personal and societal loss incurred by sudden, unexpected cardiac death.

John M. Miller, MD
Indiana University School of Medicine
Krannert Institute of Cardiology
1800 North Capitol Avenue, Room E-488
Indianapolis, IN 46202, USA

E-mail address: jmiller6@iupui.edu

CARDIOLOGY
CLINICS

Cardiol Clin 26 (2008) 321–333

The Changing Epidemiology of Ventricular Arrhythmias

Kelley P. Anderson, MD, FHRS, FACC, FACP

University of Wisconsin Medical School, Department of Cardiology, Marshfield Clinic,
1000 North Oak Avenue, Marshfield, WI 54449-5777, USA

… it is probable that fatal syncope often differs from non-fatal syncope in the supervention in the former case of fibrillar contraction (or delirium) in the ventricular muscle; this seals the fate of the depressed heart by arresting the circulation and by causing a rapid exhaustion of the ventricular energy in consequence of the violent and continued excitement of the contractile tissues. In the great majority of cases where sudden death is caused by cardiac failure, there is, no doubt, an altered and impaired state of nutrition in the cardiac tissues, sometimes rendered palpable by degenerative changes recognizable with the microscope or pointed to by the presence of disease in the coronary arteries.

—James MacWilliam, 1889 [1]

More than a century ago James MacWilliam [1] related findings from epidemiology, pathology, and the experimental laboratory when he proposed that ventricular fibrillation (VF), rather than cardiac standstill, is the mechanism of sudden cardiac death in most cases. Moreover, he recognized that death due to VF was associated with pathologic abnormalities attributable to coronary heart disease (CHD) along with other conditions, including some without evident structural heart disease [1]. Today, death caused by ventricular tachyarrhythmias (VTA) remains a problem of epidemic proportions. The incidence of VTA death is not precisely known and is estimated by the incidence of various forms of cardiac arrest or various definitions of sudden cardiac death (SCD), each of which has significant potential for error. Nevertheless, the impact of death caused by VTA can be gaged by considering statistics reported by the American Heart Association Statistics Committee [2]: (1) In 2004, 310,000 SCD (defined as CHD deaths that occurred out of hospital or in hospital emergency departments) occurred in the United States. (2) In North America the annual incidence of out-of-hospital cardiac arrest is about 55 per 100,000 population, which implies that about 166,200 out-of-hospital cardiac arrests occur annually in the United States, assuming a population of 302,196,872. (3) About two thirds of unexpected cardiac deaths occur without previous recognition of cardiac disease. (4) In a population 20 years of age or older, the incidence of out-of-hospital cardiac arrest treated by emergency medical services (EMS) is from 36 to 81 per 100,000. Of these, 20% to 38% have VTA as the first recorded rhythms (see later discussion) [2–8]. Surveys suggest that the incidence of deaths caused by VTA have been declining for several decades. Recent trends indicate a slowing of this beneficial trend, however, and a possible reversal in some groups of younger people.

Ventricular ectopic activity

Observations of accidental events and experiments performed by several teams of investigators between 1900 and 1940 led Wiggers [9] to conclude that brief, localized electrical stimuli could initiate VTA when they occurred late in systole or on the T wave during an interval that he called the "vulnerable phase". Smirk [10] noted that R waves appearing on the downslope of T waves (R-on-T) were observed in experimental studies and clinical cases to precede the onset of VTA and were associated with sudden death. These and other observations prompted clinicians and scientists to

E-mail address: kpand@att.net

postulate that ventricular ectopic activity (VEA), which refers to premature ventricular complexes (PVCs), ventricular pairs, and nonsustained ventricular tachycardia (NSVT), cause or predict VTA death. Epidemiologic studies have shown that asymptomatic ventricular arrhythmias (VA) are not unusual in healthy people, however. Hiss and Lamb [11] reported findings of resting 12-lead ECGs from 122,043 relatively young, healthy individuals entering flight training in the US Air Force from age 16 to older than 50 years. PVCs were identified in 0.78% of the subjects. In a more representative population, Chiang and colleagues [12] performed 12-lead ECGs in 5129 people composing 85% of the population of a small town in the United States, and detected PVCs in 3.6%. Longer recording durations result in detection of VEA in more subjects. In a study from the Framingham sample, Bikkina and colleagues [13] identified PVCs in 33% of subjects who did not have known CHD using 1-hour recordings. In a study of middle-aged men, both with and without known heart disease, a 6-hour monitor sampling technique identified a 62% incidence of asymptomatic VEA [14].

The prevalence of VEA is strongly related to age and sex. In healthy flight training recruits Hiss and Lamb [11] reported a prevalence of 0.47% in 16- to 19-year-olds and 1.91% in 45- to 49-year-olds. In the Tecumseh study of Chiang and colleagues [12], the prevalence rose from 1.4% in 16- to 29-year-olds to 10.7% in 60- to 69-year-olds. PVCs were recorded in 2.9% of women compared with 4.4% of men. The differences between men and women were not evident until the age of 50, however [12]. It is noteworthy that the prevalence of premature supraventricular complexes (PSVCs) was also age dependent (0.7% in 16- to 29-year-olds to 4.8% in 60- to 69-year-olds), but not different between sexes. Chiang and colleagues [12] and Hinkle and colleagues [14] found an association between VEA and CHD and subsequent SCD. In the Framingham population, Bikkina and colleagues [13] reported an association between frequent PVCs (> 30 per hour) or complex VEA (multiform PVCs, couplets, NSVT, or R-on-T PVCs) and CHD. Multivariate analysis showed that men who did not have CHD who had complex VEA or frequent PVCs were at increased risk for all-cause mortality and increased risk for myocardial infarction (MI) or death attributable to CHD. In contrast, Kennedy and colleagues [15] found that healthy subjects who had frequent or complex asymptomatic VEA had a similar mortality to that of the healthy United States population.

Coronary heart disease and ventricular ectopic activity

VA and CHD are related in many ways. PVCs are more prevalent in patients who have CHD. In the Framingham population, Bikkina and colleagues [13] reported a prevalence of 58% in men who had CHD compared with 33% in those who did not have CHD. The Tecumseh study showed a strong association between PVCs and CHD. In people older than 30 years, 15.8% of those who had PVCs had CHD, whereas only 5% of patients who did not have PVCs had CHD. Coronary risk factor levels (blood pressure, cholesterol, weight, smoking status) were no higher in people who had PVCs than in the total Tecumseh population. During follow-up, 45 people died suddenly (death within 1 hour of onset of symptoms outside the hospital). Of these, 10 had PVCs at the initial examination. Among these, only 5 had pre-existing CHD. Of those who had PVCs at the initial examination, 6.1% died suddenly compared with 1.0% of those who did not have PVCs [12]. Chiang and colleagues [12] also evaluated PSVCs. In both sexes PSVCs increased with age, similar to the trend observed with PVCs. PVCs were more frequent in men, however, a pattern that seems to become more prominent with increasing age. Moreover, in contrast to the pattern observed in subjects who had PVCs, there was no significant difference in the prevalence of CHD among people with and without PSVCs. Also, there was only 1 SCD among 78 people who had PSVCs.

In the Gruppo Italiano per lo Studio della Sopravvivenza nell'Infarto Miocardico study (GISSI), the frequency and complexity of VEA were prospectively examined in 8624 patients who had acute MI treated with thrombolytic agents [16]. Arrhythmias were present in 64% of the patients, which was somewhat lower than in studies published a decade earlier in the prethrombolytic era, such as the Multicenter Post-Infarction Research Group (MPIP) study (86%) [17] and the placebo group of the Beta-Blocker Heart Attack Trial study (84%) [18]. The prevalence of NSVT was 6.8% in the GISSI database, lower than that observed by Cats and colleagues (19.5%) [19] and the MPIP investigators (11.3%) [17]. Conversely, the 19.7% prevalence of frequent PVCs (> 10 PVCs per hour) was within the range of values reported by earlier studies, such as the MPIP (21.2%) [17], the Multicenter Investigation of the Limitation of Infarct Size (14.6%) [20], and the Beta-Blocker Heart Attack Trial study (12.9%) [18].

The mortality rate at 6 months after MI among the patients in GISSI who had 24-hour ECG recordings was 3.0%. The rate of SCD was 0.98%, or 32.8% of all deaths. The SCD rate was 0.6% in patients who did not have VA, 0.8% in those who had 1 to 10 PVCs per hour (odds ratio [OR] 1.50; 95% CI 0.85–2.64), and 2.1% in those who had 10 or more PVCs per hour (OR 4.07; 95% CI 2.30–7.20). Complex VEA was associated with an SCD rate of 1.7% (OR 3.29; 95% CI 2.08–5.19). All-cause mortality rates were 2.01% in patients who did not have VA, 2.7% in patients who had 1 to 10 PVCs per hour, 5.5% in those who had more than 10 PVCs per hour, and 4.8% in those who had complex VEA. In the multivariate Cox analysis, frequent ($\geq$ 10 per hour) PVCs and complex VEA were predictors of total mortality (relative risk [RR] 1.62; 95% CI 1.16–2.26 and RR 1.64; 95% CI 1.27–2.12, respectively) and SCD (RR 2.24; 95% CI 1.22–4.08 and RR 2.11; 95% CI 1.34–3.17, respectively). NSVT was associated with increased mortality and SCD in univariate but not multivariate analysis (RR 1.20; 95% CI 0.80–1.79 for total mortality and RR 1.42; 95% CI 0.74–2.74 for SCD). Sustained ventricular tachycardia was identified on the 24-hour ECG monitoring at predischarge in 12 patients (0.1% of the total population). At 6 months, 2 of the 12 patients had died (16.7%), whereas the mortality rate in patients who did not have sustained ventricular tachycardia was 3.0% (254 of 8540).

Death caused by ventricular tachyarrhythmias

Prevention of VTA-related deaths is one of the highest priorities of the medical community not only because it is a frequent cause of death but also because if the arrhythmia is terminated quickly, the victim may survive and live for many more years. In addition, VTA deaths are usually unexpected, often occurring in the absence of known cardiac disease and often in people in their most productive years, enhancing the disruption in the lives of family, friends, and associates of victims, and enhancing the grief and suffering. There is a profound and urgent need to better understand deaths caused by VTA to delineate the extent of the problem, to identify areas in need of research, and eventually to reduce mortality attributable to VTA. Unfortunately, barriers interfere with population studies of this

phenomenon because proof of death caused by VTA requires physiologic recordings of the onset of the events leading to death in a large, representative sample of the population. Instead, the incidence of death attributable to VTA must be based on a surrogate event in the target population. Although several surrogates for VTA deaths have been used, each has strengths and weaknesses.

A person who has cardiac arrest in whom the initial rhythm is ventricular tachycardia or VF is a possible surrogate for death caused by VTA. Cobb and colleagues [8] estimated the incidence of death due to VTA based on occurrence of VF as the initial rhythm recorded at the time of cardiac arrest in the city of Seattle and extrapolated this to the United States population. Using 2000 US Census data, the estimated age-adjusted incidence was 38 per 100,000. Extrapolation of the 2000 incidence rates of cardiac arrest for people aged 20 years or older in Seattle to a national level suggests that approximately 184,000 treated cardiac arrests could be anticipated in the United States annually. Of these, about 76,000 would have VF as the initially recorded rhythm. Cobb and colleagues observed that the age- and sex-adjusted annual incidence of VF extrapolated to the United States declined by 56% during the 20-year span between 1980 and 2000. Reductions in VF incidence rates occurred in men and women (57% and 51%, respectively) and were present in most age strata. The incidence of VF in men (60 per 100,000) far exceeded that of women (17 per 100,000), and the ratio of male/female incidence rates decreased only from 4.0 to 3.5 in 20 years. The incidence of VF cardiac arrests decreased significantly in blacks and whites but not in Asians/Pacific Islanders over the study interval. Whites experienced a decrease of 53%, from 85 to 40 per 100,000. Blacks had a 54% decrease in VF incidence. The incidence of asystole and pulseless electrical activity as the first recorded rhythms did not decrease significantly over the same period of time (Fig. 1) [8]. Decreases in the incidence of VF cardiac arrests have been observed in European cities. Kuisma and colleagues [21] reported that the incidence of out-of-hospital VF of cardiac origin decreased by 48% from 1994 to 1999 ($P = .0036$) in Helsinki, Finland. Herlitz and colleagues [22] observed a more modest decline in the proportion of patients who had VF as the initial rhythm at the time of cardiac arrest, from 39% in 1981 to 32% in 1997, whereas the number who had cardiac arrest

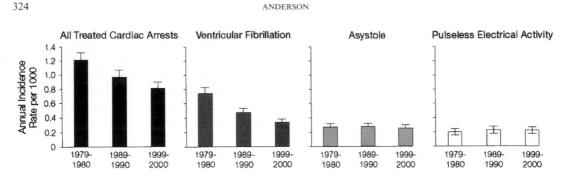

Fig. 1. Incidence rates of treated out-of-hospital cardiac arrest over a 20-year span adjusted for age and sex to the Seattle, Washington population of 2000. Error bars represent 95% CIs. Most of the reduced incidence was because of fewer cases who had ventricular fibrillation as the first identified rhythm. The proportion of cases who had ventricular fibrillation decreased from 61% in 1980 to 41% in 2000. (*From* Cobb LA, Fahrenbruch CE, Olsufka M, et al. Changing incidence of out-of-hospital ventricular fibrillation, 1980–2000. JAMA 2002;288(23):3011; with permission.)

was unchanged in Göteborg, Sweden. More striking reductions would have been identified, however, if the incidences were adjusted for the increase in number of city residents and aging of the population.

Because fatal VF often degenerates into asystole or pulseless electrical activity, using the initial recording of VF as an estimate of death due to VTA may miss episodes recorded too late to document the original rhythm. Holmberg and colleagues [23] examined the first recorded rhythm at the time of cardiac arrest in relation to the time to the first ECG recording and extrapolated backward to estimate the incidence of VF at the time of cardiac arrest. The first ECG showed VF in 43% of all patients. The investigators estimated that VF was the initial rhythm in 60% to 70% of all patients and 80% to 85% of cases who had probable heart disease.

Cardiac arrest, therefore, is a reasonable alternative event that could be used to estimate the incidence of death attributable to VTA. Several studies have prospectively examined the community incidence of primary cardiac arrest using data collected by first responders. From several studies, the annual incidence of treated primary cardiac arrest has ranged between 41 and 91 of 100,000 [8,24–27]. Cobb and colleagues [8] estimated the incidence of cardiac arrest in the United States to be 91 per 100,000 in 2000. This figure represented a significant decline of 34% since 1980.

Chugh and colleagues [28] exposed reasons that use of data from EMS could underestimate VTA-associated deaths as manifested by SCD or cardiac arrest. They identified victims of SCD or cardiac arrest in a prospectively designed study

with data from sources in addition to the EMS, including the county medical examiner's office, area hospitals, and heath care providers. SCD was defined as sudden unexpected death either within 1 hour of symptom onset (event witnessed), or within 24 hours of having been observed alive and symptom-free. Available medical records were obtained and evaluated for each case. In this study, the annual incidence of SCD was 53 per 100,000 residents, well within the range of cardiac arrests noted above. At ages older than 35 years, the lowest incidence was observed in the 35- to 44-year-old age group (17 per 100,000) and the highest incidence was observed in the 75- to 84-year-old age group (346 per 100,000). Women composed 43% of cases.

The estimation of deaths by adjudicated SCD as a representation of deaths due to VTA could be questioned. Evidence favoring a close relationship between SCD and death due to VTA has come from implantable cardioverter defibrillator (ICD) trials. In these trials the mode of each death has been determined by committees based on review of medical records and other data. In some trials committee members were blind to ICD assignment. In most trials, ICD therapy has been associated with a marked reduction in SCD in contrast to nonsudden and noncardiac deaths. This finding supports the concept that most SCD are mediated by VTA [29–32]. Although ICDs could prevent bradyarrhythmic deaths, these have been shown to represent a small component of death mechanisms in ICD trials [33].

Chugh and colleagues [28] exposed potential inaccuracies of other approaches for identifying SCD. Of all cases that met SCD criteria in their study, 64% had rhythms recorded at the time of the EMS arrival. Of these, 44% had VTA, whereas the others had pulseless electrical activity or asystole, similar to what has been reported in other trials. Some 26% of cases presenting to the EMS did not meet criteria for SCD, however. Moreover, 21% of the SCD victims were identified from sources other than EMS, including the medical examiner's office, medical providers, and hospitals, implying that accurate estimation of deaths attributable to VTA requires prospective surveillance from multiple sources and adjudication based on appropriate clinical data. Nevertheless, despite meticulous care in case ascertainment, there are chances for both underestimation and overestimation of the incidence of deaths due to VTA. Overestimation is possible because SCD attributable to bradyarrhythmias, pulseless electrical activity, or "mechanical" disorders (cardiac tamponade, aortic dissection, pulmonary embolism, and so forth) might not be distinguishable from death due to VTA. Underestimation is possible because unwitnessed deaths due to VTA that were discovered more than 24 hours after they were last seen alive have not been included. Also, county residents who suffered SCD while traveling out of state would be missed.

The methods used by Chugh and colleagues [28] could be a model for providing a reliable estimate of SCD and deaths due to VTA, but the data acquired apply only to a single year and only to a single county. The extent to which it pertains to the rest of the United States or other countries can only be assumed. To examine national trends, the US Centers for Disease Control (CDC) used national and state mortality statistics for 1999 based on data from death certificates with cardiac disease death defined as one for which the underlying cause of death was classified and coded using the International Classification of Diseases, Tenth Revision for diseases of the heart (codes I00–I09, I11, I13, and I20–I51) or congenital malformations of the heart (Q20–Q24) [34]. SCD was defined as death from cardiac disease that occurred out of hospital, in an emergency department, or one in which the decedent was reported to be "dead on arrival" at a hospital. Among 728,743 cardiac disease deaths that occurred during 1999, a total of 462,340 (63.4%) were SCDs; 120,244 (16.5%) occurred in an emergency department or were dead on arrival, and 341,780 (46.9%) occurred out of hospital. Women had a higher total number of cardiac deaths (375,243) and a higher proportion of out-of-hospital cardiac deaths

(51.9%) than men (41.7% of 353,500 deaths). Women had a lower proportion of cardiac deaths that occurred in an emergency department or were dead on arrival (12.0%) compared with men (21.2%). SCDs accounted for 10,460 (75.4%) of all 13,873 cardiac disease deaths in people aged 35 to 44 years, and the proportion of cardiac deaths that occurred out of hospital increased with age, from 5.8% in people aged 0 to 4 years to 61.0% in people aged greater than 85 years. SCDs accounted for 63.7% of all cardiac deaths among whites, 62.3% among blacks, 59.8% among American Indians/Alaska Natives, 55.8% among Asians/Pacific Islanders, and 54.2% among Hispanics. Whites had the highest proportion of cardiac deaths out of hospital, and blacks had the highest proportion of cardiac deaths in an emergency department or dead on arrival.

The SCD rate (per 100,000) was strongly related to age (3.0 in age range 0–34 years, 75.4 in 35–65 years, 1099.8 in age range 85 years or older). The overall age-adjusted rate was 175.4 per 100,000. The age-adjusted SCD rate was 47.0% higher among men than women (206.5 versus 140.7 per 100,000 population). Blacks had the highest age-adjusted rates (253.6 in men and 175.3 in women) followed by whites (204.5 in men and 138.4 in women), American Indians/Alaska Natives (132.7 in men and 76.6 in women), and Asians/Pacific Islanders (111.5 in men and 66.5 in women). Non-Hispanics (217.8 in men and 147.3 in women) had higher age-adjusted SCD rates than Hispanics (118.5 in men and 147.3 in women). In 1999, the state-specific proportion of all cardiac deaths that was SCD ranged relatively narrowly from 57.2% (Hawaii) to 72.9% (Wisconsin). In contrast, age-adjusted SCD rates in 1999 ranged widely from 114.6 (Hawaii) to 212.2 per 100,000 (Mississippi).

The death certificate data analyzed by CDC produced an age-adjusted SCD rate (175 per 100,000) more than three times greater than reported by Chugh and colleagues (55 per 100,000) [28,34]. The state with the lowest incidence of SCD was still more than twice that detected by Chugh and colleagues. To examine reasons for the differences in results based on the death certificate method, Chugh and colleagues compared results from their SCD registry to a retrospective death certificate–based analysis using methods similar to those used by the CDC. The death certificate method yielded almost three times more cases (incidence 153 per 100,000) than the prospective method and was therefore of similar magnitude to the national estimate of 175 per 100,000 reported by the CDC. Subjects identified as having SCD by retrospective death certificate review were older and more often female than subjects identified by prospective, community-based methods. Only 59% of the SCD nonsurvivors identified by prospective methods were correctly identified by retrospective review. The remaining 41% were missed by the death certificate review for several reasons, specifically inpatient location of death (25%), diabetes as cause of death (15%), and miscellaneous other noncardiac causes of death (60%). The death certificate method identified 82% non-SCDs correctly, resulting in a specificity of 86%. Of the cases designated as SCD by the death certificate method, only 19% were identified correctly. By this analysis, the death certificate method had a sensitivity of 59%, a specificity of 86%, and a positive predictive value of only 19%.

This analysis underscores the high potential for error of death certificate data for estimating VTA deaths. The accuracy of cause of death depends on the correctness of the diagnosis by the physician, medical examiner, or coroner. Furthermore, time of onset of disease symptoms and time of death are often not recorded on death certificates. Despite significant limitations, death certificate data are the only data source presently available to assess national trends in VTA-related mortality that allow comparison between states and other community units provided that the false-positive rate remains relatively constant. These methods were used by Zheng and colleagues [35] to examine mortality trends from 1989 to 1998. SCD, the VTA death surrogate, was defined as deaths occurring out of the hospital, in the emergency room, or as dead on arrival with an underlying cause of death reported as a cardiac disease (International Classification of Diseases, Ninth Revision code 390–398, 402, or 404–429). Death rates were calculated for residents of the United States aged 35 years or older and standardized to the 2000 United States population. The investigators showed that SCD rates declined between 1989 and 1998. This decline was observed in all race groups among men (Fig. 2A) and in all but American Indian/Alaska Native women, who experienced declining SCD rates until 1996, with an increase in SCD rate in 1997 and 1998 (Fig. 2B).

Overall, age-adjusted SCD rates declined 8.3% (11.7% in men and 5.8% in women) during the 10 years. The decline was less among men aged

35 to 44 years (−2.8%) compared with all other male age groups (−5.7% to −18.1%). In women, the SCD rates declined but the decrement was less than observed in the corresponding male age groups. Women aged 35 to 44 years demonstrated an increase in SCD rate of 21.1%, however. The proportion of cardiac deaths that occurred in the hospital, in the emergency room, or were dead on arrival at the emergency room declined, whereas the proportion that never made it to the hospital increased. This trend probably reflects aging of the United States population and the later onset of sudden, fatal cardiac events in the elderly, who experienced 83% of SCDs as defined in this investigation.

Death due to ventricular tachyarrhythmias related to coronary heart disease

Most VTA-related deaths are probably due to CHD. This theory is supported by retrospective death certificate data from the CDC that indicate about 70% of SCDs are attributable to CHD [34]. Chugh and colleagues [28] used a prospectively designed, multiple-source method of identification and found autopsy evidence of CHD in 76% of SCD victims. Bunch and White [36] have shown not only that a large proportion of out-of-hospital VF arrests encountered by EMS are due to CHD but also that the decline in the incidence of out-of-hospital VF is due to a decrease in VF events related to CHD (Fig. 3). Specifically, the incidence (per 100,000) of EMS-treated out-of-hospital VF in their community decreased significantly between 1991 and 2004 (1991–1994: 18.2; 1995–1999: 11.8; 2000–2004: 8.7). The incidence of out-of-hospital VF due to CHD paralleled this decline (1991–1994: 13.4; 1995–1999: 11.1; 2000–2004: 5.5). In contrast, the incidence of out-of-hospital VF not attributable to CHD increased slightly but significantly (1991–1994: 2.1; 1995–1999: 2.3; 2000–2004: 2.9) (Fig. 4) [36].

Evidence that VTA-related death due to CHD has declined has been provided by analysis from the Framingham population [37]. This sample provided advantages for studying long-term trends in CHD death and SCD because risk factors and other data were prospectively collected in uniform fashion during 50 years of observation. In particular, the mode of death was evaluated using multiple sources and adjudicated by a physician panel using prespecified criteria. SCD was defined as a CHD death that occurred within 1 hour of the onset of symptoms. This definition was

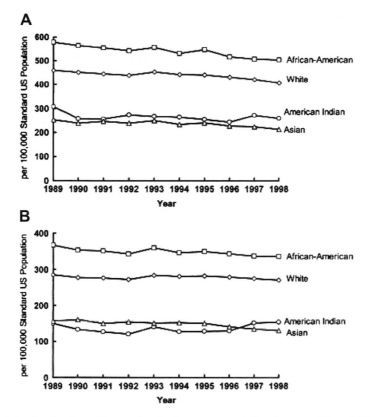

Fig. 2. Age-adjusted death rates for sudden cardiac death among men (*A*) and women (*B*) aged 35 years and older by race in the United States from 1989 to 1999. (*From* Zheng ZJ, Croft JB, Giles WH, et al. Sudden cardiac death in the United States, 1989 to 1998. Circulation 2001;104(18):2161; with permission.)

distinctive in that unwitnessed deaths were excluded unless it could be shown that the victim had been alive within the hour of discovery. Although some would be missed, deaths meeting this definition were probably dominated by fatal VTA.

Subjects between ages 40 and 79 years were analyzed in four time periods: 1950 to 1969, 1970 to 1979, 1980 to 1989, and 1990 to 1999. From 1950 to 1969 through 1990 to 1999, the overall CHD death rate decreased by 59%, SCD rates decreased by 49%, and nonsudden CHD death decreased by 64% (Fig. 5). Approximately half of the SCDs occurred in subjects who did not have a clinical history of CHD or CHF. This proportion did not change between 1950 and 1999. In subjects who did not have a prior history of CHD or CHF, the SCD risk was 39% lower in 1990 to 1999, suggesting that primary prevention participated in reductions in VTA deaths. Evidence that secondary prevention also plays a role in the reduction in deaths due to

VTA is the 57% decline in SCD victims who had a prior history of CHD or CHF during the same periods.

The decline in VTA deaths was associated with changes in the risk profile of the overall Framingham sample from the 1950 to 1969 to the 1990 to 1999 groups. Specifically, systolic blood pressure declined from 140 to 130 mm Hg, hypertension prevalence decreased from 48% to 38%, hypertension treatment increased from 7% to 20%, cholesterol declined from 241 to 207 mg/dL, and smoking prevalence declined from 44% to 27%. These findings suggest that improvements in risk factors contributed to the decrease in VTA deaths. The prevalence of diabetes increased from 3% to 8%, body mass index (BMI) increased from 26.1 to 26.9 kg/m^2, age increased from 56 to 60 years, and the proportions of male sex increased from 44% to 47%. A possible interpretation of these observations is that reduction in hypertension, cholesterol, and smoking resulted in a reduction of fatal VTA related to CHD and other types of

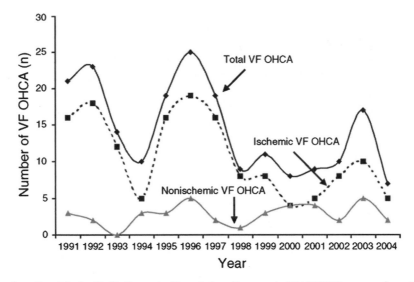

Fig. 3. The number of ventricular fibrillation out-of-hospital cardiac arrests (VF OHCA) per year from 1991 to 2004 are shown as total (*solid line with diamonds*), ischemic (*broken line with squares*), and nonischemic (*thin solid line with triangles*). (*From* Bunch TJ, White RD. Trends in treated ventricular fibrillation in out-of-hospital cardiac arrest: ischemic compared with non-ischemic heart disease. Resuscitation 2005;67(1):52; with permission.)

CHD deaths, and that reduction in these factors outweighed adverse effects of more diabetes, obesity, and older age.

The risk profile of the SCD victims differed substantially from that of the overall population in initial and final values and the magnitude of change. Comparing groups from the same two time periods (1950–1969 and 1990–1999), mean age increased from 62 to 72 years, the percentage of males decreased from 80% to 79%, systolic

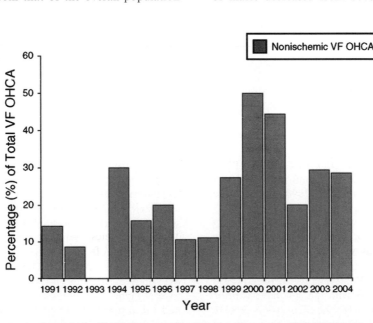

Fig. 4. The percentages of ventricular fibrillation out-of-hospital cardiac arrests (VF OHCA) per year from 1991 to 2004 attributed to nonischemic heart disease per year. (*From* Bunch TJ, White RD. Trends in treated ventricular fibrillation in out-of-hospital cardiac arrest: ischemic compared with non-ischemic heart disease. Resuscitation 2005;67(1):52; with permission.)

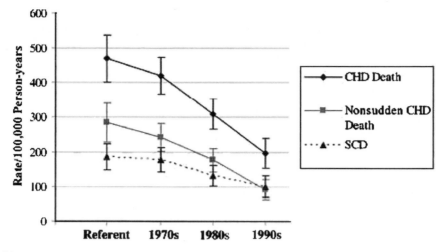

Fig. 5. Incidence rates adjusted for age and sex per 100,000 person-years for overall CHD mortality (*solid black diamonds*), nonsudden CHD death (*squares*), and SCD (*triangles*) from 1950 to 1969 (Referent) to 1990 to 1999 (1990s). Error bars represent 95% CIs. (*From* Fox CS, Evans JC, Larson MG, et al. Temporal trends in coronary heart disease mortality and sudden cardiac death from 1950 to 1999: the Framingham Heart Study. Circulation 2004;110(5):523; with permission.)

blood pressure decreased from 149 to 144 mm Hg, hypertension prevalence decreased from 67% to 63%, hypertension treatment increased from 8% to 36%, cholesterol decreased from 263 to 246 mg/dL, and smoking decreased from 52% to 26%. Diabetes increased from 9% to 19%, however, and BMI increased from 26.4 to 27.8 kg/m^2. Compared with the overall Framingham population, as might be expected, SCD victims had worse risk factors in the early (1950–1969) group (greater age, more males, higher mean blood pressure, higher cholesterol, more smokers, more diabetes, higher BMI). The changes that occurred by the time of the 1990 to 1999 cohort paralleled the changes that occurred in the overall Framingham population, but with greater risk value. Age, percentage of diabetics, and BMI increased more in the SCD victims from the 1950 to 1969 to the 1990 to 1999 groups compared with the overall Framingham sample. Mean blood pressure, prevalence of hypertension, mean cholesterol level, and percent smokers declined in the SCD victims but, with the exception of smoking, in 1990 to 1999 were still higher than in the overall Framingham sample. Although the proportion of diabetics and BMI increased in the whole Framingham sample, the SCD values were greater in the 1950 to 1969 years and increased more by 1990 to 1999. The risk profiles in the VTA death surrogate group therefore improved less with respect to hypertension and

cholesterol and worsened more with respect to age, diabetes, and BMI over the years compared with the entire Framingham sample. A possible interpretation of these risk profiles is that victims of fatal VTA were distinguished from the Framingham population as a whole as having worse risk factors at all periods of observation, as one would expect. Over time, however, as the incidence of SCD declined, deviation in risk profile seems to have increased, possibly because improved treatments have increased the intensity of certain risk factors necessary to result in VTA.

The risk profile of the nonsudden CHD victims over the course of the observation period differs little from that of the SCD victims. Specifically, age increased from 64 to 73 years, systolic blood pressure decreased from 154 to 141 mm Hg, hypertension prevalence increased slightly from 75% to 79%, hypertension treatment increased from 20% to 56%, cholesterol decreased from 268 to 240 mg/dL, and smoking decreased from 49% to 25%. Diabetes increased from 17% to 22% and BMI increased from 26.2 to 28.1 kg/m^2. The major difference was that the proportion of males was lower (62% in the 1950–1969 group to 67% in the 1990–1999 cohort) for the nonsudden CHD compared with the SCD group (see values given previously). A possible interpretation of these findings is that risk factors have similar influences on VTA-related CHD deaths and other CHD deaths.

Fox and colleagues [37] repeated the trend analyses after including 12 cases from 1990 to 1999 of participants who were resuscitated after a cardiovascular collapse and survived 1 hour or longer. These 12 cases would likely have resulted in SCD were it not for attempted resuscitation. The reduction in SCD plus resuscitated cardiovascular collapse in 1990 to 1999 compared with 1950 to 1969 was 38%, less than the reduction of 49% obtained when SCDs alone were considered. These findings suggest that measures leading to more effective resuscitation have contributed to the reduction in VTA-related deaths.

Contributors of the decline in incidence of death due to ventricular tachyarrhythmias

Elucidation of the factors that led to the decline in deaths due to VTA could provide important insights into specific treatments and direction for efficient use of health care resources. Studies discussed earlier indicate that most VTA deaths are related to CHD and that most of the decline in VTA deaths results from a decline of CHD deaths. The study of CHD deaths in the Framingham population showed that the decrease in VTA-related deaths reflects the decline in all CHD mortality over the past 50 years. Because the decrease in mortality was seen in subjects who did not have previously known CHD and subjects who had known CHD, the reduction in deaths is probably related to both primary prevention and secondary prevention. This theory was supported by a decline in several important risk factors. Conversely, other risk factors worsened and some did not seem to change. Of greater potential significance are risk factors that were not analyzed and treatments developed since the 1950s that have been shown to influence CHD mortality.

To determine the possible contributors to the decline in CHD deaths in the United States, Ford and colleagues [38] used a mortality model that incorporated risk factors and medical and surgical treatments. Their analysis included a wide array of treatments for several manifestations of CHD, including acute MI, unstable angina, secondary prevention after MI, secondary prevention after revascularization, chronic angina, and heart failure. Treatments related to acute MI, for example, included resuscitation, thrombolysis, primary angioplasty, primary coronary artery bypass grafting, beta-blocker, angiotensin-converting enzyme inhibitor, and aspirin. Inputs for each treatment included the prevalence of CHD conditions (eg,

number of people who had acute MI), the frequency of use of specific treatments (eg, aspirin), the case fatality rate, and the risk reduction due to treatment, all stratified by age and sex. The number of deaths prevented or postponed as a result of each intervention in each group of patients in the year 2000 was calculated by multiplying the number of people in each CHD condition by the proportion of those patients who received a particular treatment, by the case fatality rate over a period of 1 year, and by the relative reduction in the 1-year case fatality rate that was accounted for by the treatment.

Using United States vital statistics, Ford and colleagues [38] found that from 1980 through 2000, the age-adjusted death rate for CHD decreased from 542.9 to 266.8 deaths per 100,000 population among men and from 263.3 to 134.4 deaths per 100,000 population among women, resulting in 341,745 fewer deaths from CHD in 2000. Using their model of risk factor and treatment effects they determined that approximately 47% of this decrease in deaths could be attributed to treatments, including reductions attributable to secondary preventive therapies after MI or revascularization (11%), initial treatments for acute MI or unstable angina (10%), treatments for heart failure (9%), revascularization for chronic angina (5%), and other therapies (12%). Another 44% of the reduction in CHD deaths was attributed to changes in risk factors, including reductions in total cholesterol (24%), systolic blood pressure (20%), smoking prevalence (12%), and physical inactivity (5%), although these reductions were partially offset by increases in the BMI and the prevalence of diabetes, which accounted for an increased number of deaths (8% and 10%, respectively). Although this study did not specifically address VTA-related deaths, the evidence suggests that factors that reduce CHD deaths also reduce deaths due to VTA. This analysis implies that reduction of traditional CHD risk factors and evidence-based therapies of CHD complications have resulted in reductions in fatal VTA.

Disturbing trends

Unfortunately, there is evidence of a lessening of the decades-long decline in deaths due to VTA. Zheng and colleagues [35] reported that SCD rates decreased 8.3% (11.7% in men and 5.8% in women) during the 10-year period from 1989 to 1999. The decline was less among men aged

35 to 44 years (−2.8%) compared with all other male age groups (−5.7% to −18.1%). More alarming was the demonstrated increase in SCD rate of 21.1% among women aged 35 to 44 years.

Ford and Capewell [39] also found a lessening of the decline in CHD mortality from 1980 to 2002 in younger people. Between 1980 and 2002 they determined that the age-adjusted mortality rate declined 52% in men and 49% in women. The average annual rate of decline for men was 2.9% during the 1980s and 2.6% during the 1990s. For women, it was 2.6% and 2.4%, respectively. From 2000 through 2002, the average annual rate of decline was 4.4% for both men and women. The investigators derived the estimated annual percentage change in mortality (EAPCM), which allowed delineation and statistical evaluation of changes in slopes of time plots of CHD death incidence. Among men aged 35 to 54 years, the investigators found that EAPCM declined significantly from −6.2% during 1980 to 1989 to −2.3% during 1989 to 2000). This undesirable trend continued during 2000 to 2002 (EAPCM −0.5%). By contrast, among men 55 years and older, mortality rates improved in recent years. The investigators found that EAPCM was −2.6 between 1980 and 1990, declined significantly to −1.9 (1990–1996), but improved to −3.7 (1996–2002). The changes in CHD mortality rates were much more dramatically different between age groups in women. Among women 35 to 54 years, the EAPCM was −5.4% during 1980 to 1989, −1.2% during 1989 to 2000, and turned positive, 1.5% during 2000 to 2002. But among women 55 years and older the EAPCM increased significantly from −1.5 (1980–1999) to −4.8 (1999–2002).

Ford and Capewell [39] emphasize that the unfavorable trends in CHD mortality among young adults coincides with deterioration in several risk factors for CHD, including obesity, diabetes, and hypertension in younger adults compounded by stasis in cholesterol concentrations. The adverse trends in mortality have occurred despite continued decline in the prevalence of smoking and increasing use of evidence-based therapies, such as angioplasty, thrombolysis, angiotensin-converting enzyme inhibitors, statins, and antiplatelet agents.

Summary

Investigations of the impact of VA in populations have focused primarily on two aspects,

asymptomatic VEA and SCD. Despite a wealth of evidence that spontaneous VEA can cause fatal VTA and early reports that VEA identifies people at high risk for SCD, well-conducted studies have shown that VEA is an ambiguous signal. In people who do not have known heart disease, VEA is associated with undetected cardiac disease and as such is a risk factor for adverse events. The presence of VEA does not have an adverse prognosis in most people who do not have an identifiable cardiac disorder, however. In patients who have known heart disease, the presence of VEA is associated with more severe underlying disease and worse outcome but it is not specific for death due to VTA.

In contrast, MacWilliam's [1] speculation that SCD is caused by VTA continues to receive empiric support nearly 130 years later. MacWilliam's observation that CHD is an important background of death due to VTA remains the dominant belief today and this is supported by the observation that the decline in surrogates for fatal VTA during the past several decades parallels the decrease in CHD deaths. The reasons for the decline in fatal VTA are most likely reductions in CHD incidence and case fatality rate. There is no persuasive evidence that any specific antiarrhythmic treatment accounts for more than a small proportion of the reduced incidence of VTA deaths, and no risk factor is known to affect deaths due to VTA more than other modes of CHD deaths. Instead, the evidence supports the principle that reduction of deaths due to VTA is multifactorial and results from improved primary prevention (risk factor reduction before manifest CHD), treatment of CHD complications, and secondary prevention (risk factor control and other evidence-based treatments after manifest CHD).

Recent evidence for unfavorable trends for SCD and CHD mortality raises the specter of a reversal in the gains made against fatal VTA in recent decades. These adverse trends are all the more worrisome because they are occurring despite significant advances and wider use of preventive therapy and interventions. These dark clouds may nevertheless have a silver lining because the adverse CHD mortality trends have occurred in the context of worse control of potent risk factors and could be considered an affirmation that CHD risk factors have a crucial impact on mortality related to VTA and they provide clear targets for intervention. There is no time for complacency because there is a need to reverse the increasing incidence of risk factors, such as obesity, diabetes, and metabolic syndrome, and there is a need to interrupt the strong influence of these risk factors on fatal VTA. The demonstration that basic and clinical research and public education have contributed to large reductions in fatal VTA, along with reductions in other forms of morbidity and mortality, is an achievement that should not be discounted at this critical time, because it illuminates the path to be followed to address the new challenges.

Acknowledgments

The author thanks Marshfield Clinic Research Foundation for its support through the assistance of Linda Weis and Alice Stargardt in the preparation of this article.

References

[1] McWilliam J. Cardiac failure and sudden death. Br Med J 1889;1:6–8.

[2] Rosamond W, Flegal K, Furie K, et al. Heart disease and stroke statistics 2008 Update. A report from the American Heart Association Statistics Committee and Stroke Statistics Subcommittee. Circulation 2008;117(4):e25–146.

[3] Vital statistics of the U.S., data warehouse. National Center for Health Statistics. Available at: http://www.cdc.gov/nchs/datawh.htm. Accessed December 7, 2007.

[4] Vaillancourt C, Stiell IG. Canadian Cardiovascular Outcomes Research Team. Cardiac arrest care and emergency medical services in Canada. Can J Cardiol 2004;20(11):1081–90.

[5] Rea TD, Eisenberg MS, Sinibaldi G, et al. Incidence of EMS-treated out-of-hospital cardiac arrest in the United States. Resuscitation 2004;63(1):17–24.

[6] Monthly postcensal resident population (8/1/2005). U.S. Census data. Available at: http://www.census.gov. Accessed December 7, 2007.

[7] Myerburg RJ, Kessler KM, Castellanos A. Sudden cardiac death: epidemiology, transient risk, and intervention assessment. Ann Intern Med 1993; 119(12):1187–97.

[8] Cobb LA, Fahrenbruch CE, Olsufka M, et al. Changing incidence of out-of-hospital ventricular fibrillation, 1980–2000. JAMA 2002;288(23):3008–13.

[9] Wiggers CJ. The mechanism and nature of ventricular fibrillation. Am Heart J 1940;20:399–412.

[10] Smirk FH. R waves interrupting T waves. Br Heart J 1949;11(1):23–6.

[11] Hiss RG, Lamb LE. Electrocardiographic findings in 122,043 individuals. Circulation 1962;25:947–61.

[12] Chiang BN, Perlman LV, Ostrander LD Jr, et al. Relationship of premature systoles to coronary heart disease and sudden death in the Tecumseh epidemiologic study. Ann Intern Med 1969;70(6): 1159–66.

[13] Bikkina M, Larson MG, Levy D. Prognostic implications of asymptomatic ventricular arrhythmias: the Framingham Heart Study. Ann Intern Med 1992;117(12):990–6.

[14] Hinkle LE Jr, Carver ST, Stevens M. The frequency of asymptomatic disturbances of cardiac rhythm and conduction in middle-aged men. Am J Cardiol 1969;24(5):629–50.

[15] Kennedy HL, Whitlock JA, Sprague MK, et al. Long-term follow-up of asymptomatic healthy subjects with frequent and complex ventricular ectopy. N Engl J Med 1985;312(4):193–7.

[16] Maggioni AP, Zuanetti G, Franzosi MG, et al. Prevalence and prognostic significance of ventricular arrhythmias after acute myocardial infarction in the fibrinolytic era. GISSI-2 results. Circulation 1993;87(2):312–22.

[17] Bigger JT Jr, Fleiss JL, Kleiger R, et al. The relationships among ventricular arrhythmias, left ventricular dysfunction, and mortality in the 2 years after myocardial infarction. Circulation 1984;69(2): 250–8.

[18] Kostis JB, Byington R, Friedman LM, et al. Prognostic significance of ventricular ectopic activity in survivors of acute myocardial infarction. J Am Coll Cardiol 1987;10(2):231–42.

[19] Cats VM, Lie KI, Van Capelle FJ, et al. Limitations of 24 hour ambulatory electrocardiographic recording in predicting coronary events after acute myocardial infarction. Am J Cardiol 1979;44(7): 1257–62.

[20] Mukharji J, Rude RE, Poole WK, et al. Risk factors for sudden death after acute myocardial infarction: two-year follow-up. Am J Cardiol 1984;54(1):31–6.

[21] Kuisma M, Repo J, Alaspää A. The incidence of out-of-hospital ventricular fibrillation in Helsinki, Finland, from 1994 to 1999. Lancet 2001; 358(9280):473–4.

[22] Herlitz J, Andersson E, Bång A, et al. Experiences from treatment of out-of-hospital cardiac arrest during 17 years in Göteborg. Eur Heart J 2000; 21(15):1251–8.

[23] Holmberg M, Holmberg S, Herlitz J. Incidence, duration and survival of ventricular fibrillation in out-of-hospital cardiac arrest patients in Sweden. Resuscitation 2000;44(1):7–17.

[24] Westfal RE, Reissman S, Doering G. Out-of-hospital cardiac arrests: an 8-year New York City experience. Am J Emerg Med 1996;14(4):364–8.

[25] Lombardi G, Gallagher J, Gennis P. Outcome of out-of-hospital cardiac arrest in New York City. The Pre-Hospital Arrest Survival Evaluation (PHASE) study. JAMA 1994;271(9):678–83.

[26] Kass LE, Eitel DR, Sabulsky NK, et al. One-year survival after prehospital cardiac arrest: the Utstein style applied to a rural-suburban system. Am J Emerg Med 1994;12(1):17–20.

[27] Fredriksson M, Herlitz J, Nichol G. Variation in outcome in studies of out-of-hospital cardiac arrest: a review of studies conforming to the Utstein guidelines. Am J Emerg Med 2003;21(4): 276–81.

[28] Chugh SS, Jui J, Gunson K, et al. Current burden of sudden cardiac death: multiple source surveillance versus retrospective death certificate-based review in a large U.S. community. J Am Coll Cardiol 2004;44(6):1268–75.

[29] AVID Investigators. Causes of death in the Antiarrhythmics Versus Implantable Defibrillators (AVID) trial. J Am Coll Cardiol 1999;34(5): 1552–9.

[30] Bigger JT Jr, Whang W, Rottman JN, et al. Mechanisms of death in the CABG patch trial: a randomized trial of implantable cardiac defibrillator prophylaxis in patients at high risk of death after coronary artery bypass graft surgery. Circulation 1999;99(11):1416–21.

[31] Greenberg H, Case RB, Moss AJ, et al. Analysis of mortality events in the Multicenter Automatic Defibrillator Implantation Trial (MADIT-II). J Am Coll Cardiol 2004;43(8).1459–65.

[32] Anderson KP. Sudden cardiac death unresponsive to implantable defibrillator therapy: an urgent target for clinicians, industry and government. J Interv Card Electrophysiol 2005;14(2):71–8.

[33] Packer DL, Bernstein R, Wood F, et al. Impact of amiodarone versus implantable cardioverter defibrillator therapy on the mode of death in congestive heart failure patients in the SCDHeFT Trial [abstract AB20-2]. Heart Rhythm 2005;2(5):S38.

[34] Centers for Disease Control and Prevention (CDC). State-specific mortality from sudden cardiac death— United States, 1999. MMWR Morb Mortal Wkly Rep 2002;51(6):123–6.

[35] Zheng ZJ, Croft JB, Giles WH, et al. Sudden cardiac death in the United States, 1989 to 1998. Circulation 2001;104(18):2158–63.

[36] Bunch TJ, White RD. Trends in treated ventricular fibrillation in out-of-hospital cardiac arrest: ischemic compared to non-ischemic heart disease. Resuscitation 2005;67(1):51–4.

[37] Fox CS, Evans JC, Larson MG, et al. Temporal trends in coronary heart disease mortality and sudden cardiac death from 1950 to 1999: the Framingham Heart Study. Circulation 2004;110(5): 522–7.

[38] Ford ES, Ajani UA, Croft JB, et al. Explaining the decrease in U.S. deaths from coronary disease, 1980-2000. N Engl J Med 2007;356(23):2388–98.

[39] Ford ES, Capewell S. Coronary heart disease mortality among young adults in the U.S. from 1980 through 2002: concealed leveling of mortality rates. J Am Coll Cardiol 2007;50(22):2128–32.

ELSEVIER
SAUNDERS

Cardiol Clin 26 (2008) 335–353

CARDIOLOGY
CLINICS

Genetic Basis of Ventricular Arrhythmias

Tim Boussy, MD[a],*, Gaetano Paparella, MD[a], Carlo de Asmundis, MD[a],
Andrea Sarkozy, MD[a], Gian Battista Chierchia, MD[a],
Josep Brugada, MD, PhD[b], Ramon Brugada, MD, PhD[c],
Pedro Brugada, MD, PhD[a]

[a]Heart Rhythm Management Institute, University hospital Brussels, Belgium,
Laarbeeklaan 101 - 1090 Brussels, Belgium
[b]Thorax Institute, Hospital Clinic, University of Barcelona, C. Villaroel, Barcelona, Spain
[c]Montreal Heart Institute, 5000 reu Belanger, Montreal QC HiT iC8, Canada

Sudden cardiac death caused by malignant ventricular arrhythmias is the most important cause of death in the industrialized world. Most of these lethal arrhythmias occur in the setting of ischemic heart disease. A significant number of sudden deaths, especially in young individuals, are caused by inherited ventricular arrhythmic disorders, however. Genetically induced ventricular arrhythmias can be divided in two subgroups: the primary electrical disorders or channelopathies, in which no apparent structural heart disease can be identified, and the secondary arrhythmogenic cardiomyopathies. In these "single gene disorders," mutations are restricted to one gene, rendering a predictable mendelian fashion of transmission. The highly variable phenotypic expression of these monogenic mutations (even within the same family) makes risk assessment of a single individual difficult, if not impossible. This article focuses on the genetic background of these electrical disorders and the current knowledge of genotype-phenotype interactions.

Monogenic modes of transmission

Protein-coding sequences comprise less than 1.5% of the human genome [1]. The rest contain RNA genes, regulatory sequences, introns, and so-called "junk DNA." Each individual has two copies of each gene (called alleles), which are localized along 23 chromosome pairs (22 pairs of autosomes, 1 pair of sex chromosomes). Each parent contributes one member of each chromosome pair, thus providing one copy of each gene. An individual is considered "homozygous" for a specific gene locus when both gene loci are occupied by two identical alleles or "heterozygous" when both alleles differ. According to Mendel's first law, each of the two alleles separates independently and is passed on to the next generation. Most of the single gene disorders are caused by point mutations (alteration of a single nucleotide), in which a nucleotide is substituted, resulting in formation of a different amino acid (missense mutation), a truncated protein (caused by mutation to a stop codon), or an elongated protein (caused by elimination of a stop codon). If the phenotype is expressed in the presence of only one mutated allele, the inheritance is called dominant. When phenotype expression requires both alleles to be mutant, the pattern of inheritance is called recessive (Fig. 1).

Autosomal dominant inheritance

The phenotype can be expressed in a heterozygous setting, in which only one of the two alleles is affected. In the presence of identical mutations, different individuals may express different clinical features because of a different degree of expressivity, which is amenable to environmental and genetic factors. In an autosomal dominant trait,

* Corresponding author.
  E-mail address: tboussy@yahoo.com (T. Boussy).

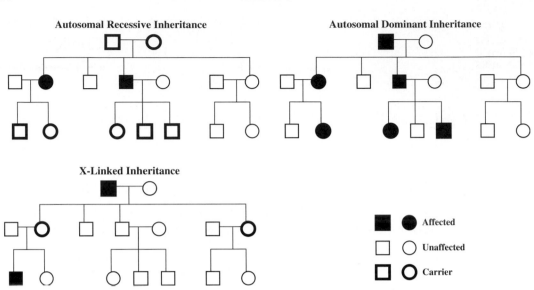

Fig. 1. Monogenic patterns of inheritance.

men and women are equally prone to inherit the mutation, and each child has a 50% chance of being affected by receiving the mutant allele. Each affected person has an affected parent. Normal children of an affected parent are noncarriers and cannot pass on the disease. In most autosomal dominant inherited diseases, the onset of the first phenotypic expression is delayed.

Autosomal recessive inheritance

In autosomal recessive disorders, the phenotype can only manifest when both alleles are mutated at the locus responsible for the disease. Because 1 of the 22 autosomes is involved, there is an equal distribution between male and female subjects. Because of the early onset of expression, recessive disorders are mainly diagnosed during childhood. Each child has a 25% chance of being affected, and heterozygote parents are clinically normal.

X- linked inheritance

Disorders caused by genes located on the sex chromosomes (X-linked) demonstrate a significantly different pattern of transmission with a different clinical outcome between both sexes. In women, one or both X chromosomes can be affected, with dominant or recessive properties. Because men only carry one X chromosome, the probability that the disease will manifest in the presence of a mutant gene is much higher. Mutant X genes can be received

from the affected father or the homozygote (affected) or heterozygote mother. No male-to-male transmission is possible (genetic material from father to son is located on the Y chromosome), and all daughters of affected men are carriers.

Channelopathies

The genetic background and detailed pathogenic mechanisms of these primary electrical disorders have been studied extensively in the last two decades [2]. At first, because of a lack of systematic investigation and low patient numbers, information was obtained from animal models, which were extrapolated to humans. Later, genetic linkage techniques and long-term information of multigenerational families increased our understanding of these relatively new diseases. Currently, several genes have been identified coding for the expression of ion channel proteins, located in the membrane of the cardiomyocyte. The principal function of these cardiac channels is the formation of an electrical potential. Ion currents are regulated by synchronized opening and closing of these channels. Gene mutations alter their pore-forming capacities and gate function, which results in an impaired depolarization or repolarization. This results in an increased vulnerability of the cardiomyocyte for dangerous arrhythmias. The channelopathies show a pronounced genetic heterogeneity, with dispersion of gene mutations within the affected gene.

Voltage-gated sodium channelopathies

The cardiac sodium channel

Voltage-gated sodium channels are responsible for the upstroke of the action potential and play an important role in the propagation of the electrical impulse in all excitable tissues (eg, muscle, nerve, and heart). The opening of sodium channels in the heart underlies the QRS-complex on the electrocardiogram (ECG) and enables a synchronous ventricular ejection. Because the upstroke of the electrical potential primarily determines the speed of conduction between adjacent cells, sodium channels can be found in tissues in which speed is of importance [3–5]. Cardiac Purkinje cells contain up to 1 million sodium channels, which illustrates the importance of rapid conductance in the heart.

Sodium channels consist of a pore-forming α-subunit and one or two β-subunits (Figs. 2 and 3). The α-subunit is a large transmembrane protein encoded by nine genes, in which the SCN5A gene (chromosome 3p21) is the only one coding for the cardiac isoform (Table 1). Mutations in the Na− channel α-subunit gene SCN5A result in multiple cardiac arrhythmia syndromes.

Mutations leading to a voltage-gated sodium channel dysfunction can result in Brugada syndrome, progressive cardiac conduction disturbances (PCCD) or Lenègre disease, and long QT syndrome. Several different types of mutations have been identified, including missense, deletions, insertions, and splicing errors, resulting in a decreased or increased function of the sodium channel. Combinations of all three phenotypes have been documented [6]. Certain mutations may manifest different phenotypes in different individuals of the same family.

Loss of sodium channel function disorders

The Brugada syndrome. Since 1992, Brugada syndrome (BS) has been known as one of the genetically transmittable cardiac channelopathies, characterized by a susceptibility for lethal ventricular arrhythmias in the presence of typical ST-segment changes in the right precordial leads [7]. In patients who have BS, no structural heart disease can be identified despite thorough invasive and noninvasive exploration. The baseline ECG deviations show a dynamic character, with possible transient normalization [8]. They seem to be based on an impaired function of cardiac sodium channels, creating an altered morphology of the cardiac action potential associated with increased arrhythmic vulnerability.

More than 70 gene mutations have been identified in only 20% to 25% of all patients who have BS (most are located in the cardiac SCN5A gene), which suggests that other gene mutations may be responsible [9]. All SCN5A mutations modify the sodium channel function by either creating a truncated protein or increasing the channel inactivation. This results in a shortening of the action potential because of faster phase 1 depolarization. In 2002, Weiss and colleagues [10] located a second locus linked to BS on chromosome 3, and recently the same group identified the causative mutation in the glycerol-3-phosphate dehydrogenase 1-like gene (GPD1L) [11]. Patients who have BS, particularly with an SCN5A mutation, show clinical signs of slowed conduction by means of PR, HV, and QRS prolongation, which illustrates the overlap with Lenègres syndrome.

Recently, remarkable genetic data were published regarding the importance of single

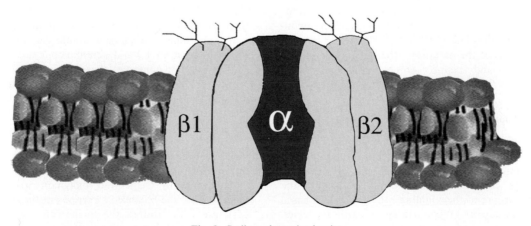

Fig. 2. Sodium channel subunits.

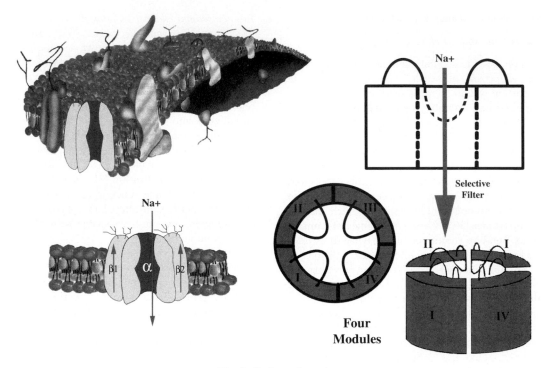

Fig. 3. Sodium channel.

nucleotide polymorphisms, which might possibly explain the different clinical phenotypes and incidence of BS in diverse geographic regions [12]. Ethnic-specific single nucleotide polymorphism distributions in the SCN5A promoter region were reported. A certain combination of six single nucleotide polymorphisms (designated as haplotype B variant) only occurred in Asian subjects (at an allele frequency of 22%) and was absent in the other ethnic groups. This haplotype variant resulted in decreased sodium channel expression and function. In the last years, several case reports proved that certain SCN5A polymorphism in the presence of a BS-causing SCN5A mutation can influence the clinical phenotype and clinical consequences of the mutation. The polymorphism can rescue and restore or—by contrast—further worsen the sodium channel function [13].

Pathophysiology

Antzelevitch [14] performed extensive research on possible pathophysiologic mechanisms explaining the ST-segment changes and the vulnerability for ventricular arrhythmias in BS. According to their findings, the disorder is based on an impaired repolarization of cardiomyocytes. There is a striking difference in action potential morphology in the epicardial, endocardial, and M cells, especially during phases 2 and 3 of the action potential. Whereas the epicardial action potential shows a prominent notch and dome immediately after phase 0 depolarization, the endocardial action potential has a steadier shape during early repolarization. The transmural gradient that originates from this shape difference corresponds to the ST segment on the surface ECG. Alterations of spike and dome morphology (phase 1), in particular in the epicardium, are predominantly mediated by the transient outward current (I_{to}). In BS, the loss of right ventricular outflow tract (RVOT)-epicardial (not endocardial) action potential dome and plateau amplitude, caused by an increase in I_{to} and simultaneous decrease in (inward) I_{Na}, underlies the prominent J-wave and ST-segment elevation (mimicking right bundle branch block morphology). The conduction of the action potential dome from sites at which it is maintained to sites at which it is lost allows local pre-excitation via a phase 2 re-entry mechanism when a closely coupled extra systole occurs in the vulnerable window. These premature beats might eventually trigger the malignant arrhythmia. Because the balance of currents at the onset of phase 2 determines the maintenance of the action potential dome, acquired forms of BS can

Table 1
Overview of sodium channel genes, tissue specificity, and clinical features associated with channelopathies

Gene	Channel	Location	Tissue	Associated disorders
SCN1A	$Na_v1.1$	2q24	Brain, CNS	Brain sodium channelopathies: epilepsy, familial hemiplegic migraine, familial autism
SCN2A	$Na_v1.2$	2q23–q24.3	Brain, CNS	Severe myoclonic epilepsy, familial neonatal- infantile seizures
SCN3A	$Na_v1.3$	2q24	Brain, CNS	Epilepsy, familial hemiplegic migraine, familial autism
SCN4A	$Na_v1.4$	17q23.1–q25.3	Adult skeletal muscle	Muscle sodium channelopathies: hyperkalemic periodic paralysis, paramyotonia congenital, potassium aggravated myotonia
SCN5A	$Na_v1.5$	3p21	Heart muscle, skeletal muscle	Cardiac sodium channelopathies (see text)
SCN6A/SCN7A	Na_x	2q21–q23	PNS, heart muscle, skeletal muscle, uterus	
SCN8A	$Na_v1.6$	12q13	CNS, brain	Cerebellar atrophy, ataxia, mental retardation
SCN9A	$Na_v1.7$	2q24	PNS	Peripheral nerve sodium channelopathies: pain sensitization
SCN10A	$Na_v1.8$	3p24.2–p22	PNS	Peripheral nerve sodium channelopathies
SCN11A	$Na_v1.9$	3p24–p21	PNS	Peripheral nerve sodium channelopathies
SCN1B	$Na_v\beta1$	19q13.1	Brain, heart muscle, skeletal muscle	Brain sodium channelopathies: generalized epilepsy with febrile seizures
SCN4B	$Na_v\beta4$	11q23	Brain, PNS, heart muscle, skeletal muscle	Cardiac sodium channelopathies: long QT syndrome

Abbreviation: PNS, peripheral nerve system.
Data from Koopmann TT, Bezzina CR, Wilde AA. Voltage-gated sodium channels: action players with many faces. Ann Med 2006;38:472–82.

originate from an increase in outward currents (I_{to}, I_{K-ATP}, IKs, and I_{Kr}) or a decrease in inward currents (I_{Ca-L}, I_{Na}). Case reports over the last 13 years described ST changes as in BS caused by drugs, ischemia, electrolyte disturbances, hyper- and hypothermia, elevated insulin levels, and mechanical compression of the RVOT.

Recently, Meregalli and colleagues [15] presented an alternative "depolarization disorder" theory, providing another possible explanation for the Brugada ECG abnormalities. This model is based on a conduction delay in the RVOT. Because of action potential differences between the RVOT and the rest of the right ventricle, a closed-loop current originates between these two regions and creates an initial ST elevation followed by a negative T wave at the level of the right precordial leads. It is also possible that both of the mechanisms operate in the pathophysiology of the Brugada ECG pattern and the ventricular arrhythmias.

Lev-Lenègre syndrome

Lev-Lenègre's disease or PCCD is characterized by an age-related alteration of electrical conductance through the His-Purkinje system. This disorder, first described in 1964 [16,17], initially was thought to be degenerative, is caused by selective and progressive fibrosis of the His-Purkinje system. Genetic familial screening of these patients reveals causative gene mutations. Clinically, PCCD manifests as a progressive blockage of the atrioventricular conduction (requiring pacemaker implantation) or—on an infra-hissian level—as a fascicular or bundle branch block. Multiple reports have shown a familial clustering of patients with chronic bundle branch block and various degrees of atrioventricular block (suggesting a genetic origin) [18,19].

In 1995, a South African study group genotyped a large family of 86 members, in which 39 were affected with PCCD [20]. They mapped the first locus to 19q13.2–13.3 in near proximity of the myo-tonic dystrophy locus, which explained the occur-rence of conduction abnormalities in these patients. Another gene locus mapped on 1q32.2–q32.3 was linked to cardiac conduction defects in combination with dilated cardiomyopathy [21]. Probst and colleagues [21] were the first to identify mutations responsible for isolated cardiac conduc-tion defects. They were located on the cardiac so-dium channel gene (SCN5A) and segregated in an autosomal dominant fashion. Sequencing the en-tire SCN5A coding region in a large French family (with 15 affected family members), they identified a $T \geq C$ substitution (IVS22 + 2 $T \geq C$) that resulted in an impaired gene product, lacking the voltage sensitive segment of the sodium channel. In a smaller Dutch family, another SCN5A mutation cosegregated with a nonprogressive conduction deficit. A second, thorough, and more complete in-vestigation of the same French pedigree demon-strated that PCCD related to SCN5A mutations is based on the combination of haploinsufficiency of the cardiac sodium channel gene and an addi-tional unknown mechanism (altering cardiac con-duction in relation to aging) [22].

Disorders associated with a gain of function of cardiac sodium channels

Long QT3 syndrome. In contrast to most long QT-syndrome phenotypes, which are based on mutations that modify the cardiac potassium currents, long QT3 mutations are located on the cardiac sodium channel gene SCN5A. These mutations cause a sustained reopening of sodium channels and result in a small inward current that adds up to the peak upstroke of the ventricular action potential. This additional inward current prolongs cardiac repolarization by selective alter-ation of phase 1 or the early repolarization phase. The surface ECG manifests a long QT interval with late onset of the T wave. Arrhythmic events occur more commonly during rest or sleep. Beta-blockers are contraindicated in this group because inhibition of the sympathetic activity enhances the risk of arrhythmic events.

Potassium channelopathies

The cardiac potassium channel

Potassium channels, which mediate the out-ward K^+ currents, play a major role in the forma-tion of the cardiac action potential by enabling repolarization currents to counteract the depolar-ization front (phases 1 through 4) [23–27].

Different expression of voltage-gated potassium channels in the different layers of the cardiac mus-cle and in different cardiac tissues seems to be responsible for the changes in morphology of the cardiac action potential. The cardiac volt-age-gated potassium channel consists of four al-pha-subunits ($K_V\alpha$), which together represent a pore-forming unit (see Fig. 2). The assembly of a functional tetramer can only occur in the presence of multiple auxiliary units. The slow and fast component of the transient outward cur-rent I_{to} is created through the assembly of four α-subunits from the K_v1-K_v4 subfamilies (KCNA to D gene), while joining of the *HERG* (*human ether-a-go-go*–related) gene and K_vLQT1 α-subunits underlie the delayed rectifier current (I_{Kr} and I_{Ks}). Disorders associated with an impaired func-tion of these potassium channels are the long and the short QT syndrome.

Loss of sodium potassium channel function disorders

The long QT syndrome. In its idiopathic or congenital form, long QT syndrome refers to a group of genetically transmittable disorders that affect cardiac ion channels in a way that results in slowed ventricular repolarization with prolongation of the QT interval. This can lead to early after-depolarizations and life-threatening torsade de pointes. The incidence of long QT syndrome has been estimated to be approximately 1 per 10,000 without apparent ethnic or geo-graphic predilection. Through the last two de-cades, eight genotypes (LQT1–8) have been described (with up to 500 mutations and 130 polymorphisms). Each subgroup affects the mor-phology of the ventricular action potential in a different way and shows minor differences in clinical manifestations. Because most of these repolarization disorders involve the cardiac po-tassium currents (I_{Ks}, I_{Kr}, I_{Ki}), an overview of the potassium-dependent long QT syndrome sub-groups is presented in this section (Table 2).

Long QT 1. Long QT 1 syndrome, caused by KCNQ1 mutations, is the most common form of long QT syndrome [27] Mutations in the KCNQ1-gene (α-subunit K_vLQT1) can cause autosomal-dominant Romano-Ward syndrome and autosomal-recessive Jervell and Lange-Nielsen syndrome. KCNQ1 and KCNE1 (minK) form the slowly activating component of the de-layed rectifier K^+ current (I_{Ks}), which contributes to cardiac repolarization. Functional expression

Table 2
Long QT-syndrome genotype groups with associated pathophysiologic and clinical features

LQT subgroup	Gene	Locus	Encoded protein	Ion current affected	Effect of mutation	Triggers	ECG findings
LQT1	KvLQT1, KCNQ1	11p15.5	Alpha subunit of potassium channel	I_{Ks}	Loss of function	Exercise, swimming, emotional stress	Broad based T wave, late-onset T wave
LQT2	HERGKCNH2	7q35–36	Alpha subunit of potassium channel	I_{Kr}	Loss of function	Rest, sleep, auditory stimuli, emotional stress, postpartum	Split, notched T wave, low amplitude T wave
LQT3	SCN5A	3p21–24	Alpha subunit of sodium channel	I_{Na}	Gain of function	Rest/sleep	Late onset, peaked, biphasic T wave
LQT4	ANKB, ANK2	4q25–27	Membrane anchoring protein	Na^+, K^+ and Ca^{2+} exchange	Loss of function	Exercise, emotional stress	Inverted or low amplitude T wave, inconsistent QT prolongation, prominent U wave
LQT5	mink,I_sK, KCNE1	21q22.1–2	Beta subunit to KCNQ1	I_{Ks}	Loss of function	Unknown	Unknown
LQT6	MiRP1, KCNE2	21q22.1	Beta subunit to HERG	I_{Kr}	Loss of function	Unknown	Unknown
LQT7	Kir2.1, KCNJ2	17q23	Kir2.1 subunits	I_{K1}	Loss of function	Accompanied by alterations in serum K^+ levels	Prominent U wave, prolonged terminal T downslope
LQT8	CACNA1C	12p13.3	Alpha subunit	$I_{Ca,L}$	Gain of function	Hypoglycemia, sepsis	Severe QT-prolongation, 2:1 atrioventricular block, overt T-wave alternans

Data from Modell SM, Lehmann MH. The long QT syndrome family of cardiac ion channelopathies: a HuGE review. Genet Med 2006;8(3):143–55.

of mutant KCNQ1 α-subunits results in a loss of channel function. More than 100 mutations have been identified and associated with a variety of ion channel dysfunction mechanisms. The net effect of these mutations is a decrease in outward K^+ current during the plateau phase of the cardiac action potential. The channel remains open longer, ventricular repolarization is delayed, and the QT interval is prolonged [28].

Long QT 2. The second most common cause of congenital long QT syndrome is mutation in the *HERG* (*human-ether-a-go-go*–related) gene, which generates the long QT 2 phenotype (35%–45%) [29]. Currently, more than 80 mutations, mostly single amino acid substitutions, have been described. *HERG* encodes the voltage-gated potassium channels that produce the rapidly activating rectifier K^+ current (I_{Kr}). Similar as the I_{Ks} in long QT 1, the I_{Kr} plays an important role in controlling the balance of membrane currents during the plateau phase (phase 2) of the cardiac action potential. Long QT 2 is an autosomal-dominant inherited disease in which normal and mutant *HERG* genes are present. Experiments performed by Sanguinetti and Keating [30,31] contributed to our understanding in possible assembly mechanisms of the α-subunits. They concluded that the presence of a single mutant subunit (in a tetramer) conveys a dysfunctional channel phenotype. They called this the "dominant negative effect," which results in a channel function reduction of much more than the expected 50%. Because the *HERG* channel is considered a target for various cardiovascular and noncardiovascular drugs, it is partly responsible for the striking similarities between congenital and acquired or drug-induced forms of long QT syndrome.

Long QT 5. The congenital long QT5 phenotype has been linked to mutations in the minK gene *KCNE1* [32]. MinK is one of the auxiliary units that coassemble with K_v LQT1 to produce the slow delayed rectifier K^+ current I_{Ks}. As in previous long QT groups, the impaired repolarization prolongs the duration of the action potential by influencing phase 2 and, to a lesser degree, phase 3 of the action potential. The function of the regulatory subunit minK may not be restricted to K_vLQT1 alone in its interactions with the voltage-gated potassium channel. Recently, it has been shown to affect the amplitude and gating properties of the *HERG* subunits, raising the possibility that both I_{Ks} and I_{Kr} currents are altered in the long QT 5 syndrome. Currently, only five mutations have been identified [33].

Long QT 6. Another regulatory protein MiRP1, which is the product of the *KCNE2* gene, is dysfunctional in long QT 6 syndrome [27]. This gene bears many similarities to the *KCNE1* gene, which suggests a common evolutionary origin. Both genes are located next to each other on the same chromosome, and both encode an auxiliary unit of the voltage-gated potassium channel. The *MiRP1* gene product *KCNE2* coassembles as a β-subunit with the *HERG* α-subunits to regulate the I_{Kr} currents. Because it predominantly alters the I_{Kr} currents, it phenotypically mimics the long QT 2 syndrome. The long QT 6 variant is an uncommon variant ($<1\%$) of the disease and is usually associated with minor clinical manifestations (because of its incomplete penetrance).

Long QT 7. The long QT 7 syndrome—or the Andersen-Tawil syndrome—is a skeletal muscle disease associated with periodic paralysis, prolonged QT intervals, and fluctuations in plasma potassium levels [34]. It has been linked to mutations in the *KCNJ2* gene (chromosome 17), encoding for the inward rectifier potassium channel (I_{K1}or Kir2.1). The alterations in action potential morphology occur during phase 3, because the I_{K1} current is predominantly active during late repolarization. Clinically, patients typically present with the triad of periodic paralysis, cardiac arrhythmias, and developmental dysmorphisms. Possible triggers for arrhythmias are hypokalemia and concomitant infections.

Disorders associated with a gain of function of cardiac potassium channels

Short QT syndrome. In 2000, Gussak and colleagues [35] first described a clinical syndrome that linked a short QT interval to an increased risk for malignant ventricular arrhythmias. Two years later, Gaita and colleagues [36] reported two families with short QT syndrome and a high incidence of sudden death, providing evidence for a genetic origin. As in long QT syndrome, mutations are located in genes that encode for subunits of the cardiac potassium channel. In contrast to the long QT syndrome, the gain of function of potassium channels results in faster repolarization with shortening of the action potential duration. Currently, three genes have been associated with the syndrome: *KCNH2*, *KCNQ1*, and *KCNJ2* [37].

KCNH$_2$ gene mutations. Brugada and colleagues [38] identified two different missense mutations in the *KCNH$_2$* or *HERG* gene in two unrelated families. *HERG* encodes the voltage-gated potassium channels that produce the rapidly activating rectifier K$^+$ current (I$_{Kr}$). *HERG* mutations associated with short QT syndrome block the inactivation of the *HERG* channels, which results in an increase in I$_{Kr}$. Coexpression of the *KCNE$_2$* gene does not alter these changes. The same group showed that *HERG* mutations cause a selective shortening of the ventricular action potentials that is not present in the Purkinje fibers. These differences in duration of action potentials and refractory periods could possibly create a substrate for re-entry arrhythmias. Because atrial fibrillation is frequently correlated with the same mutations, this heterogeneity probably extends to the atrial tissue [39]. This was demonstrated by identification of another family with short QT syndrome, in which atrial fibrillation was the only clinical manifestation.

KCNQ$_1$ gene mutations. To date, only two mutations in the *KCNQ$_1$* gene have been identified [40]. The first one exhibited a voltage-dependent character. A gain of function in the outward potassium current (and subsequent shortening of the action potential) could only be demonstrated at more negative potentials. The second mutation was identified in a newborn, who phenotypically showed atrial fibrillation with slowed ventricular response and a short QT interval. A de novo missense mutation revealed a voltage-independent alteration of the potassium currents, which resulted in shortened ventricular repolarization.

KCNJ$_2$ gene mutations. Recently, Priori and colleagues [41] described a third form of short QT syndrome linked to mutations in the *KCNJ$_2$* gene on chromosome 17, which is encoded for the inward rectifier potassium channel (I$_{K1}$ or Kir2.1). Similarly as in long QT 7, the alterations in action potential morphology occur during phase 3, because the I$_{K1}$ current is predominantly active during late repolarization. This phenotypically manifests as asymmetrical T waves with a rapid terminal phase on the surface ECG. Simulation of the effects of the mutated gene in animal models confirms this selective acceleration of phase 3 of the ventricular action potential.

Calcium channelopathies

The voltage-gated cardiac calcium channel

Cardiac calcium channels play a crucial role in the proper functioning of excitable cardiac cells. The heart expresses different types of voltage-gated Ca^{2+} channels that enable the coupling of electrical signaling to intracellular biochemical changes. In 2000 [42], a new classification model was introduced (Table 3) that presented the

Table 3
Ca^{2+}-dependent arrhythmia syndromes

Timothy syndrome

Gene	Locus	Syndrome	Protein	Functional abnormality
CACNA1CA	12p13.3	Timothy syndrome1, autism	Ca$_v$1.2 α$_{1C}$	I$_{Ca-L}$ ↑
CACNA1C	12p13.3	Timothy syndrome1, autism	Ca$_v$1.2 α$_{1C}$	I$_{Ca-L}$ ↑
Catecholaminergic polymorphic ventricular tachycardia				
RyR2	1q42	CPVT1, SIDS	RyR2α	SR Ca^{2+} leak ↑
RyR2	1q42–q43	CPVT1, QT prolongation	RyR2α	SR Ca^{2+} leak ↑
RyR2	1q42–q43	CPVT1, ARVC2	RyR2α	SR Ca^{2+} leak ↑
CASQ2	1p13.3	CPVT2	Calsequestrin	SR Ca^{2+} leak ↑
KCNJ2	17q23	CPVT3	Kir2.1α	I$_{K1}$ ↑
ANK2	4q25	CPVT?	Ankyrin-B	SR Ca^{2+} leak ↑
Dilated cardiomyopathy				
ABCC9	12p12.1	DCM, VT	SUR2Aβ	Ca^{2+} − overload
PLN	6q22.1	DCM, HF, LVH	PLNβ	Ca^{2+} − overload

Abbreviations: ARVC, arrhythmogenic right ventricular dysplasia; CPVT, catecholaminergic polymorphic ventricular tachycardia; DCM, dilated cardiomyopathy; HF, heart failure; LVH, left ventricular hypertrophy; SIDS, sudden infant death syndrome; SR, sarcoplasmatic reticulum; VT, ventricular tachycardia.

Data from Splaswski I, Timothy KW, Sharpe LM, et al. Ca(V)1.2 calcium channel dysfunction causes a multisystem disorder including arrhythmia and autism. Cell 2004;119:19–31.

results of recent genetic, molecular, and biochemical studies. All voltage-gated $Ca^{2}+$ channels are large heteromers that contain a minimum of three core units: α1, α2/δ, and β. The pore-forming α1 subunits contain the gating machinery required for adequate channel function. A wide spectrum of inherited calcium channelopathies results from mutations in these pore-forming α-subunits [44].

The most prominent extracellular cardiac calcium channels (located in the cell membrane or in the sarcolemma) are the high voltage–activated $Ca_v1.2/Ca_v1.3$ or slow calcium channels (L-type) (Fig. 4), which trigger the release and refilling of calcium in the sarcoplasmatic reticulum (SR). They predominantly affect phase 0 of the action potential in slow fibers (SA and atrioventricular node) or phase 2 in ventricular and atrial muscle cells (fast fibers). The resulting SR- calcium outflow in these cells can induce early after-depolarizations. L-type calcium channels act as a target for various drugs (calcium antagonists) that are aiming for a decrease in excitability of the cardiomyocytes (Fig. 5).

The low voltage activated $Ca_v3.1$ and $Ca_v3.2$ fast T-type channels show a relative prominence in pacemaker cells and conductive tissue and activate at more hyperpolarizing potentials. Based on these findings, T channels are presumed to play a vital role in atrial pacemaking.

Timothy syndrome

Timothy syndrome is a recently described form of long QT syndrome (long QT 8) [43,45]. Extracardiac features of this disease include syndactyly, facial dysmorphy, myopia, immunodeficiency, and generalized cognitive impairment. It results from a de novo, gain-of-function missense mutation in splice exon 8A of CACNA1C that encodes

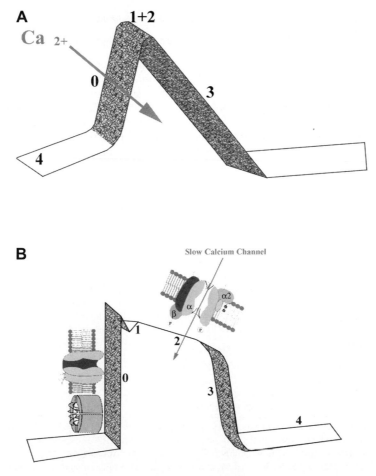

Fig. 4. Calcium channels.

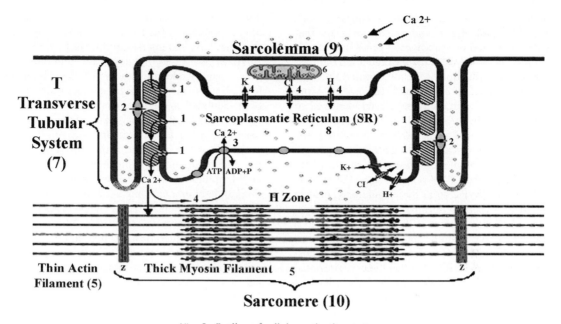

Fig. 5. Outline of cellular activation system.

for the pore-forming subunit ($Ca_v1.2$) of the cardiac L-type Ca^{2+} channel. The causative mutation G406R results in loss of voltage-dependent channel inactivation leading to maintained inward Ca^{2+} currents and prolongation of the action potential. Because the combination of neurologic and cardiac phenotypes has been reported in CACNA1-mutations, special interest for neurologic evaluation is indicated in these cases.

The ryanodine receptor (or intracellular calcium release channel)

Activation of the contractile elements of the cardiac muscle is mainly governed by mobilization of calcium out of the sarcoplasmatic reticulum into the cytosol [46]. An increase in intracellular calcium concentration is obtained through complex interaction between different calcium channels (eg, Ca-ATPase, voltage-gated calcium channels) and auxiliary proteins. The ryanodine receptor (RyR) plays a crucial role in this process and has been identified in the membrane of the sarcoplasmatic reticulum of different excitable cells (RyR1 in skeletal muscle, RyR2 in cardiac muscle, and RyR3 in brain tissue). Depolarization of the cell membrane at the level of the T tubules triggers the voltage-gated L-type calcium channels to release a small amount of calcium. This small rise in intracellular calcium triggers the activation

or opening of the RyR2 with subsequent massive release of calcium out of the SR. A cluster of approximately 100 RyR2 channels and 25 L-type calcium channels form a "junction." The systolic contraction of the heart is the result of the simultaneous activation of hundreds of thousands of these junctions.

Cardiac calsequestrin

Calsequestrin is the most important calcium storage protein in the sarcoplasmatic reticulum. It is able to bind luminal calcium during diastole to prevent Ca^{2+} precipitation and reduce the ionic calcium concentration. In the heart, RyR2 does not act alone but is part of a macromolecular complex that contains several proteins, including calsequestrin, triadin, junctin, and junctophilin, which make up the calcium release unit.

Catecholaminergic polymorphic ventricular tachycardia

Catecholaminergic polymorphic ventricular tachycardia (CPVT) is a familial arrhythmogenic disorder characterized by adrenergically mediated polymorphic or bidirectional ventricular tachycardia [47]. Two genetic variants of CPVT have been identified as an autosomal-dominant trait caused by mutation in the gene encoding for the RyR2 receptor and one recessive form caused by mutations in the cardiac isoform of the calsequestrin gene (*CASQ2*) [48]. These findings demonstrate that CPVT is caused by mutations of genes that encode for proteins responsible for the regulation of intracellular calcium. Both genes are located on chromosome one (1q42–Q43 and 1p13–p21). More than 70 RyR2 mutations have been identified so far. All are single base pair substitutions, which are mainly located at the carboxy terminus of the protein. Wehrens and colleagues [49] suggested that the common mechanism by which RyR2 mutations cause CPVT is by reducing the binding affinity of RyR2 for the regulatory protein FKBP12.6 (peptidyl-propyl isomerase). The depressed affinity of mutant RyR2 for FKBP12.6 is present in the resting state and worsens when beta-adrenergic stimulation leads to PKA phosphorylation of RyR2. Another theory, proposed by Jiang and colleagues, claims that CPVT is caused by an increased sensitivity to luminal calcium activation. The exaggerated spontaneous calcium release from the SR facilitates the development of delayed after-depolarizations and triggered arrhythmias.

Arrhythmogenic cardiomyopathies

Hypertrophic cardiomyopathy

The prevalence of unexplained left ventricular hypertrophy (LVH) in the general population is estimated to be 1 in 500 [50,51]. Hypertrophic cardiomyopathy (HCM) is a common autosomal-dominant genetic disorder caused by sarcomere mutations; it may account for up to 60% of unexplained cases of LVH, making HCM the most common genetic cardiovascular disorder [52–54]. This clinical entity was first described in 1958 by a pathologist, Donald Teare, as a "benign muscular hamartoma of the heart" [55]. Actually HCM is a well-defined cardiomyopathy characterized macroscopically by LVH, which may be asymmetrical or symmetric. The symmetric form of HCM accounts for more than one third of cases and is characterized by concentric thickening of the left ventricle with a small ventricular cavity dimension. The asymmetrical variant implies thickening of the basal anterior septum, which bulges beneath the aortic valve and causes narrowing of the left ventricular outflow tract; however, HCM may affect any portion of the left ventricle [56]. Another common variant of the asymmetrical form is HCM with apical hypertrophy, which was first described in Japan in 1970 but has been increasingly

diagnosed in western populations. The main pathologic hallmark is the triad of myocyte hypertrophy, disarray, and interstitial fibrosis [57,58].

HCM is caused by dominant mutations in genes that encode constituents of the sarcomere [59]. More than 400 individual mutations have been identified in 11 sarcomere genes, including cardiac α- and β-myosin heavy chains, cardiac troponins T, I, and C, cardiac myosin-binding protein C, α-tropomyosin, actin, titin, and essential and regulatory myosin light chains [60–62]. HCM mutations do not show specific predilections and are unique. Only a few sarcomere mutations have demonstrated a high incidence of premature death or end-stage heart failure, which defines their mutations as potentially "malignant." There are numerous exceptions, however, which indicates the importance of genetic modifiers and the environment on ultimate phenotypic development. Most mutations are single point missense mutations or small deletions or insertions. The most frequent causes of HCM are mutations in cardiac β-myosin heavy chain, cardiac troponin T, cardiac troponin I, and myosin-binding protein C genes [57].

For each gene, several different mutations have been identified, and specific mutations are associated with different severity and prognosis. For example, mutations in troponin T cause only mild or subclinical hypertrophy associated with a poor prognosis and high risk of sudden death (SD). In contrast, mutations in myosin-binding protein C are associated with mild disease and onset in middle age or late adult life. HCM also exhibits intrafamilial phenotypic variation, whereby affected individuals from the same family with an identical genetic mutation display distinct clinical and morphologic manifestations. This finding suggests that lifestyle factors or modifier genes are likely to influence the hypertrophic response [57].

The first pathologic gene identified as responsible for HCM has been the gene encoding for β-myosin heavy chain, mapped on chromosome 14q11 [52]. Cardiac myosin is formed of two heavy chains, two essential and two regulatory light chains. The heavy chains contain two sites for actin interaction and for ATPase activity, respectively. Each heavy chain is compounded by two isoforms: α and β. The first one is predominantly expressed in the atrium, whereas the β isoform preferentially expresses in the ventricle. The genes that encode the β and α isoforms are MYH7 and MYH6, respectively [63,64]. The identified mutations of the first gene number more than

80 and are responsible for HCM in 30% to 40% of patients. These mutations seem to be associated with a severe form of HCM with early onset, complete penetrance, and increased risk of cardiac sudden death. Mutations of MYH6 are rare; most of these mutations are "missense" [65].

Another gene involved in the pathogenesis of HCM is *MYBPC3*, which encodes cardiac myosin-binding protein C; it is located on chromosome 11q1. More than 50 mutations of *MYBPC3* have been identified; they are responsible for an abnormal protein that is unable to interact with myosin and titin. Mutation of cardiac myosin-binding protein C has been found in 30% to 40% of patients [66,67].

HCM also could be caused by a mutation of genes that code for the troponin complex. The gene of troponin T (*TNNT2*) contains 17 exons; "missense" mutations have been found in 15% to 20% of patients with HCM [65]. On the other side, the gene that encodes troponin I (*TNNI3*) is a small gene that is compounded by only 6 exons. It is responsible for a rare asymmetrical HCM characterized by a LV apical hypertrophy; actually only 6 missense mutations have been reported [68].

Mutant essential light chains are responsible for 2% to 3% of HCM; these proteins have a crucial role for calcium linking. *MYL3* is the gene that encodes the isoform light slow ventricular chain (MLC-1 s/v). One single missense mutation (Met 149Val) has been found in this gene causing a form of obstructive HCM [69]. The gene *MYL2* encodes the ventricular isoform regulatory myosin light chain (MLC-2s); 5 different mutations have been reported as causing a phenotype similar to *MYL3* mutation [69].

Cardiac actin has several isoforms also expressed in the skeletal muscle; its gene is *ACTC*. Mutation of this gene causes a mutant product that is not able to interact with β-myosin [54,70,71]. Finally, mutation of gene of α-tropomyosin named *TPM1* is also responsible for 3% of cases of HCM.

Recently genetic studies of familial and sporadic unexplained LVH accompanied by conduction disturbances (progressive atrioventricular block, Wolff-Parkinson-White syndrome, atrial fibrillation) have identified metabolic cardiomyopathies. These genetic forms of hypertrophy reflect mutations in γ2 regulatory subunit (PRKAG2) of AMP-activated protein kinase, an enzyme involved with glucose metabolism, or in the X-linked lysosome-associated membrane protein (LAMP2) gene 22, 23. These clinical entities are distinct from HCM caused by sarcomere protein mutations, despite the shared feature of LVH. A high prevalence of conduction system dysfunction (with the requirement of permanent pacing in 30% of patients) characterizes PRKAG2 mutations. LAMP2 mutations are X linked, which results in male predominance. LAMP2 mutations are associated with early-onset LVH (often in childhood) with rapid progression of heart failure and poor prognosis.

Arrhythmogenic right ventricular dysplasia

Arrhythmogenic right ventricular dysplasia (ARVD) is a disease characterized by the progressive loss of myocytes, and it affects mainly the right ventricular myocardium [72]. It is caused by either massive or partial replacement of myocardium by fatty or fibro-fatty tissue advancing from the epicardium to the endocardium. This infiltration provides a substrate for electrical instability and leads to sustained arrhythmias and sudden death [73].

There are several current concepts surrounding the pathogenesis of ARVD, including the progressive loss of myocytes by programmed cell death (apoptosis) as a consequence of cardiac injury. In some cases of ARVD, myocarditis has been implicated, and entero- and adenoviruses have been identified as potential etiologic agents [72]. There is a strong familial incidence (approximately 50% of cases) with autosomal-dominant inheritance, variable penetrance, and polymorphic phenotypic expression, which suggests that a genetically determined loss of myocytes may account for many cases of the disease. An autosomal-recessive form of ARVD also has been identified. It is associated with palmoplantar keratoderma and woolly hair (Naxos disease). This type of ARVD is caused by a mutation of the plakoglobin gene, the product of which is a component of desmosomes and adherens junctions [73]. The search for the genes responsible for autosomal-dominant ARVD is still underway, and gene linkage analysis of large pedigree has revealed multiple chromosomal loci involved in the pathogenesis of this cardiomyopathy. According to these gene mutations, several different phenotypes of ARVD have been defined.

Arrhythmogenic right ventricular dysplasia 1. This phenotype is caused by mutation in the transforming growth factor beta-3 gene (TGFβ3) on chromosome 14q23–q24. The coding region encodes for a protein of 849 amino acids with a single transmembrane domain and a short stretch of intracellular domain [25]. Beta-type TGFs are polypeptides that act like hormones and control the proliferation and differentiation of multiple cell types. Rampazzo and colleagues [74] performed linkage studies in two large Italian families, one of which had 19 affected members in four generations. They found that 14q23–q24 locus was frequently involved. They also identified in four affected patients two types of mutations of the TGFβ3 gene: 36 G-A transition in the 5′-UTR and 1723 C-T transition in the 3′ UTR.

Arrhythmogenic right ventricular dysplasia 2. ARVD 2 is an autosomal dominant cardiomyopathy characterized by partial degeneration of right ventricular myocardium, electrical instability, and SD [75]. This disease and catecholaminergic polymorphic ventricular tachycardia (CPVT) can be caused by mutation in the cardiac RyR 2 gene located on chromosome 1q42.1–q43. The channel is a tetramer compounded by 4 RyR2 polypeptides and 4 FK506-binding proteins [76]. In myocardial cells, RyR2 proteins—activated by calcium—induced the release of this ion from the sarcoplasmatic reticulum into the cytosol. Tiso and colleagues [75] have demonstrated that RyR2 mutations provide different effects: ARVD 2-associated mutations increase RyR2-mediated calcium release to the cytoplasm and increase intracellular calcium level. RyR2 is the cardiac counterpart of RyR1, which is located in the skeletal muscle and is involved in malignant hyperthermia susceptibility and in central core disease (CCD).

Studies in a family with a "concealed" form of ARVD demonstrated that affected members did not show any structural heart disease, but they consistently presented effort-induced polymorphic ventricular tachycardias. In this family, however, a linkage to 1q42–q43 was demonstrated. In two other families, linkage to 1q42–q43 and 14q23–q24 (ARVD 1) was excluded, which provided evidence of further genetic heterogeneity [77].

ARVD 3. The existence of a novel ARVD locus on chromosome 14, in addition to ARVD 1 at 14q23–q24, was suggested by Severini and colleagues [78] that studied the linkage in three small different families. They found linkage to markers on the proximal part of 14q, named 14q12–q22. This locus is mapped on the long arm of chromosome 14; the gene responsible for ARVD is still unknown.

ARVD 4. In studies of three families, Rampazzo and colleagues [79] mapped a novel ARVD locus to 2q32.1–q32.3. Affected members of the three

families showed clinical characteristics of ARVD according to the diagnostic criteria. Two episodes of SD in young patients were observed. These families were considered unusual in the finding of localized involvement of the left ventricle with left bundle branch block in some affected members. The gene responsible for ARVD 4 is still unknown.

ARVD 5, 6. By linkage analysis in a large North American family, Ahmad and colleagues [80] identified a novel locus for ARVD on 3p23. Asano and colleagues [81] implicated the laminin receptor-1 gene (LAMR1) as responsible for ARVD. An in vitro study of cardiomyocytes expressing the product of mutated Lamr1 showed early cell death accompanied by alterations of chromatine architecture. Asano found that Lamr1 mapped to 3p21, and its mutant product was able to cause degeneration of cardiomyocytes. This mutation is associated with patients affected by ARVD 5.

After exclusion of the five previously known loci, Li and colleagues [82] identified a novel locus on 10p14–p12; they investigated the involvement of the protein tyrosine phosphatase-like gene in a North American family with early-onset ARVD and high penetrance. Protein tyrosine phosphatases mediate the dephosphorylation of phosphotyrosine and are known to be involved in many signal transduction pathways leading to cell growth, differentiation, and oncogenic transformation. Li and colleagues found a missense mutation in gene encoding for protein tyrosine phosphatases; this is the cause of ARVD6.

ARVD 7. Desmin-related myopathy is another term referring to myofibrillar myopathy in which there are intrasarcoplasmic aggregates of desmin. ARVD 7, which maps to chromosome 10q22.3, is another desmin-related myopathy. This is characterized by skeletal muscle weakness associated with cardiac conduction blocks, arrhythmias, heart failure, and intracytoplasmatic accumulation of desmin-reactive deposits in cardiac and skeletal muscle cells [83]. Approximately one third of desmin-related myopathies are thought to be caused by mutations in the desmin gene. The DES gene encodes desmin, a muscle-specific cytoskeletal protein found in the smooth, cardiac, and heart muscles. Melberg and colleagues [84] identified mutations in the ZASP gene, which is located on 10q22.3; patients affected by this mutation showed myopathy, supraventricular arrhythmias, and bradyarrhythmias. Several patients were found to have dilatation of the right ventricle and showed fibro-fatty replacement of myocardium.

ARVD 8. ARVD 8 is caused by a mutation in the gene encoding desmoplakin, which is the most abundant protein of the desmosomes with two isoforms produced by alternative splicing. The gene mentioned previously is on chromosome 6p24. ARVD 8 seems to be caused by a missense mutation in exon 7 of the desmoplakin gene [85]; another mutation has been identified in exon 23. The first mutation is interesting because a homozygous desmoplakin missense mutation had been reported to cause a dilative cardiomyopathy associated with keratoderma and woolly hair. These data suggest that ARVD 8 results from defects in intercellular connections.

ARVD 9. This form of ARVD is caused by heterozygous mutations in the *PKP2* gene, which encodes plakophilin-2 gene, an essential protein of cardiac desmosome [86]. Desmosomes are a complex of multiprotein structures of the cell membrane and provide structural and functional integrity to adjacent cells. The plakophilins are located in the dense plaque of desmosomes, but they are also found in the nucleus, where they have a role in transcriptional regulation. Gerull and colleagues [87] examined 120 patients with diagnosis of ARVD according the criteria proposed by McKenna. They found a high prevalence of mutation of *PKP2* gene, which was mapped to chromosome 12p11. Gerull and colleagues concluded that lack of plakophilin-2 or incorporation of mutant plakophilin-2 in the cardiac desmosomes impairs cell-cell contacts and provides intrinsic variation in conduction properties that may lead to life-threatening arrhythmias.

ARVD 10. The desmosomal cadherins are cell adhesion molecules, and two classes of desmosomal cadherins are known: the desmogleins and the desmocollins (DSC). The desmogleins gene is mapped to chromosome 18q12.1–q12.2 [88]. ARVD 10 is an autosomal-dominant disorder with reduced penetrance characterized by fibrofatty replacement of cardiac myocytes. The more frequent mutation identified is a transition G-to-A at the nucleotide 134 in exon 3. Another mutation, which causes a premature termination of codon, is a 915G-A transition in exon 8 [89].

ARVD 11. This form is caused by a mutation of the *DSC2* gene on chromosome 18q21. Syrris and colleagues [90] identified two different heterozygous mutations in the *DSC2* gene. Both mutations resulted in frame shifts and premature truncation of the DSC protein.

Familial dilated cardiomyopathy

Idiopathic dilated cardiomyopathy (DCM) is the most common cause of congestive heart failure and is characterized by an increase in myocardial mass and a reduction in ventricular wall thickness. The heart assumes a globular shape, and there is a pronounced ventricular chamber dilatation and atrial enlargement, often with thrombi in the appendages. It has been estimated that up to 35% of individuals with idiopathic DCM have a familial disease [59]. This estimate has been shown by detailed pedigree analyses of relatives of patients with DCM coupled with the identification of single gene mutations in structural proteins of the myocyte cytoskeleton or sarcolemma [91]. It has been proposed that familial DCM (FDCM) is a form of "cytoskeletalopathy."

The pattern of inheritance of FDCM is variable and includes autosomal-dominant, X-linked, autosomal-recessive, and mitochondrial inheritance [90]. The autosomal form of FDCM is the most frequent and can be further grouped into either a pure CMP phenotype or DCM with cardiac conduction system disease. Major progress has been made in the identification of candidate disease loci and the genes responsible for FDCM, including mutations in the genes that encode cardiac actin, desmin, δ-sarcoglycan, β-sarcoglycan, cardiac troponin T, and α-tropomyosin. Four candidate genetic loci also have been mapped for DCM with cardiac conduction system disease, but to date there has been identification of only one gene, the lamin A/C gene [91,92]. Mutations in the lamin A/C gene also cause autosomal-dominant FDCM with mild skeletal myopathy and autosomal-dominant Emery-Dreifuss muscular dystrophy. Most molecular causes of autosomal DCM are still unknown; linkage analysis allows mapping many mutations in different chromosomes, such as 1p1–1q1, 9q13–q22, and 3p22–p25. The single mutant gene responsible has not been identified, however. Recently, a missense mutation of gene encoding cardiac actin has been localized on 3p22–p25. In these patients a defect of actin-Z band was evidenced [70].

The X-linked forms of DCM include X-linked DCM and Barth syndrome. The first one is a type of DCM that occurs in boys during adolescence or early adulthood with a rapidly progressive clinical course. Female carriers develop a mild form of DCM with onset in middle age. X-linked DCM is associated with raised concentrations of creatine kinase but without signs of skeletal myopathy and is caused by mutations in the dystrophin gene [91]. Mutations of this gene are also responsible for Duchenne's and Becker's muscular dystrophies. The infantile form of X-linked DCM or Barth syndrome typically affects male infants and is characterized by neutropenia, growth retardation, and mitochondrial dysfunction [93]. One mutant gene, responsible for DCM, is the G4.5, which has been mapped on Xq28. Mutation of this gene causes Barth syndrome, and it seems to be involved in left ventricular noncompaction [91].

Summary

Sudden cardiac death and its devastating consequences still affect millions of individuals throughout the world. Over the last three decades, a tremendous amount of research has focused on possible contributing pathophysiologic mechanisms. The discovery of inherited primary and secondary electrical disorders caused by alterations in our genetic material opened a whole new era of understanding. The knowledge obtained should be incorporated into our new, contemporary approach to malignant ventricular arrhythmias. In the past, the diagnosis of an idiopathic ventricular arrhythmia (without clear cause) was all too readily made. The search for any other plausible explanations ceased whenever structural heart disease could be excluded. Careful familial screening and genetic analysis should be performed in all of these cases. Cardiac channelopathies represent a group of recently discovered arrhythmogenic disorders in structurally normal hearts. In this field, only a fraction of the causative gene mutations have so far been identified. Prognostic assessment of each member of an affected family calls for an individual approach based on clinical features, family analysis, and genetic results.

References

[1] Birney E, Stamatoyannopoulos JA, Dutta A, et al. Identification and analysis of functional elements in 1% of the human genome by the ENCODE pilot project. Nature 2007;447(7146):799–816.

[2] Towbin JA, Bowles NE. Human molecular genetics and the heart. In: Zipes DP, Jalife J, editors. Cardiac electrophysiology, from cell to bedside. 4th edition: Saunders; 2004. p. 444–61.

[3] Noda M, Shimizu S, Tanabe T, et al. Primary structure of electrophorus electricus sodium channel deduced form cDNA sequence. Nature 1984;312: 121–7.

[4] Marban ET, Yamagisji T, Tomaselli GF. Structure and function of voltage gated sodium channels. J Physiol 1998;508(3):647–57.

[5] Balser JR. The cardiac sodium channel: gating function and molecular pharmacology. J Mol Cell Cardiol 2001;33(4):599–613.

[6] Grant AO, Carboni MP, Neplioueva V, et al. Long QT-syndrome, Brugada syndrome and conduction disease are linked to a single sodium channel mutation. J Clin Invest 2002;110:1201–9.

[7] Brugada P, Brugada J. Right bundle branch block, persistent ST-segment elevation and sudden cardiac death: a distinct clinical and electrocardiographic syndrome. A multicenter report. J Am Coll Cardiol 1992;20:1391–6.

[8] Antzelevitch C, Brugada P, Borggrefe M, et al. Brugada syndrome: report of the second consensus conference. Circulation 2005;111:659–70.

[9] Chen Q, Kirsch GE, Zhang D, et al. Genetic basis and molecular mechanism for idiopathic ventricular fibrillation. Nature 1998;392:293–6.

[10] Weiss R, Barmada MM, Nguyen T, et al. Clinical and molecular heterogeneity in the Brugada syndrome: a novel gene locus on chromosome 3. Circulation 2002;105:707–13.

[11] London B, Sanyal S, Michalec M, et al. A mutation in the glycerol-3-phosphate dehydrogenase 1-like gen (GPD1L) causes Brugada syndrome. Circulation 2007;116(20):2260–8.

[12] Bezzina CR, Shimizu W, Yang P, et al. Common sodium channel promoter haplotype in Asian subjects underlies variability in cardiac conduction. Circulation 2006;113:338–44.

[13] Poelzing S, Forleo C, Samodell M, et al. SCN5A polymorphism restores trafficking of a Brugada syndrome mutation on a separate gene. Circulation 2006;114:368–76.

[14] Antzelevitch C. The Brugada syndrome: ionic basis and arrhythmia mechanisms. J Cardiovasc Electrophysiol 2001;12:268–72.

[15] Meregallli PG, Wilde AA, Tan HL. Pathophysiological mechanisms of Brugada syndrome: depolarization disorder, repolarization disorder, or more? Cardiovasc Res 2005;67:367–78.

[16] Lenègre J, Moreau PH. Le bloc auriculo-ventriculaire chronique: etude anatomique, clinique et histologique. Arch Mal Coeur Vaiss 1963;56:867–88.

[17] Lev M. Anatomic basis of atrioventricular block. Am J Cardiol 1964;37:742–8.

[18] Combrink JM, Davis WH, Snyman HW, et al. Familial bundle branch block. Am Heart J 1962;64:397–400.

[19] Steenkamp WF. Familial trifascicular block. Am Heart J 1972;84:758–60.

[20] Brink PA, Ferreira A, Moolman JC, et al. Gene for progressive familial heart block type I maps to chromosome 19q13. Circulation 1995;91:1633–40.

[21] Scott JJ, Alshinawi C, Kyndt F, et al. Cardiac conduction defects associate with mutations in SCN5A. Nat Genet 1999;23:20–1.

[22] Probst V, Kyndt F, Potet F, et al. Haploinsufficiency in combination with aging causes SCN5A-linked hereditary Lenègre disease J Am Coll Cardiol 2003; 41(4):643–52.

[23] Rivolta I, Abriel H, Tateyama M, et al. Inherited Brugada and LQT3-syndrome mutations of a single residue of the cardiac sodium channel confer distinct channel and clinical phenotypes. J Biol Chem 2001; 276:30623–30.

[24] Deal KK, England SK, Tamkun MM. Molecular physiology of cardiac potassium channels. Physiol Rev 1996;76:49–67.

[25] Pongs O, Leicher T, Berger M, et al. Functional and molecular aspects of voltage-gated K-channel B subunits. Ann N Y Acad Sci 1999;868:344–55.

[26] Yellen G. The voltage-gated potassium channels and their relatives. Nature 2002;419:36–42.

[27] Modell SM, Lehmann MH. The long QT syndrome family of cardiac ion channelopathies: a HuGE review. Genet Med 2006;8(3):143–55.

[28] Yoshiyasu A, Kazuo U, Fabiana S, et al. A novel mutation in KCN1 associated with a potent dominant negative effect as the basis for the LQT1 form of the long QT syndrome. J Cardiovasc Electrophysiol 2007;18:972–7.

[29] Craig TJ, Qiuming G, Zhou Z, et al. Long QT syndrome: cellular basis and arrhythmia mechanism in LQT2. J Cardiovasc Electrophysiol 2000; 11:1413–8.

[30] Sanguinetti MC, Keating MT. Role of delayed rectifier potassium channels in cardiac repolarization and arrhythmias. News Physiol Sci 1997;12:152–7.

[31] Sanguinetti MC, Jiang C, Curran ME, et al. A mechanistic link between an inherited and an acquired cardiac arrhythmia: HERG encodes the Ikr potassium channel. Cell 1995;81:299–307.

[32] Laura B, Zhijun S, Dennis AT, et al. Cellular dysfunction of LQT5-minK mutants: abnormalities of Iks, Ikr and trafficking in long QT syndrome. Hum Mol Genet 1999;8:1499–507.

[33] Curran ME, Splawski I, Timothy KW, et al. A molecular basis for cardiac arrhythmias: HERG mutations cause long QT syndrome. Cell 1995;80:795–803.

[34] Tsuboi M, Antzelevitch C. Cellular basis for electrocardiographic and arrhythmic manifestations of Andersen-Tawil syndrome (LQT7). Heart Rhythm 2006;3:328–35.

[35] Gussak I, Brugada P, Brugada J, et al. Idiopathic short QT-interval: a new clinical syndrome? Cardiology 2000;94:99–102.

[36] Gaita F, Cuistetto C, Bianchi F, et al. Short QT-syndrome: a familial cause of sudden death. Circulation 2003;108:965–70.

[37] Brugada R, Hong K, Cordeiro JM, et al. Short QT-syndrome. CMAJ 2005;173(II):1349–54.

[38] Brugada R, Hong K, Dumaine R, et al. Sudden death associated with short-QT syndrome linked to mutations in HERG. Circulation 2004;109:30–5.

[39] Hong K, Bjerregaard P, Gussak I, et al. Short QT-syndrome and atrial fibrillation caused by mutation in KCNH2. J Cardiovasc Electrophysiol 2005; 16:394–6.

[40] Hong K, Piper DR, Diaz-Valdecantos A, et al. De novo KCNQ1-mutation responsible for atrial fibrillation and short QT syndrome in utero. Cardiovasc Res 2005;68(3):1310–25.

[41] Priori SG, Pandit SV, Rivolta I, et al. A novel form of short QT syndrome (SQT3) is caused by a mutation in the KCNJ2 gene. Circ Res 2005;96:800–7.

[42] Ertel EA, Campbell KP, Harpold MM, et al. Nomenclature of voltage-gated calcium channels. Neuron 2000;25:533–5.

[43] Splawski I, Timothy KW, Sharpe LM, et al. Ca(V)1.2 calcium channel dysfunction causes a multisystem disorder including arrhythmia and autism. Cell 2004;119:19–31.

[44] Mckeown L, Robinson P, Jones T. Molecular basis of inherited calcium channelopathies: role of mutations in pore forming units. Acta Pharmacol Sin 2006;27(7):799–812.

[45] Lehnart SE, Ackerman MJ, Benson DW, et al. Inherited arrhythmias: a National Heart, Lung, and Blood Institute and Office of Rare Diseases workshop consensus report about the diagnosis, phenotyping, molecular mechanisms, and therapeutic approaches for primary cardiomyopathies of gene mutations affecting ion channel dysfunction. Circulation 2007;116:2325–45.

[46] Pitt GS, Dun W, Boyden P. Remodeled cardiac calcium channels. J Mol Cell Cardiol 2006;41:373–88.

[47] Mohamed U, Napolitano C, Priori SG. Molecular and electrophysiological bases of catecholaminergic polymorphic ventricular tachycardia. J Cardiovasc Electrophysiol 2007;18:791–7.

[48] Liu N, Colombi B, Raytcheva-Buono E, et al. Catecholaminergic polymorphic ventricular tachycardia. Herz 2007;32:212–7.

[49] Wehrens XH, Lenhart SE, Huang F, et al. FKBP12.6 deficiency and defective calcium release channel (ryanodine receptor) function linked to exercise induced sudden cardiac death. Cell 2003;113:829–40.

[50] Maron BJ, Gardin JM, Flack JM, et al. Prevalence of hypertrophic cardiomyopathy in a general population of young adults: echocardiographic analysis of 4111 subjects in the CARDIA study. Circulation 1995;92:785–9.

[51] Zou Y, Song L, Wang Z, et al. Prevalence of idiopathic hypertrophic cardiomyopathy in China: a population-based analysis of 8080 adults. Am J Med 2004;116:14–8.

[52] Van Driest SL, Ellsworth EG, Ommen SR, et al. Prevalence and spectrum of thin filament mutations

in outpatient referral population with hypertrophic cardiomyopathy. Circulation 2003;108:445–51.

[53] Richard P, Charron P, Carrier L, et al. Hypertrophic cardiomyopathy: distribution of disease genes, spectrum of mutations and implications for a molecular diagnosis strategy. Circulation 2003;107:2227–32.

[54] Arad M, Maron BJ, Gorham JM, et al. Glycogen storage diseases presenting as hypertrophic cardiomyopathy. N Engl J Med 2005;352:362–72.

[55] Teare D. Asymmetrical hypertrophy of the heart in young adults. Br Heart J 1958;20:1–8.

[56] Maron BJ. Sudden death in young athletes. N Engl J Med 2003;349:1064–75.

[57] Maron BJ. Hypertrophic cardiomyopathy: a systematic review. JAMA 2002;287:1308–20.

[58] Hughes SJ. The pathology of hypertrophic cardiomyopathy. Histopathology 2004;44:412–27.

[59] Towbin JA, Bowles NE. The failing heart. Nature 2002;415:227–33.

[60] Seidman JG, Seidman C. The genetic basis for cardiomyopathy: from mutation identification to mechanistic paradigms. Cell 2001;104:557–67.

[61] Charron P, Heron D, Gargiulo M, et al. Genetic testing and genetic counseling in hypertrophic cardiomyopathy: the French experience. J Med Genet 2002;39:741–6.

[62] Geisterfer-Lowrance AA, Kass S, Tanigawa G, et al. A molecular basis for familial hypertrophic cardiomyopathy: a β-myosin heavy chain gene missense mutation. Cell 1990;62(5):999–1006.

[63] Jaenicke T, Diederich KW, Haas W, et al. The complete sequence of the human β myosin heavy chain gene and a comparative analysis of its product. Genomics 1990;8:194–7.

[64] Liew CC, Sole MJ, Yamauchi-Takihara K, et al. Complete sequence and organization of the human cardiac β myosin heavy chain gene. Nucleic Acids Res 1990;18:3647–52.

[65] Watkins H, McKenna WJ, Thierfelder L, et al. Mutations in the genes for cardiac troponin T and α tropomyosin in hypertrophic cardiomyopathy. N Engl J Med 1995;332:1058–63.

[66] Nimura H, Bachinski LL, Sangwatanaroj S, et al. Mutations in the gene for cardiac myosin binding protein C and late onset familial hypertrophic cardiomyopathy. N Engl J Med 1998;338:1248–53.

[67] Rottbauer W, Gautel M, Zehelein J, et al. Novel splice donor site mutation in the cardiac myosin binding protein C gene in familial hypertrophic cardiomyopathy: characterization of cardiac transcript and protein. J Clin Invest 1997;100:475–8.

[68] Moolman JC, Corfield VA. Sudden death due to troponin T mutations. J Am Coll Cardiol 1997;29: 549–54.

[69] Poetter K, Jiang H, Hassanzadeh S, et al. Mutations in either the essential or regulatory light chains of myosin are associated with a rare myopathy in human heart and skeletal muscle. Nat Genet 1996;13: 63–6.

[70] Olson TM, Michels VV, Thibodeau SN, et al. Actin mutations in dilated cardiomyopathy, a heritable form of heart failure. Science 1998;280:750–2.

[71] Blair E, Redwood C, Ashrafian H, et al. Mutations in the gamma(2) subunit of AMP-activated protein kinase cause familial hypertrophic cardiomyopathy: evidence for the central role of energy compromise in disease pathogenesis. Hum Mol Genet 2001;10: 1215–20.

[72] Basso C, Thiene G, Corrado D, et al. Arrhythmogenic right ventricular cardiomyopathy: dysplasia, dystrophy or myocarditis? Circulation 1996;94: 983–91.

[73] Corrado D, Fontine G, Marcus FI, et al. Arrhythmogenic right ventricular dysplasia/cardiomyopathy: need for international registry. Study group on arrhythmogenic right ventricular dysplasia/cardiomyopathy of the working groups of myocardial and pericardial disease and arrhythmias of the European Society of Cardiology and of the Scientific Council of Cardiomyopathies of the World Heart Federation. Circulation 2000;101:E101–6.

[74] Rampazzo A, Beggagna G, Nava A, et al. Arrhythmogenic right ventricular cardiomyopathy type 1 (ARVD1): confirmation of locus assignment and mutation screening of four candidate genes. Eur J Hum Genet 2003;11:69–76.

[75] Tiso N, Stephan DA, Nava A, et al. Identification of mutations in the cardiac ryanodine receptor gene in family affected by arrhythmogenic right ventricular cardiomyopathy type 2 (ARVD2). Hum Mol Genet 2001;10:189–94.

[76] Marx SO, Reiken S, Hisamatsu Y, et al. PKA phosphorylation dissociates FKBP12,6 from the calcium release channel (ryanodine receptor): defective regulation in failing hearts. Cell 2000;101:365–76.

[77] Moren A, Ichijo H, Miyazono K. Molecular cloning and characterization of the human and porcine transforming growth factor beta-type III receptors. Biochem Biophys Res Commun 1992; 189:356–62.

[78] Severini GM, Krajinovic M, Pinamonti B, et al. A new locus for arrhythmogenic right ventricular dysplasia on the long arm of chromosome 14. Genomics 1996;31:193–200.

[79] Rampazzo A, Nava A, Miorin M, et al. ARVD4, a new locus for arrhythmogenic right ventricular cardiomyopathy, maps to chromosome 2 long arm. Genomics 1997;45:259–63.

[80] Ahmad F, Li D, Karibe A, et al. Localization of a gene responsible for arrhythmogenic right ventricular dysplasia to chromosome 3p23. Circulation 1998;98:2791–5.

[81] Asano Y, Takashima S, Asakura M, et al. Lamr1 functional retroposon causes right ventricular dysplasia in mice. Nat Genet 2004;36:123–30.

[82] Li D, Ahmad F, Gardner MJ, et al. The locus of a new gene responsible for arrhythmogenic right ventricular dysplasia characterized by early onset

and high penetrance maps to chromosome 10p12-p14. Am J Hum Genet 2000;66:148–56.

[83] Ferreiro A, Ceuterick-de Groote C, Marks JJ, et al. Desmin-related myopathy with Mallory body-like inclusions is caused by mutations of the selenoprotein N gene. Ann Neurol 2004;55(5):676–86.

[84] Seicen D, Engel AG. Mutations in ZASP define a novel form of muscular dystrophy in humans. Ann Neurol 2005;57:269–76.

[85] Rampazzo A, Nava A, Malacrida S, et al. Mutation in human desmoplakin domain binding to plakoglobin causes a dominant form of arrhythmogenic right ventricular dysplasia. Am J Hum Genet 2002;71:1200–6.

[86] Grossmann KS, Grund C, Huelsken J, et al. Requirement of plakophilin 2 for heart morphogenesis and cardiac junction formation. J Cell Biol 2004;167:149–60.

[87] Gerull B, Heuser A, Wichter T, et al. Mutations in the desmosomal protein plakophilin-2 are common in arrhythmogenic right ventricular cardiomyopathy. Nat Genet 2004;36:1162–4.

[88] Arnemann J, Spurr NK, Magee AI, et al. The human gene (DSG2) coding for HDGC, a second member of the desmoglein subfamily of the desmosomal cadherins, is like DSG1coding for desmoglein DGI, assigned to chromosome 18. Genomics 1992;13:484–6.

[89] Awad MM, Dalal D, Cho E, et al. DSG2 mutations contribute to arrhythmogenic right ventricular dysplasia/cardiomyopathy. Am J Hum Genet 2006;79:136–42.

[90] Syrris P, Ward D, Evans A, et al. Arrhythmogenic right ventricular dysplasia/cardiomyopathy associated with mutations in the desmosomal gene desmocollin-2. Am J Hum Genet 2006;79:978–84.

[91] Sinagra G, Di Lenarda A, Brodsky GL, et al. Current perspectives: new insights into the molecular basis of familial dilated cardiomyopathy. Ital Heart J 2001;2:280–6.

[92] Kass S, MacRae C, Graber HL, et al. A gene defect that causes conduction system disease and dilated cardiomyopathy maps to chromosome 1p1-1q1. Nat Genet 1994;7:546–51.

[93] Bowles NE, Bowles KR, Towbin JA. The "final common pathway" hypothesis and inherited cardiovascular disease. The role of cytoskeletal proteins in dilated cardiomyopathy. Herz 2000;25:168–75.

ELSEVIER
SAUNDERS

Cardiol Clin 26 (2008) 355–366

CARDIOLOGY
CLINICS

Risk Factor Assessment: Defining Populations and Individuals at Risk

Stefan H. Hohnloser, MD, FHRS, FACC, FESC

Department of Medicine, Division of Cardiology, Section Clinical Electrophysiology,
J.W. Goethe University, Theodor-Stern-Kai 7, D-60590 Frankfurt, Germany

Sudden cardiac death (SCD) is defined as the unexpected natural death from cardiac causes within a short time period in a person without a cardiac condition that would appear fatal [1]. SCD is responsible for approximately 300,000 fatalities in the Unites States alone [2,3]. It is estimated that 50% of all cardiac deaths are sudden, and this proportion has remained constant despite the overall decline in cardiovascular mortality during the last decades [3]. In approximately three fourths of cases, SCD is caused by ventricular tachycardia (VT) and fibrillation (VF) [4–6], although in patients who have underlying congestive heart failure (CHF), a significant proportion of SCD is the consequence of bradycardic events or electromechanical dissociation [7].

This article summarizes the current knowledge on risk stratification in patients who have structural heart disease, notably coronary artery disease and nonischemic cardiomyopathy. Although other types of structural heart disease and inherited ion channel abnormalities are also associated with a risk of SCD, the risk stratification strategies and data in these entities are diverse and beyond the scope of this article.

Epidemiologic considerations for risk stratification

The magnitude of the problem in specific subgroups of patients prone to SCD was addressed by Myerburg in a review of the population impact of emerging implantable cardioverter/defibrillator (ICD) trials [8]. The highest incidence of SCD occurred in survivors of out-of-hospital cardiac death and high-risk post infarction subgroups, but the greatest absolute number of SCD events (population attributable risk) occurred in larger subgroups of patients at somewhat lower risk, including patients with left ventricular dysfunction, CHF, or any prior coronary events. The challenge is to identify risk factors for SCD among the large group of patients at relatively low risk, which applies, for example, directly to survivors of myocardial infarction, in an era when the prognosis has improved substantially in comparison with prior series antedating the widespread use of reperfusion therapy.

Among patients suffering from cardiac arrest, most have some form of structural heart disease, with most patients suffering from coronary artery disease [9,10], but acute myocardial infarction is seen in less than half [10,11]. In a series of 151 hearts from men who died from sudden cardiac death, the presence of acute thrombus/plaque rupture or erosion was noted in 67% of patients aged 30 to 39, but this proportion declined with age and was present in only 31% of patients ages 60 to 69 [12]. In another series of patients surviving a cardiac arrest who underwent angiography, recent coronary occlusions were noted in 48% [13].

Risk stratification aims at identifying quantitative and qualitative measurements that can serve as sensitive and specific predictors of cardiac, particularly arrhythmogenic mortality in patients with coronary disease or other cardiovascular diseases [14]. Although risk stratification is always a topic of interest from an intellectual perspective, its clinical relevance depends on the availability of a therapeutic intervention that reduces the risk of

E-mail address: hohnloser@em.uni-frankfurt.de

arrhythmogenic death. Its current relevance is greatly enhanced by the availability of medical therapies and the ICD that have been shown to reduce total and SCD mortality in selected high-risk patients [15–19].

Several potentially useful modalities can be used to stratify postinfarction patients according to their risk of an arrhythmogenic death. To exert an impact on SCD from an epidemiologically meaningful point of view, prognostic tests need to achieve a high positive predictive accuracy together with a reasonable degree of sensitivity. Otherwise, the test or the combination of tests would be too specific to have any significant impact on the epidemiologic problem of SCD simply because they yield positive findings only in a small minority of the postinfarction population. The first step toward this goal requires knowledge of the total number of sudden deaths within a specific patient population expressed as a fraction of total mortality within this group. For example, in patients who have CHF, Kjekshus [20] demonstrated that in studies in which the mean functional New York Heart Association (NYHA) class was between I and II, the overall death rate was relatively low, but 67% of deaths were sudden. In contrast, among studies with a mean functional class of IV, there was a high total mortality, but the fraction of sudden deaths was only 29%. For an intervention specific for the problem of SCD, it is important not only to identify patients at high risk of death but also to predict the most likely mode of death (ie, arrhythmic or nonarrhythmic death) because such a distinction would have a major influence on the treatment strategy. Patients with a high propensity for arrhythmic death may benefit from preventive antiarrhythmic interventions, whereas such treatment may provide no advantage or even increase the risk of mortality in patients more likely to die from nonarrhythmic death. Similarly, the likelihood of a significant benefit from an ICD would only be present in the former group. Accordingly, the various risk stratifiers currently in clinical use need to be examined not only in regard to their ability to predict total mortality but also with respect to their potential to predict specific causes of death.

A pivotal aspect of the clinical impact of risk stratification is that the methodology be applicable not only to specialized referral centers but also to the community hospital setting in which most patients with acute myocardial infarction receive care. For these reasons, invasive procedures are unlikely to gain widespread acceptance. Accordingly, current investigations focus on the development of newer methods of noninvasive risk stratification. Another prerequisite for the process of risk stratification for arrhythmic death is that it be initiated in the predischarge period. The highest risk for sudden cardiac death is within the first 12 months after the index infarction, and most events occur within the first few months [21,22]. Most recently, a substudy from the VALIANT trial reemphasized this finding clearly [23]. This trial enrolled more than 14,000 infarct survivors with left ventricular dysfunction (left ventricular ejection fraction [LVEF] ≤ 40%). These authors clearly demonstrated that the period of highest risk for SCD or cardiac arrest was the first month after myocardial infarction (event rate 1.4%), with a dramatic drop to a fairly constant rate of 0.14% to 0.18% per month thereafter.

Relation between the pathophysiology of sudden cardiac death and risk stratification methods

The conditions that lead to VT/VF may occur transiently or develop during the course of healing from injury to ventricular myocardium and persist. Perhaps as the most important prerequisite, death of myocardial cells results in scar formation, alterations in chamber geometry, and electrical and anatomic remodeling. Trigger or modulating factors of life-threatening arrhythmias include changes in autonomic nervous system activity, metabolic disturbances, myocardial ischemia, electrolyte abnormalities, acute volume and pressure overload of the ventricles, ion channel abnormalities, and proarrhythmic actions of cardiac and noncardiac drugs. The electrophysiologic alterations induced by these conditions initiate and maintain VT/VF most likely via re-entrant mechanisms, although abnormal automaticity, triggered activity, or combinations of these mechanisms may be operative.

Noninvasive approaches have been developed to detect the presence of arrhythmogenic factors that initiate and maintain VT or VF in patients with ischemic and nonischemic heart disease (Fig. 1). For instance, the specific techniques aim to detect extent of myocardial damage and scar formation (LVEF, regional wall motion abnormalities), ventricular ectopy (Holter monitoring), slowed conduction (QRS duration, signal-averaged electrocardiogram [ECG]), heterogeneities

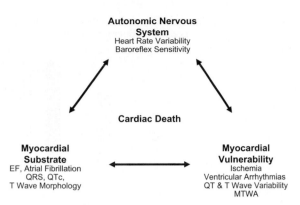

Fig. 1. Factors contributing to cardiac death and respective Holter-derived ECG parameters.

in ventricular repolarization (microvolt T-wave alternans [MTWA]), or imbalances in autonomic tone (heart rate variability [HRV], heart rate turbulence [HRT]).

Approaches to risk stratification

Clinical and demographic data

The GISSI-II Trial of 10,219 hospital survivors after thrombolytic therapy identified several clinical variables that were independently predictive of 6-month mortality. In order of importance, they were the ineligibility for an exercise test (for cardiac or noncardiac reasons), early left ventricular failure, left ventricular dysfunction in the recovery phase, age older than 70 years, electrical instability, late left ventricular failure, prior myocardial infarction, and a history of hypertension [24]. For example, in a recent study of 103,164 patients with myocardial infarction who were 65 years or older, a single-risk model (including older age, comorbidity, heart failure, reduced LVEF, and peripheral vascular disease) effectively stratified patients according to their risk of death 1 year after discharge [25].

Recently, Goldenberg and colleagues [26] attempted to develop a simple risk stratification score for primary ICD therapy based on the MADIT II population. Using best-subset proportional-hazards regression analysis, the following five risk factors for all-cause mortality were identified: age, NYHA class, blood urea nitrogen level, atrial fibrillation, and QRS duration. The risk score was constructed as a count of risk factors identified in each patient. Almost one third of the entire patient population had a risk score of 0;

in this group, crude mortality was similar in the conventional and the ICD groups. By contrast, among patients with one or more risk score factors, crude mortality rates were lower in ICD patients than among patients in the control arm of the study (2-year mortality rate in the ICD group 15% versus 27% in the control arm, $P < .001$). On the other hand, among patients with three or more risk factors, mortality rates were similar in both groups. Based on these findings, the authors noted that a U-shaped pattern for ICD efficacy exists in a population of coronary patients with reduced LV function (Fig. 2). The ICD was found to have a pronounced benefit in the intermediate-risk patients but attenuated efficacy in lower and higher risk subsets. These observations may have important clinical implications when deciding on ICD therapy in individual patients.

Ventricular function

Ventricular function as defined by the predischarge LVEF has been recognized as a major determinant of late mortality for decades [14,22,27,28]. Although the proportion of patients with impaired left ventricular function has declined after reperfusion therapy, the correlation between impaired LVEF and late mortality persists [27]. In comparison with earlier studies, recent series suggest that the curve relating mortality to LVEF has "shifted to the left," implying that for a given degree of left ventricular dysfunction, the increase in mortality is somewhat less than previously reported. A recent study of 313 patients, all of whom had a patent infarct-related artery at the time of discharge, identified that an LVEF of 35% or less still had a positive predictive value of

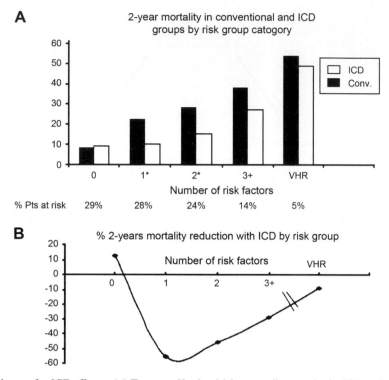

Fig. 2. U-shaped curve for ICD efficacy. (*A*) Two-year Kaplan-Meier mortality rates in the ICD and conventional ther-apy groups. (*B*) The corresponding 2-year mortality rate reduction with an ICD, by risk score, and in very high risk (VHR) patients. * = $P < .05$ for the comparison between the conventional therapy and the ICD groups. (*Adapted from* Goldenberg I, Vyas AK, Hall WJ, et al. Risk stratification for primary implantation of a cardioverter-defibrillator in patients with ischemic left ventricular dysfunction. J Am Coll Cardiol 2008;51:288–96; with permission.)

28% for cardiac death or sustained ventricular ar-rhythmias during follow up [29].

In another series of patients with an anterior myocardial infarction, all of whom underwent primary percutaneous transluminal coronary an-gioplasty, the presence of restrictive diastolic fill-ing as defined by deceleration time on echocardiography of less than 130 msec was asso-ciated with a 2-year mortality rate over a mean of 32 months of 21% versus only 3% in patients without restrictive features [30]. Data such as these point to the presence of smaller patient sub-groups (30% of the total in this series) who may benefit from further risk stratification. On the other hand, these data also suggest that the re-maining 70% of patients with an excellent prog-nosis might not require any additional risk stratification, given a mortality rate of only 3% at 2 years. What is important in this study is that the predictive power of diastolic dysfunction was independent of LVEF.

The use of LVEF as the predominant risk stratifier has serious limitations, however,

because LVEF lacks sensitivity for prediction of SCD. This is emphasized by the fact that less than 50% of infarct survivors who die suddenly have a LVEF of 30% or less. In a recent analysis of the MUSTT data [31], the relationship be-tween 25 variables and total and arrhythmic mortality was examined in 674 patients not re-ceiving antiarrhythmic therapy. In multivariate analysis, the variables with the greatest prognos-tic impact were NYHA class, history of heart failure, nonsustained VT, enrollment as inpa-tient, and atrial fibrillation. From this analysis, it could be shown that patients whose only risk factor is LVEF 30% or less have a predicted 2-year arrhythmic death risk of less than 5% [31]. Importantly, approximately 25% of patients whose LVEF was 30% or less did not have addi-tional risk factors. The conclusion of this study was that in these patients the ICD does not dem-onstrate significant benefit, whereas patients with a LVEF more than 30% but with additional risk factors may derive more benefit from device therapy.

Ambulatory electrocardiographic monitoring

Holter monitoring is a comprehensive tool for identifying and quantifying factors that might contribute to the mechanism of SCD (see Fig. 1). Historically, detecting and quantifying Holter-recorded ventricular arrhythmias was the first ECG-based approach to determine the risk of patients and implement antiarrhythmic therapy [1]. There is clear association between the detection of ventricular arrhythmias (ventricular premature beats [VPBs], non-sustained ventricular tachycardia [NSVT]) on Holter ECG in patients after myocardial infarction with left ventricular dysfunction and the risk for mortality. Primary prevention of sudden death with ICD therapy was introduced by the MADIT and MUSTT trials in patients with documented nonsustained VT and inducibility of ventricular tachyarrhythmias [15,16]. After the MADIT II [18] and SCD-HeFT [32] trials, however, LVEF of 30% or less is considered a sufficient risk stratifier without the need for documenting Holter-detected ventricular arrhythmias or inducible VT. Accordingly, the incremental risk stratification value provided by the finding of spontaneous ventricular arrhythmias in patients with LVEF of 35% or less is unclear. On the other hand, patients with LVEF between 35% and 40% may warrant Holter ECG recordings to assess for nonsustained VT, because this group has been shown to benefit from an ICD if VT is induced at electrophysiologic study. Patients with preserved left ventricular function after myocardial infarction are generally at low risk, and current data suggest that they would not benefit from undergoing risk stratification using Holter ECG recording.

QRS width, signal-averaged electrocardiogram

A broad QRS complex is associated with an increased risk of mortality, and patients with conduction disturbances do not benefit much from signal-averaged ECG (SAECG) analyses. The presence of late potentials or prolonged filtered QRS duration in SAECG in patients with normal QRS duration on standard ECG indicates increased risk of cardiac events, however. Data from MUSTT trial [33] in 1925 patients demonstrated that filtered QRS duration longer than 114 msec was significantly associated with the primary study endpoint (arrhythmic death or cardiac arrest) after adjustment for clinical covariates. Patients with an abnormal SAECG had a 28% incidence of primary endpoints in comparison to

17% in patients with normal SAECG ($P < .001$) during 5-years' follow-up. Cardiac death and total mortality also were significantly higher. In this study, combination of prolonged filtered QRS duration longer than 114 msec and LVEF less than 30% identified a high-risk subset of patients. This finding was of particular importance because the clinical usefulness of inducible ventricular tachycardia was found to be limited in this study.

Data also indicate that the combination of abnormalities in SAECG with positive results of T-wave alternans test might be useful in identifying high-risk individuals in the early postinfarction period [34,35]. Bayley et al [36] suggested the use of SAECG together with LVEF as first steps of risk stratification process in postinfarction patients. Patients with normal SAECG and preserved left ventricular function have a low risk of arrhythmic events (approximately 2% over 5-year period), whereas patients with abnormal SAECG and depressed LVEF have a high risk of such events (approximately 38%). Intermediate groups, with either test abnormal, require further stratification using Holter-based HRV and ventricular arrhythmia analysis or programmed ventricular stimulation. Ultimately, this strategy is likely to identify most patients eligible for ICD therapy and patients who may not need this treatment. In summary, ample data show that an abnormal SAECG may identify patients with prior myocardial infarction at risk for SCD. Given the high negative predictive value of this test, it may be useful for identifying patients at low risk. Routine use of SAECG for identifying patients at high risk for SCD seems to be not adequately supported at this time, however.

Microvolt T-wave alternans

The presence of subtle beat-to-beat changes in the in the amplitude of the T-wave in the surface ECG, which is termed microvolt T-wave alternans (MTWA), has been shown to be associated with an increased risk of SCD or other serious ventricular tachyarrhythmic events [34,35,37]. Particularly in patients with ischemic and nonischemic cardiomyopathy, assessment of MTWA has been shown to be useful for prediction of arrhythmic complications during the subsequent course of these patients. For instance, a report on 129 patients with ischemic cardiomyopathy found that over 24 months' follow-up, no major arrhythmic event or SCD occurred in patients who tested negative; on the other hand, in MTWA-positive patients or patients with an indeterminate test result, the event rate was 15.6% [38].

Bloomfield and coworkers [39] recently reported their findings in 177 MADIT II-like patients in whom they assessed MTWA and whom they followed for 2 years. They found that a positive MTWA was associated with a higher mortality rate than that associated with a prolonged QRS duration of more than 120 msec. The actuarial mortality rate was 17.8% in patients with a positive MTWA compared with only 3.8% in patients who tested negative for MTWA (hazard ratio 4.8, 95% confidence interval 1.1–20.7, $P = .02$). Several additional studies confirmed these early findings (Fig. 3). It is of particular note that in all studies evaluating MTWA for arrhythmic risk stratification, MTWA carried a high negative predictive value of between 96% and 100%. This finding indicates that analysis of MTWA may be particularly helpful to avoid unnecessary ICD implantations in patients with depressed LV function who test negative for MTWA.

Similarly, there are at least four prospective studies about the predictive value of MTWA after myocardial infarction. In all but one of these studies, assessment of a positive (abnormal) MTWA carried prognostic implications with respect to future arrhythmic events and SCD [34,40–42]. One of these studies deserves more detailed considerations because currently, risk stratification after acute myocardial infarction relies predominantly on the presence of reduced LV function. Little is known about the value of risk markers in infarct survivors with preserved LV function. Accordingly, Ikeda and colleagues [42] measured MTWA in 1014 patients with a LVEF of 0.40 or more at 48 ± 66 days after an acute myocardial infarction along with 10 other commonly used risk variables. Over a mean of 32 ± 14 months, a positive MTWA, nonsustained VT, and ventricular late potentials were predictors of SCD or ventricular tachyarrhythmias (primary study endpoint). On multivariate analysis, a positive MTWA test result was the most significant predictor (HR 19.7).

In conclusion, these studies indicate that MTWA assessment may yield prognostic information regarding ventricular tachyarrhythmic events in infarct survivors even in patients with preserved LV function. It seems clear, however, that MTWA evolves during the subacute phase of myocardial infarction, indicating that its determination should be postponed until some weeks after the index event.

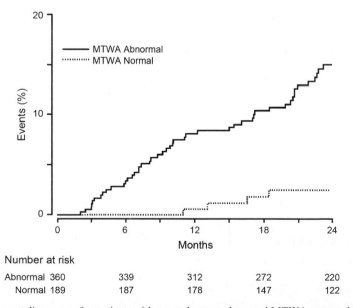

Fig. 3. Kaplan-Meier mortality curves for patients with normal versus abnormal MTWA test results. During the 2-year follow-up period, only four events occurred in 189 patients with a negative MTWA compared with 47 in the nonnegative group. Nonnegative test results comprised positive tests ($n = 162$, 2-year event rate 12.3%) and indeterminate test ($n = 198$, 2-year event rate 17.5%). (*From* Bloomfield D, Bigger J, Steinman R, et al. Microvolt T-wave alternans and the risk of death or sustained ventricular arrhythmias in patients with left ventricular dysfunction. J Am Coll Cardiol 2006;47:460; with permission.)

Measures of autonomic control

Numerous studies explored the prognostic value of HRV parameters for predicting outcomes in postinfarction patients [43–47]. They consistently showed that depressed HRV is associated with increased mortality. Limited data are available regarding the prognostic significance of HRV parameters for predicting sudden or arrhythmic death. The limited evidence for the association between depressed HRV parameters and SCD might be caused by the difficulty in categorizing sudden or arrhythmic nature of death but also could be because of lack of strong evidence for this association. HRV also operates differently in different patient populations depending not only on the disease but also on advancement of the disease process. HRV parameters predict well CHF worsening and total mortality in CHF patients, whereas the predictive value of HRV for SCD is limited. Similarly, there are no studies linking HRV with inducibility at electrophysiologic testing, which further indicates that HRV might not be the right approach to identify susceptibility to arrhythmias. Reported associations with arrhythmic events are most likely driven by CHF, which predisposes to SCD itself.

HRT is a new method to evaluate the response of sinus beats to single ventricular premature beats [48]. The normal response to VPBs consists of immediate acceleration with subsequent deceleration of heart rate, whereas a blunted response, which does not show such a reaction, is considered as a noninvasive sign of impaired baroreflex sensitivity. Schmidt and coworkers [48] demonstrated that HRT quantified using two parameters that describe turbulence onset and turbulence slope was an independent predictor of total or cardiovascular mortality in two large post infarction populations. This observation was further substantiated by recent analysis of data in postinfarction patients from the ATRAMI study [49] and the ISAR study [50], with most patients treated with primary coronary interventions. As with HRV parameters, there is no support for direct association between HRT parameters and sudden death. Finally, the method of HRT assessment was recently even more refined by characterizing the deceleration and acceleration of heart rate [51]. This finding led to the determination of deceleration capacity, which could be shown to be a significant predictor of mortality after myocardial infarction.

In summary, strong evidence links depressed HRV and abnormal HRT with cardiac mortality. These methods should be used in the risk stratification process, however, with full realization that their predictive value might not be directly related to sudden death or arrhythmic events.

Invasive electrophysiological testing

Testing inducibility of ventricular tachycardia in postinfarction patients became a standard modality for identifying high-risk individuals prone to sudden death. MADIT and MUSTT were designed to enroll postinfarction patients with depressed LVEF who presented with nonsustained VT and inducibility of ventricular tachyarrhythmias during invasive electrophysiologic testing [15,16]. These primary prevention trials with the use of ICDs demonstrated that the risk stratification algorithm was able to select a subset of postinfarction patients with high mortality risk. Secondary analysis from MUSTT [52] revealed that despite significant difference in outcome between inducible patients enrolled in the trial and noninducible patients enrolled in a registry, electrophysiological (EP) inducibility was found of limited use because the 5-year mortality rate in inducible patients was 48% compared with 44% in noninducible patients.

Later, data from MADIT II showed that there is no need for additional risk stratifiers (including EP testing) when LVEF is so low. In more than 80% of patients randomized to the ICD arm of MADIT II, invasive EP testing with attempt to induce tachyarrhythmias was performed at the time of ICD placement. VT inducibility, observed in 40% of studied patients, was not effective in identifying patients with cardiac events defined as ventricular tachycardia, ventricular fibrillation, or death. These observations from both MUSTT and MADIT II subanalyses suggest that in patients with substantially depressed left ventricular function, EP inducibility should not be considered a useful predictor of outcome. It is possible, however, that inducibility might have much better predictive value in postinfarction patients with LVEF more than 30% or more than 35%.

Risk stratification in nonischemic cardiomyopathy

The previous sections focused on postinfarction patients, whereas a growing number of patients who have CHF and nonischemic

Table 1
Prospective studies using microvolt T-wave alternans for risk stratification in patients with dilated cardiomyopathy

Study (reference)	Patient population	Patients (N)/follow-up (mo)	Primary study endpoint	% patients with nonnegative MTWA	Main result
Klingenheben [56]	CHF, LVEF < 0.45, ICMP 70%, NICMP 30%	107 14.6 mo	Arrhythmic death or VT/VF	70%	MTWA = predictor of PEP (HR ∞)
Hohnloser [38]	ICMP, LVEF <0.35	129 24 mo	Arrhythmic death	73%	MTWA = predictor of PEP (HR ∞)
Bloomfield [39]	ICMP, LVEF < 0.35	177 20 ± 6 mo	2 year all-cause mortality	68%	MTWA = predictor of PEP (HR 4.8)
Hohnloser [53]	NICMP	137 14 ± 6 mo	Arrhythmic death or resuscitated VF/VT	75%	MTWA = predictor of PEP (HR 3.4)
Grimm [54]	NICMP	343 52 ± 21	Arrhythmic death or resuscitated VF/VT	NA	MTWA not predictive of PEP
Bloomfield [57]	ICMP (49%), NICMP (51%)	549 20 ± 6 mo	All-cause mortality or non-fatal VT/VF	66%	MTWA = predictor of PEP (HR 6.5)
Chow [58]	ICMP, LVEF < 0.35	768 18 ± 10 mo	All-cause mortality	67%	MTWA = predictor of all-cause (HR 2.2) and arrhythmic mortality (HR 2.3)
Salerno-Uriarte [55]	NICMP, LVEF < 0.40	446 NA	Cardiac death, life-threatening ventricular arrhythmias	65%	MTWA = predictor of PEP (HR 4.0)

Abbreviations: CHF, congestive heart failure; HR, hazard ratio; ICMP, ischemic cardiomyopathy; NICMP, nonischemic cardiomyopathy; PEP, primary endpoint.

cardiomyopathy is being seen by cardiologists and is considered for prophylactic ICD therapy. DEFINITE [19] was a recent trial that evaluated the effects of ICD therapy on mortality in patients with nonischemic cardiomyopathy. Approximately half of patients enrolled in SCD-HeFT [32] had nonischemic cardiomyopathy. Both these studies indicated that ICD therapy reduces mortality in nonischemic cardiomyopathy patients. Following these findings, new indications for ICD in the United States include nonischemic cardiomyopathy with LVEF of 30% or less.

The question remains as to how to identify patients with nonischemic cardiomyopathy who might benefit from ICD therapy more than other individuals. Invasive EP testing with inducibility of ventricular arrhythmias is not useful as a risk stratification method. Several noninvasive techniques were explored, including presence of nonsustained VT, abnormal signal averaged ECG, HRV, and recently, MTWA. Among these noninvasive modalities, MTWA seems to be of increasing interest in dilated cardiomyopathy patients. For instance, Hohnloser et al [53] studied 137 dilated cardiomyopathy patients followed for a mean 14 months and found that decreased baroreflex sensitivity and presence of MTWA were the only two significant predictors of arrhythmic events outperforming other tested parameters, including NSVT, SAECG, LVEF, and HRV. At least one other study could not confirm these observations, however [54].

Several other studies have examined the prognostic yield of MTWA determination in this population (Table 1). Recently, the largest prospective study on the use of MTWA for risk stratification in nonischemic cardiomyopathy was published [55]. In an Italian multicenter study, 464 patients were tested for MTWA and subsequently followed for 18 to 24 months for the primary endpoint of cardiac death and life-threatening arrhythmias. For patients who tested MTWA positive, the unadjusted and adjusted hazard ratios were 4.0 (95% confidence interval 1.4–11.4; $P = .002$) and 3.2 (1.1–9.2; $P = .013$). Importantly, the negative predictive value of the test was more than 97%. The authors concluded that an abnormal MTWA test result in patients with nonischemic cardiomyopathy, NYHA II/III CHF, and a LVEF less than 40% selects a group of patients at high risk for SCD. Conversely, patients with unremarkable test results have a benign prognosis and are not expected to derive much benefit from ICD therapy.

Summary

Vigorous efforts have been made in developing noninvasive stratification methods. Unfortunately, a coherent strategy for intervention based on data integrating the results of these techniques is still lacking. Currently, the primary technique for stratifying risk to determine who are appropriate candidates for an ICD for primary prevention of SCD is the LVEF. It is reasonable to place patients with LVEF of 30% to 35% or less in the highest risk group that can be identified currently. This applies to patients with coronary artery disease and dilated cardiomyopathy. Future studies will assess whether further risk stratification within this population can be achieved. More randomized intervention trials based on the results of risk stratification techniques (ie, assessment of MTWA or HRT) are needed. Although the lack of a dominant strategy using these techniques is caused partly by the absence of clinical trial data, it is also important to consider that there may be limitations to the current techniques. Most of these techniques focus on the evaluation of electrical, autonomic, or anatomic substrates of the patient at rest, when the risk of SCD is low. Some of the techniques involve evaluations during exercise and the post-exercise recovery period—times of relatively increased risk for SCD and ventricular arrhythmias. Other factors may be implicated in the pathophysiology of SCD. Newer approaches that encompass a more general evaluation of "vulnerability" to sudden death, including genetic profiling, serum markers, and new imaging approaches, are necessary. Finally, if risk stratification is to be applied to a population with an overall low risk of SCD to identify a subgroup with more significant risk, it is likely that multiple tests will need to be incorporated into a risk stratification strategy. A single test, even with good sensitivity and specificity, when applied to a population with a low incidence of SCD has has poor positive predictive value. Although it is possible that multiple positive test results could be used to identify particularly high-risk individuals, it is also possible that such a strategy would limit the proportion of the "at-risk" population that can be identified.

References

[1] Zipes DP, Wellens HJJ. Sudden cardiac death. Circulation 1998;98:2334–22351.

[2] Gillum RF. Sudden coronary deaths in the Unites States 1980–1985. Circulation 1989;79:756–65.

[3] Myerburg RJ, Kessler KM, Catellanos A. Sudden cardiac death: structure, function, and time-dependence of risk. Circulation 1992;85(Suppl I):I1–10.

[4] Schaffer WA, Cobb LA. Recurrent ventricular fibrillation and modes of death in survivors of out-of-hospital ventricular fibrillation. N Engl J Med 1975;293:259–62.

[5] Wilber DJ, Garan H, Finkelstein D, et al. Out-of-hospital cardiac arrest: use of electrophysiologic testing in the prediction of long-term outcome. N Engl J Med 1988;318:19–24.

[6] Meissner AD, Akhtar M, Lehman MH. Nonischemic sudden tachyarrhythmic death in artheroscleratic heart disease. Circulation 1991;84:905–12.

[7] Liu M, Stevenson WG, Stevenson LW, et al. Diverse mechanisms of unexpected cardiac arrest in advanced heart failure. Circulation 1989;80:1675–80.

[8] Myerburg RJ, Mitrani R, Interian A, et al. Interpretation of outcomes of antiarrhythmic clinical trials: design features and population impact. Circulation 1998;97:1514–21.

[9] Liberthson RR, Nagel EL, Hirschman JC, et al. Pathophysiologic observations in prehospital ventricular fibrillation and sudden cardiac death. Circulation 1974;49:790–7.

[10] Reichenbach DD, Moss NS, Meyer E. Pathology of the heart in sudden cardiac death. Am J Cardiol 1977;39:865–9.

[11] Kannel WB, Thomas HE. Sudden coronary death: the Framingham study. Ann N Y Acad Sci 1982;382:3–21.

[12] Farb A, Burke AP, Kolodgie FD, et al. Risk profiles are more abnormal and acute thrombi more frequent in young men with sudden death [abstract]. J Am Coll Cardiol 1999;33:324.

[13] Spaulding CM, Joly LM, Rosenberg A, et al. Immediate coronary angiography in survivors of out-of-hospital cardiac arrest. N Engl J Med 1997;336:1629–33.

[14] Camm AJ, Katrisis DG. Risk stratification of patients with ventricular arrhythmias. In: Zipes DP, Jalife J, editors. Cardiac electrophysiology: from cell to bedside. Philadelphia: W.B. Saunders Co.; 2000. p. 808–28.

[15] Moss AJ, Hall WJ, Cannom DS, et al. Improved survival with an implanted defibrillator in patients with coronary disease at high risk for ventricular arrhythmias. N Engl J Med 1996;335:1933–40.

[16] Buxton AE, Lee KL, Fischer JD, et al. A randomized study of the prevention of sudden death in patients with coronary artery disease: Multicenter Unsustained Tachycardia Trial Investigators. N Engl J Med 1999;341:1882–90.

[17] The Antiarrhythmics Versus Implantable Defibrillators (AVID) Investigators. A comparison of antiarrhythmic-drug therapy with implantable defibrillators in patients resuscitated from near-fatal ventricular arrhythmias. N Engl J Med 1997;337:1576–83.

[18] Moss AJ, Zareba W, Hall WJ, et al, Multicenter Automatic Defibrillator Implantation Trial II investigators. Prophylactic implantation of a defibrillator in patients with myocardial infarction and reduced ejection fraction. N Engl J Med 2002;346:877–83.

[19] Kadish A, Dyer A, Daubert JP, et al. Prophylactic defibrillator implantation in patients with nonischemic dilated cardiomyopathy. N Engl J Med 2004;350:2151–8.

[20] Kjekshus J. Arrhythmias and mortality in congestive heart failure. Am J Cardiol 1990;65:421–8.

[21] Myerburg Kessler M, Castellanos A. Sudden cardiac death: epidemiology, transient risk, and intervention assessment. Ann Intern Med 1993;119:1187–97.

[22] Hohnloser SH, Klingenheben T, Zabel M. Identification of patients after myocardial infarction at risk of life-threatening arrhythmias. Eur Heart J 1999;1(Suppl C):C11–20.

[23] Solomon SD, Zelenkofske S, McMurray JJ, et al. Sudden death in patients with myocardial infarction and left ventricular dysfunction, heart failure, or both. N Engl J Med 2005;352:2581–8.

[24] Tavazzi L, Volpi A. Remarks about postinfarction prognosis in light of the experience with the Gruppo Italiano per lo Studio della Sopravivenza nell' Infarto Miocardico (GISSI) Trials. Circulation 1997;95:1341–5.

[25] Krumholz HM, Chen J, Chen YT, et al. Predicting one-year mortality among elderly survivors of hospitalization for an acute myocardial infarction: results from the cooperative cardiovascular project. J Am Coll Cardiol 2001;38:453–9.

[26] Goldenberg I, Vyas AK, Hall WJ, et al. Risk stratification for primary implantation of a cardioverter-defibrillator in patients with ischemic left ventricular dysfunction. J Am Coll Cardiol 2008;51:288–96.

[27] Rouleau JL, Talajic M, Sussex B, et al. Myocardial infarction patients in the 1990s: their risk factors, stratification and survival in Canada. The Canadian Assessment of Myocardial Infarction (CAMI) Study. J Am Coll Cardiol 1996;27:1119–27.

[28] Gomes JA, Winters SL, Martison M, et al. The prognostic significance of quantitative signal-averaged variables related to clinical variables, site of myocardial infarction, ejection fraction and ventricular arrhythmias: a prospective study. J Am Coll Cardiol 1988;1:377–84.

[29] Klingenheben T, Sporis S, Mauss O, et al. Value of autonomic markers for noninvasive risk stratification in post infarction patients with a patent infarct-related artery [abstract]. Pacing and Clinical Electrophysiology 2000;23(II):733.

[30] Cerisano G, Bolognese L, Buonamici P, et al. Prognostic implications of restrictive left ventricular filling in reperfused anterior acute myocardial infarction. J Am Coll Cardiol 2001;37:793–9.

[31] Buxton AE, Lee KL, hafley GE, et al. Limitations of ejection fraction for prediction of sudden death risk in patients with coronary artery disease. J Am Coll Cardiol 2007;50:1150–7.

[32] Bardy GH, Lee KL, Mark DB, et al. Amiodarone or an implantable cardioverter-defibrillator for congestive heart failure. N Engl J Med 2005;352: 225–37.

[33] Gomes Gomez JA, Caine ME, Buxton AE. Prediction of long-term outcomes by signal-averaged electrocardiography in patients with unsustained ventricular tachycardia, coronary artery disease, and left ventricular dysfunction. Circulation 2001; 104:436–41.

[34] Ikeda T, Sakata T, Takami M, et al. Combined assessment of T-wave alternans and late potentials used to predict arrhythmic events after myocardial infarction: a prospective study. J Am Coll Cardiol 2000;35:722–30.

[35] Gold MR, Bloomfield DM, Anderson KP, et al. Comparison of T-wave alternans, signal averaged electrocardiography and programmed ventricular stimulation for arrhythmia risk stratification. J Am Coll Cardiol 2000;36:2247–53.

[36] Bailey JJ, Berson AS, Handelsman H, et al. Utility of current risk stratification tests for predicting major arrhythmic events after myocardial infarction. J Am Coll Cardiol 2001;38:1902–11.

[37] Hohnloser SH. T wave alternans. In: Zipes DP, Jalife J, editors. Cardiac electrophysiology: from cell to bedside. 4th edition. Philadelphia: WB Saunders Co.; 2004. p. 839–47.

[38] Hohnloser SH, Ikeda T, Bloomfield DM, et al. T-wave alternans negative coronary patients with low ejection fraction and benefit from defibrillator implantation. Lancet 2003;362:125–6.

[39] Bloomfield DM, Steinman RC, Namerow PB, et al. Microvolt T-wave alternans distinguishes between patients likely and patients not likely to benefit from implanted cardiac defibrillator therapy. Circulation 2004;110:1885–9.

[40] Tapanainen JM, Still AM, Airaksinen KEJ, et al. Prognostic significance of risk stratifiers of mortality, including T-wave alternans, after acute myocardial infarction: results of a prospective follow-up study. J Cardiovasc Electrophysiol 2001; 12:645–52.

[41] Ikeda T, Saito H, Tanno K, et al. T-wave alternans as a predictor for sudden cardiac death after myocardial infarction. Am J Cardiol 2002;89: 79–82.

[42] Ikeda T, Yoshino H, Sugi K, et al. Predictive value of microvolt T-wave alternans for sudden cardiac death in patients with preserved cardiac function after acute myocardial infarction. J Am Coll Cardiol 2006;48:2268–74.

[43] Kleiger RE, Miller JP, Bigger JT Jr, et al. Decreased heart rate variability and its association with increased mortality after acute myocardial infarction. Am J Cardiol 1987;59:256–62.

[44] Bigger JT Jr, Fleiss JL, Kleiger R, et al. The relationships among ventricular arrhythmias, left ventricular dysfunction, and mortality in the 2 years after myocardial infarction. Circulation 1984;69: 250–8.

[45] Bilchick KC, Fetics B, Doukeng R, et al. Prognostic value of heart rate variability in chronic congestive heart failure (Veterans Affairs' Survival Trial of Antiarrhythmic Therapy in Congestive Heart Failure). Am J Cardiol 2002;90:24–8.

[46] Nolan J, Batin PD, Andrews R, et al. Prospective study of heart rate variability and mortality in chronic heart failure: results of the United Kingdom heart failure evaluation and assessment of risk trial (UKHeart). Circulation 1998;98:1510–6.

[47] Fauchier L, Babuty D, Cosnay P, et al. Prognostic value of heart rate variability for sudden death and major arrhythmic events in patients with idiopathic dilated cardiomyopathy. J Am Coll Cardiol 1999; 33:1203–7.

[48] Schmidt G, Malik M, Barthel P, et al. Heart-rate turbulence after ventricular premature beats as a predictor of mortality after acute myocardial infarction. Lancet 1999;353:1390–6.

[49] Ghuran A, Reid F, La Rovere MT, et al. The ATRAMI Investigators: heart rate turbulence-based predictors of fatal and nonfatal cardiac arrest. The Autonomic Tone and Reflexes After Myocardial Infarction substudy. Am J Cardiol 2002;89: 184–90.

[50] Barthel P, Schneider R, Bauer A, et al. Risk stratification after acute myocardial infarction by heart rate turbulence. Circulation 2003;108:1221–6.

[51] Bauer A, Kantelhardt JW, Barthel P, et al. Deceleration capacity of heart rate as a predictor of mortality after myocardial infarction. Lancet 2006;367: 1674–81.

[52] Buxton AE, Lee KL, DiCarlo L, et al. Electrophysiologic testing to identify patients with coronary artery disease who are at risk for sudden death. N Engl J Med 2000;342:1937–45.

[53] Hohnloser SH, Klingenheben T, Bloomfield D, et al. Usefulness of microvolt T-wave alternans for prediction of ventricular tachyarrhythmic events in patients with dilated cardiomyopathy: results from a prospective observational study. J Am Coll Cardiol 2003;41:2220–4.

[54] Grimm W, Christ M, Bach J, et al. Noninvasive arrhythmia risk stratification in idiopathic dilated cardiomyopathy: results of the Marburg Cardiomyopathy Study. Circulation 2003;108: 2883–91.

[55] Salerno-Uriarte JA, De Ferrari GM, Klersy C, et al. Prognostic value of T-wave alternans in patients with heart failure due to nonischemic cardiomyopathy. J Am Coll Cardiol 2007;50:1896–904.

[56] Klingenheben T, Zabel M, D'Agostino RB, et al. Predictive value of T-wave alternans for arrhythmic events in patients with congestive heart failure. Lancet 2000;356:651–2.

[57] Bloomfield D, Bigger J, Steinman R, et al. Microvolt T-wave alternans and the risk of death or sustained ventricular arrhythmias in patients with left ventricular dysfunction. J Am Coll Cardiol 2006;47:456–63.

[58] Chow T, Kereiakes D, Bartone C, et al. Prognostic utility of microvolt T-wave alternans in risk stratification of patients with ischemic cardiomyopathy. J Am Coll Cardiol 2006;47:1820–7.

Ventricular Arrhythmias in Normal Hearts

Shuaib Latif, MD, Sanjay Dixit, MD, David J. Callans, MD*

*Department of Medicine, Cardiovascular Medicine Division, Section of Electrophysiology,
Hospital of the University of Pennsylvania, 9129 Founders Pavilion,
3400 Spruce Street, Philadelphia, PA 19104, USA*

Despite advances in the treatment of ventricular tachyarrhythmias, their management continues to challenge clinicians. Ventricular tachyarrhythmias are most commonly seen in patients who have structural heart disease; however, 10% of patients presenting with ventricular tachyarrhythmias have no apparent structural heart disease. These patients are said to have idiopathic ventricular tachycardia (VT) and have been segregated into subtypes defined by QRS morphology, ventricular origin, and response to pharmacologic agents. The management and the prognosis of idiopathic VT differ considerably from VT in the setting of identifiable structural abnormalities.

The diagnosis of idiopathic VT is made after a thorough cardiac evaluation yields normal results. The initial evaluation often consists of the resting ECG and evaluation of ventricular function, both of which are normal between episodes of tachycardia. Further evaluation by signal-averaged ECG also demonstrates normal findings between episodes of tachycardia [1]. An evaluation of coronary perfusion should be considered in appropriate patients to exclude possible coronary artery disease as an etiology of VT. Further studies such as right ventricular (RV) perfusion imaging [2] and RV biopsy [3–5] are rarely performed but may be of use in differentiating between idiopathic VT and VT in the setting of organic heart disease. It is important to note that although the classic definition of idiopathic VT continues to refer to a structurally normal

heart, techniques for assessing myocardial structure and function continue to evolve and provide further insight into possible mechanisms of these arrhythmias. Cardiac MRI may reveal mild structural abnormalities, the significance of which is still debated [6–8]. In addition, positron emission tomography has been used to demonstrate functional autonomic differences in patients who have idiopathic VTs [9,10]. I-131 meta-iodobenzylguanidine imaging staining has inconsistently shown abnormalities in the outflow tract region of some patients manifesting idiopathic VT [11,12]. As the resolution of testing continues to increase to the cellular and molecular level, it is likely that these arrhythmias will be found to have associated abnormalities.

Although subtle abnormalities may be seen on advanced imaging studies in idiopathic VTs, it may be difficult to distinguish normal myocardium from pathologic substrates early in their course. Pathologic conditions such as arrhythmogenic RV cardiomyopathy/dysplasia (ARVC/D) demonstrate electrical abnormalities on signal-averaged ECG [13,14], voltage mapping [15], and inducible VT with programmed stimulation. In addition, there are identifiable genetic mutations in desmosomal proteins in some patients who have ARVC/D [16]; however, patients initially diagnosed with idiopathic VT then found to develop ARVC/D have been reported, demonstrating the potential difficulty in differentiating between the two diagnoses [17].

The syndrome of idiopathic VT refers specifically to monomorphic VTs. Polymorphic VTs and ventricular fibrillation have been described in structurally normal hearts but differ from idiopathic VT mechanistically and prognostically.

---

* Corresponding author.

E-mail address: david.callans@uphs.upenn.edu
(D.J. Callans).

0733-8651/08/$ - see front matter © 2008 Elsevier Inc. All rights reserved.
doi:10.1016/j.ccl.2008.03.011

Idiopathic VT can be subclassified based on several criteria (eg, mechanism, location, response to pharmacologic therapy). Most commonly, these arrhythmias are subgrouped as outflow tract tachycardias, idiopathic left VTs (ILVTs), and automatic VTs.

Outflow tract tachycardia

VTs originating from the outflow tracts account for most cases [18]. The outflow tract region typically encompasses the RV region between the pulmonary and tricuspid valves, the basal left ventricle including the outflow tract under the aortic valve, the aortic cusps, and the basal left ventricular (LV) epicardium. The clinical presentation of tachycardias originating from these sites includes isolated monomorphic frequent ventricular premature complexes (VPCs), repetitive nonsustained runs of VT, and less commonly sustained VT [19,20]. Paroxysmal sustained VT is typically precipitated by exercise or emotional stress. Repetitive nonsustained VT is also seen with exercise testing and usually occurs during recovery, often with a reproducible relationship to heart rate. In female patients, there is also a strong association of the occurrence of tachycardia related to the menstrual cycle [21].

Based on seminal studies by Lerman and colleagues [22,23] delayed afterdepolarization (DAD)-mediated triggered activity is believed to be the mechanism underlying these arrhythmias. DAD-triggered activity is typically mediated by intracellular calcium overload. As a result, outflow tract tachycardias are frequently precipitated by catecholaminergic stimulation, resulting in an increase in intracellular cAMP and calcium. Thus, these rhythms are usually induced by rapid stimulation with or without isoproterenol infusion. Furthermore, this dependence on cAMP explains their sensitivity to β-blockade, calcium channel blockade, and adenosine.

Although the outflow tract occupies a relatively narrow anatomic zone, the ECG manifestations of tachycardias originating from this region can have a wide range. Nevertheless, the ECG morphologies of these arrhythmias are often predictable, making this an important tool in accurately localizing their site of origin even before the patient is brought to the electrophysiology laboratory. Determining this site is important for procedural planning and for discussion of specific risks with the patient.

RV outflow tract (RVOT) tachycardias are the most common form of outflow tract VTs, accounting for approximately 75% of cases. RVOT VTs have a characteristic left bundle branch block (LBBB) pattern with an inferior axis and a QRS transition (ie, from negative to positive) in the precordial lead V_3 or V_4 (Fig. 1). Several studies have demonstrated that the 12-lead ECG can be used to further localize the site of origin of these tachycardias. Jadonath and colleagues [24] divided the RVOT region into nine regions and used QRS morphology in leads I and aVL in addition to R wave transition to differentiate anterior from posterior RVOT sites. Anterior sites demonstrated a Q wave (Q or qR) in lead I and a QS in lead aVL. Posterior sites demonstrated an R wave in lead I and an early precordial transition (R > S in V_3). In all patients, a QS was noted in aVR, and monophasic R waves were seen in the inferior leads. Further refinement in these observations was made by Dixit and colleagues [25] to more accurately differentiate septal from free wall RVOT VTs. Typically, RVOT VTs originating from septal locations manifests taller, narrower monophasic R waves in the inferior leads compared with the corresponding free wall locations. Furthermore, free wall RVOT VTs demonstrate notching in the inferior leads and a later transition in the precordial leads (>V_3) compared with septal RVOT VTs. Further localization of VT originating in the superior RVOT can be aided by the QRS morphology in lead I. RVOT VTs originating from posterior locations manifest predominantly positive QRS complexes in lead I, and anterior sites manifest predominantly negative complexes. RVOT VTs originating between the anterior and posterior locations typically demonstrate a multiphasic QRS morphology in this lead (Fig. 2).

LVOT tachycardias manifest clinical features similar to RVOT VTs, probably because they share the same underlying mechanism [26,27]. The ECG has again been shown to help differentiate RVOT tachycardias from LVOT tachycardias. VT arising from the LVOT has been shown to manifest two patterns on ECG: (1) a right bundle inferior axis with a dominant R wave in V_1 and lack of precordial transition with or without a late appearing S wave in V_6 and V_2; and (2) a left bundle inferior axis morphology with an early precordial R wave transition ($\geq V_2$) [28,29]. Further localization of VT originating from this region can be aided by the QRS morphology in lead I, R wave morphology in lead

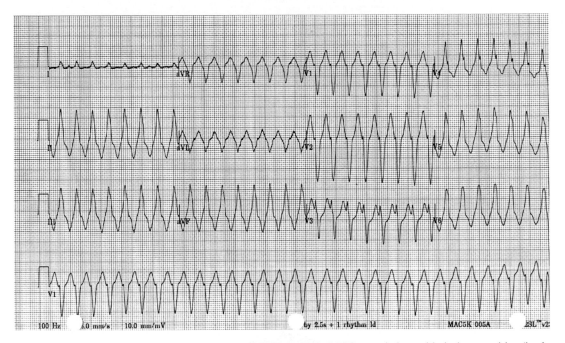

Fig. 1. Twelve-lead ECG of VT originating from the RVOT. Note the LBBB morphology with the late transition (ie, the QRS complex is not positive until lead V₄) in the precordial leads and an inferior axis in the limb leads.

V₁, and the ratio of R waves in limb leads II and III [18].

Tachycardia manifesting clinical features similar to RVOT and LVOT has also been demonstrated from the aortic cusp region (Fig. 3). Depending on the site of origin from the right or left coronary cusp, these tachycardias produce right bundle branch block (RBBB) or LBBB morphology. In the authors' experience, the QRS morphology in leads I and V₁ can help differentiate VT originating from the cusps and the aortomitral continuity. VT originating from the left coronary cusp or the aortomitral continuity often demonstrates a terminal S wave in lead I [30]. Furthermore, Ouyang and colleagues [31] described quantitative ECG measurements to discriminate RVOT tachycardia from aortic cusp tachycardia. In their study, R wave duration and the R/S wave amplitude ratio in leads V₁ and V₂ were greater in tachycardias originating from the cusp compared with the RVOT. In addition, precordial lead transition was earlier in cusp VT, occurring before lead V₃ (Fig. 4). Other investigators have also reported features that may help with this differentiation, such as the absence of an S wave in V₅ or V₆, which has demonstrated a specificity of 88% for cusp VT compared with RVOT VT [32]. Although VT can arise from the right

coronary cusp or noncoronary cusp, most VTs seem to arise from the left cusp and specifically from the junction of the left and right cusps. Given the proximity of the right coronary cusp to the RVOT, it is not surprising that ECG-based differentiating algorithms may not be consistently accurate. Ultimately, localization must be based on the earliest intracardiac activation or on pace mapping (Fig. 5).

Infrequently (9%–13% of idiopathic VT), outflow tract VT can originate from epicardial locations [33,34]. Often, the focus arises from the proximal coronary venous vasculature [33]. The ECGm may be useful in suggesting an epicardial origin (Fig. 6). Tada and colleagues [34] found that R wave amplitude was significantly greater in the inferior leads, that lead I had an S wave as part of an rS or QS pattern, and that Q wave amplitude was greater in aVL compared with aVR (ratio >1.4) in the epicardial group compared with an RV endocardial or an LV endocardial group. In addition, the LV epicardial group had a distinct R wave in V₁ with a greater amplitude than in the RV endocardial group and significant S waves in V₁ (>1.2 mV) and V₂. The authors' data demonstrate that a Q wave in lead I more commonly identifies VT from an epicardial site compared with an endocardial site; however,

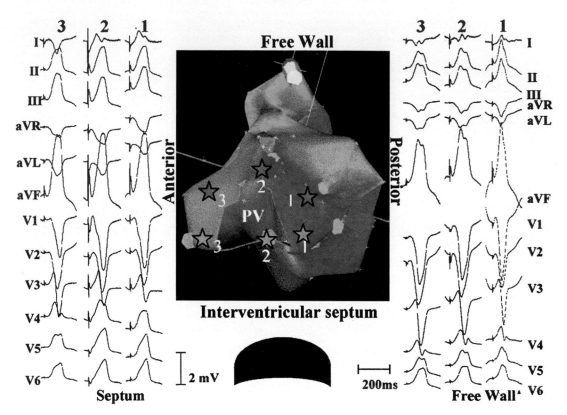

Fig. 2. Twelve-lead ECG pace maps from anterior, intermediate, and posterior sites (3, 2, and 1, respectively) of the RVOT septum and free wall. All pace maps show an LBBB morphology and inferior frontal plane axis. Lead I is negative in the anterior sites (site 3) and positive in the posterior sites (site 1). R waves in the inferior leads are broader, shorter, and notched in free wall pace map sites. (*From* Dixit S, Gerstenfeld EP, Lin D, et al. Electrocardiographic patterns of superior right ventricular outflow tract tachycardias: distinguishing septal and free wall sites of origin. J Cardiovasc Electrophysiol 2003. p. 3; with permission.)

other morphologic criteria are site specific, reflecting local ventricular activation. Furthermore, ECG features distinguishing epicardial VT arising from the left ventricle do not reliably diagnose epicardial VT from the right ventricle [35,36]. In an attempt to increase the reliability of ECG criteria in diagnosing epicardial VT, Daniels and colleagues [33] demonstrated that a precordial maximum deflection index greater than 0.55 reliably localized VT to the epicardium with a sensitivity of 100% and a specificity of 98%.

Thus, if carefully analyzed, the 12-lead ECG remains a powerful tool in localizing the site of origin of outflow tract tachycardias and can greatly facilitate accurate localization and successful ablation of these arrhythmias.

Outflow tract VT has good prognosis with a benign course in most patients [19,20,37,38]; however, patients identified with RVOT VPCs have developed spontaneous ventricular

fibrillation or polymorphic VT. Typically, polymorphic VT is caused by unusually short–coupled RVOT VPCs; these patients appear to respond well to successful VPC ablation [38–40]. In addition, frequent VPCs may cause a tachycardiamediated cardiomyopathy with LV dysfunction; LV function may recover following VPC ablation [41,42]. Finally, it is important to differentiate outflow tract VT from ARVC/D because ARVC/D is associated with a significantly worse prognosis, including sudden cardiac death [17,43,44].

Management of outflow tract VTs may encompass medical therapy or catheter ablation. The initial decision to treat is dictated by frequency and severity of symptoms. Attention to the coupling interval of extrasystoles may offer clues to a potentially more malignant prognosis and may suggest catheter ablation as the initial choice of therapy [45]. Because triggered activity is

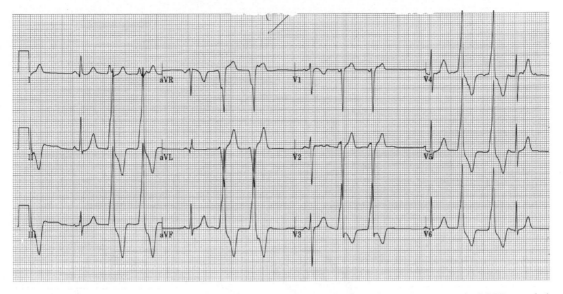

Fig. 3. Twelve-lead ECG of premature ventricular contraction originating from the coronary cusp. An LBBB morphology with transition by V_3, tall R waves in the inferior leads, and an s wave in lead I suggest the VPC arises from the left coronary cusp.

the cause of most outflow tract tachycardias, adenosine, verapamil, β-blockers, and carotid sinus massage often terminate the tachycardia acutely. β-blockers and calcium channel blockers may be used for chronic suppressive therapy; the efficacy in clinical studies has been variable, with success rates of up to 67% in patients who have typical RVOT tachycardia [46]. In some patients who have breakthrough tachycardia on β-blocker or calcium channel blockers, class I antiarrhythmic or class III antiarrhythmic therapy has been shown to be effective [1,47].

Although medical therapy may be effective in patients who have mild to moderate symptoms, it is frequently ineffective in patients who have severe symptoms [48]. Catheter ablation using radiofrequency energy has evolved significantly and currently has a high success rate (>80%) in treating these arrhythmias [49–54]. In planning ablation, the 12-lead ECG is used to localize the site of origin of tachycardia. Tachycardia localization involves intracardiac activation and pace mapping. Pace mapping is useful because typically the site of origin is focal and, because the underlying tissue is normal, pacing is performed with a low output, resulting in a small discrete area of depolarization. Thus, when pace mapping is performed at the site of origin of the clinical arrhythmia, the ECG should mimic the clinical arrhythmia perfectly (12/12, including notches)

[53]. Activation mapping is another approach. Because these arrhythmias are mediated by triggered activity, the electrogram at the site of origin typically precedes the onset of the QRS by approximately 20 milliseconds. An exception to this may be in cusp VT, in which impressive prepotentials (~50 milliseconds) may be seen during VPCs that correspond to late potentials during sinus rhythm [31]. Electroanatomic re-creation of the three-dimensional anatomy can be very helpful for catheter mapping and can facilitate accurate localization of the site of origin. If incessant, the three-dimensional anatomy should ideally be created during the tachycardia, which should be able to localize the earliest site to a small region (<5 mm) with centrifugal activation; typically, pace mapping from this region should achieve a perfect match. Rarely, there may be lack of congruence between the activation and pace map localization because the latter can occasionally be satisfactory over a large area. Predictors for successful ablation include a single VT morphology, accurate pace maps, the absence of a deltalike wave at the beginning of the QRS during tachycardia, and the ability to use pace mapping and activation mapping [54,55]. Although ablation of outflow tract tachycardias may be performed successfully in many cases, some tachycardias arise from the epicardium, necessitating ablation from the great cardiac vein [56] or the epicardium itself

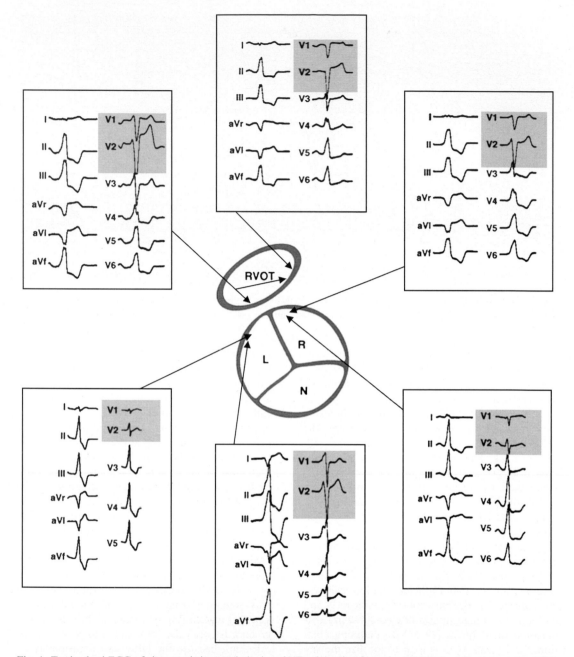

Fig. 4. Twelve-lead ECG of characteristic morphologies of VT originating from the RVOT, the left coronary cusp (L), and the right coronary cusp (R). N, noncoronary cusp. (*From* Ouyang F, Fotuhi P, Ho SY, et al. Repetitive monomorphic ventricular tachycardia originating from the aortic sinus cusp: electrocardiographic characterization for guiding catheter ablation. J Am Coll Cardiol 2002;39(3):503; with permission.)

using a pericardial puncture technique [57]. Coronary angiography is performed before ablation on the epicardium or in the aortic sinus because damage to the coronary arteries may occur [58]. Complications during outflow tract VT ablation are rare but can include development of RBBB (1%) and cardiac perforation, which may or may not result in tamponade. There are rare case reports of damage to the coronary artery (left anterior descending) during ablation in the cusp region [59].

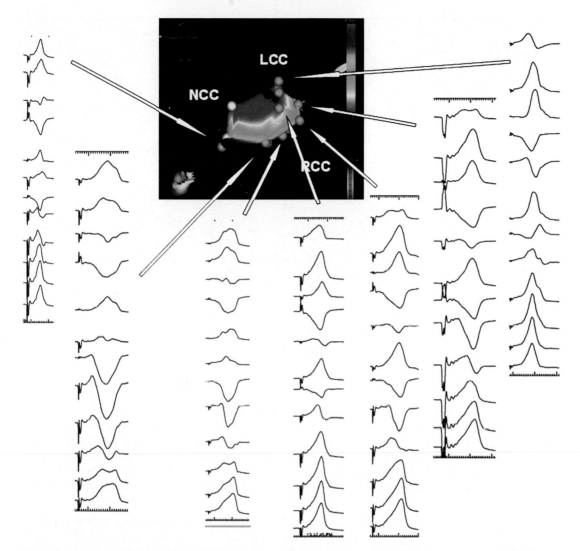

Fig. 5. Pace map morphologies of VT originating from the left coronary cusp (LCC), right coronary cusp (RCC), and noncoronary cusp (NCC).

Long-term cure rates after a successful initial ablation are high, and the overall recurrence rate is approximately 10% [54,60,61].

Idiopathic left ventricular tachycardia

VTs in the normal heart may also arise from the left ventricle. The most common form of ILVT is verapamil-sensitive tachycardia (Fig. 7). First described by Zipes and colleagues [62] in 1979, the tachycardia had the following triad: (1) induction with atrial pacing, (2) RBBB morphology with left axis deviation, and (3) occurrence in patients who did not have structural heart disease. Belhassen and colleagues [63] demonstrated verapamil sensitivity of the tachycardia.

ILVT is seen most often in patients between 15 and 40 years old. Typical symptoms include palpitations, fatigue, and presyncope. Syncope and sudden cardiac death are rare but have been described [64]. Incessant tachycardia leading to a tachycardia-induced cardiomyopathy has also been described but is unusual because episodes are typically infrequent [65]. Most episodes occur at rest, making exercise testing unreliable in assessing the tachycardia.

The anatomic basis for ILVT is unclear. By endocardial activation mapping during tachycardia,

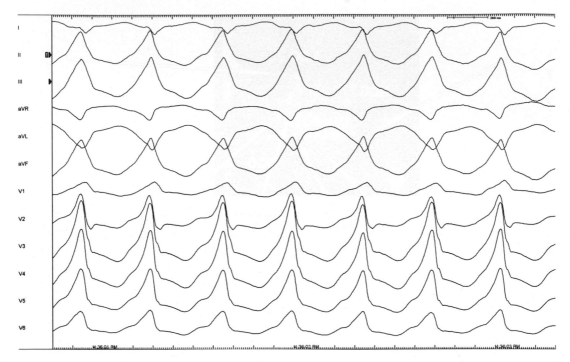

Fig. 6. Twelve-lead ECG of VT originating from the epicardium. There is a Q wave in lead I and a terminal S wave in V_2 (Paper speed 100 mm/s).

the earliest site of activation is in the region of the inferoposterior LV septum. Nakagawa and colleagues [66] recorded high-frequency potentials preceding the earliest ventricular activation in sinus rhythm and during tachycardia thought to represent activation of a component of the left posterior fascicle. Late diastolic potentials (LDPs) have been identified more recently that precede the Purkinje potentials seen by Nakagawa and colleagues [66] and appear to be located nearer the main portion of the left bundle branch (Fig. 8) [67]. Some data, however, suggest that the

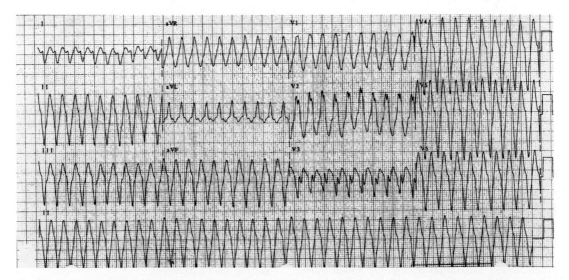

Fig. 7. Twelve-lead ECG of VT with an RBBB, a right superior axis in the frontal plane, and a late precordial transition consistent with origination from the left posterior fascicle.

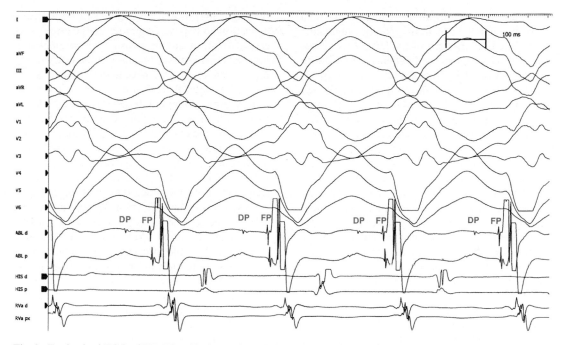

Fig. 8. Twelve-lead ECG of VT. The ablation catheter is in the region of the left posterior fascicle. Intracardiac electrograms demonstrate a middiastolic potential (DP) and a fascicular potential (FP) (*Courtesy of* H. Hsia, MD, Stanford, CA).

tachycardia originates from a false tendon that extends from the posteroinferior left ventricle to the basal septum, with resection of the tendon or ablation at the septal insertion site eliminating tachycardia [68–70]. Furthermore, one study found a false tendon on transthoracic echocardiography extending from the posteroinferior LV free wall to the septum in 15 of 15 patients who had ILVT, whereas only 5% of control subjects were found to have a false tendon. The exact role the tendon plays in the tachycardia remains unclear because the specificity may be low, another study confirmed the presence of a false tendon in 17 of 18 patients who had fascicular VT but also identified false tendons in 35 of 40 control subjects [71].

Most evidence indicates localized reentry as the predominant mechanism in verapamil-sensitive ILVT. Tachycardia can be initiated and terminated with programmed atrial or ventricular stimulation, it demonstrates an inverse relationship between the coupling interval of the initiating extrastimulus and the initial tachycardia QRS, and it can be entrained [63,64,72,73]. Okumura and colleagues [74] further characterized the nature of the tachycardia circuit. They demonstrated entrainment with a zone of slow conduction between the RVOT (pacing site) and the earliest

site of activation in the LV (compared with the RV apex). Tsuchiya and colleagues [67] further localized the zone of slow conduction to the interval between the LDP and the Purkinje potential. Furthermore, variations in VT cycle length are preceded by variations in the LDP–Purkinje potential interval. In addition, the zone of slow conduction is dependent partly on calcium channel–dependent conduction and partly on depressed sodium channel–dependent conduction because intravenous verapamil and lidocaine lead to prolongation of the tachycardia cycle length that was entirely due to prolongation in the zone of slow conduction. The entrance site to the zone of slow conduction is thought to be near the base of the left interventricular septum, near the site of the LDP. Taken together, the data suggest a reentrant circuit with an entrance near the LDP, a zone of slow conduction between the LDP and the Purkinje potential, and an exit site distal to the Purkinje potential.

Because ILVT affects patients who have structurally normal hearts, the baseline 12-lead ECG is normal in most patients. Corresponding to its LV origin, ILVT has a right bundle, left superior frontal plane axis morphology with a relatively narrow QRS duration (typically no longer than

140 milliseconds), and an RS interval less than 80 milliseconds [75] in most patients, suggesting an exit site near the area of the left posterior fascicle. A small proportion of patients have VT with a right bundle, right frontal plane axis morphology, suggesting an exit near the area of the left anterior fascicle [76]. Because of the relatively narrow, complex QRS and the response to verapamil, ILVT may be confused with supraventricular tachycardia with aberrancy.

As with outflow tract VTs, the long-term prognosis of patients who have ILVT is very good [48,77]. Patients who have incessant tachycardia, however, may develop a tachycardia-related cardiomyopathy [65]. Intravenous verapamil is effective in acutely terminating VT [48,72]. Patients who have mild to moderate symptoms may be treated chronically with verapamil, but this medical therapy is often ineffective in patients who have severe symptoms [48].

Patients who have ILVT associated with significant symptoms or who are intolerant or resistant to medical therapy should be considered for radiofrequency ablation. Numerous strategies have been employed to identify the ideal site for ablation, including pace mapping, endocardial activation mapping [78–80], identifying Purkinje potentials [66], and identifying late diastolic

potentials [67]. Initial attempts using endocardial activation and pace mapping characterized successful ablation sites as areas of activation 30 milliseconds earlier than the onset of the QRS during tachycardia and with a pace map similar to tachycardia. Of note, there is not a consistent correlation between mapping based on pace mapping (which identifies the circuit exit) and activation mapping (which identifies more proximal portions of the circuit) because the circuit in ILVT has a significant size. Others have described successful ablation sites as being marked by areas of high-frequency Purkinje potentials that precede the earliest ventricular activation during tachycardia and may be located away from the site of earliest ventricular activation. Ablation at such an area terminates VT and prevents re-induction; however, these potentials are not always seen during VT [54]. More recent data have suggested that ablation of the reentrant circuit at the site of the late diastolic potential also terminates VT successfully without recurrence [67,78]. These studies depend on the induction of tachycardia, which may be difficult in the electrophysiology laboratory in some patients. Ouyang and colleagues [81] demonstrated an abnormal potential signifying a retrograde Purkinje potential identified during sinus rhythm in patients who had ILVT. In three

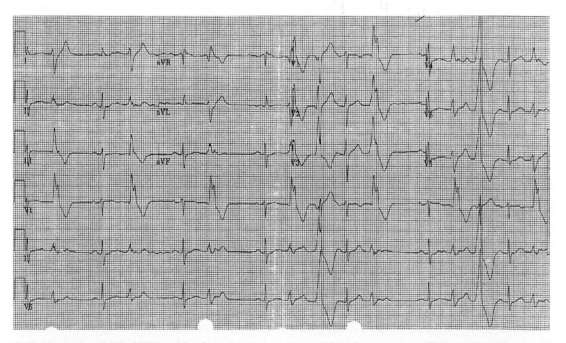

Fig. 9. Twelve-lead ECG of VPCs arising from the coronary cusp and from the anterior papillary muscle consistent with automatic VPCs.

patients, ablation was performed during sinus rhythm at the site of the retrograde Purkinje potential, resulting in freedom from symptoms on no antiarrhythmic therapy during a mean follow-up of 9 months. More recently, Lin and colleagues [82] demonstrated that an empiric linear lesion placed in the area of posterior fascicle and guided by Purkinje potentials was successful in patients who could not be tachycardia induced during the procedure. Long-term success after catheter ablation is more than 90%, with rare complications.

Automatic ventricular tachycardia

Also referred to as adrenergic or propranolol-sensitive VT, automatic VT is usually seen in patients younger than 50 years and is often precipitated by exercise. Automatic VT can arise from anywhere within the right or left heart, although there are several areas that appear to be more common, such as around the mitral annulus, the papillary muscles, the para-Hisian area, and the RV inflow tract (Fig. 9). Thus, the ECG may demonstrate an RBBB or LBBB morphology and may present as monomorphic or polymorphic VT. It is important to recognize that VT with these "atypical" (ie, nonoutflow tract) signatures does not necessarily imply the presence of structural heart disease, particularly ARVC/D. It is thought to result from adrenergically mediated automaticity because it is induced with exercise and catecholamines, is sensitive to β-blockers, is unresponsive to calcium channel blockers, and cannot be initiated with programmed stimulation [83]. Although the underlying mechanism of this arrhythmia has not been studied extensively, it is thought that some forms of this entity may be caused by automaticity from within the Purkinje fibers mediated by I_f [84]. Reports of incessant VT have been reported to cause cardiomyopathy, with one report of VT in a patient who had pheochromocytoma resolving with resection of the tumor [85].

Summary

VT in the structurally normal heart accounts for approximately 10% of cases. Although the overall prognosis is relatively good, with a benign course in most patients, these arrhythmias can lead to significant symptoms. Our understanding of these arrhythmias has progressed significantly, leading to effective therapies targeting their underlying mechanism. In many cases, catheter ablation is successful and the therapy of choice in patients who have sufficient symptoms.

References

[1] Buxton AE, Waxman HL, Marchlinski FE, et al. Right ventricular tachycardia: clinical and electrophysiologic characteristics. Circulation 1983;68(5): 917–27.

[2] Eguchi M, Tsuchihashi K, Nakata T, et al. Right ventricular abnormalities assessed by myocardial single-photon emission computed tomography using technetium-99m sestamibi/tetrofosmin in right ventricle-originated ventricular tachyarrhythmias. J Am Coll Cardiol 2000;36(6):1767–73.

[3] Mehta D, Odawara H, Ward DE, et al. Echocardiographic and histologic evaluation of the right ventricle in ventricular tachycardias of left bundle branch block morphology without overt cardiac abnormality. Am J Cardiol 1989;63(13):939–44.

[4] Mehta D, McKenna WJ, Ward DE, et al. Significance of signal-averaged electrocardiography in relation to endomyocardial biopsy and ventricular stimulation studies in patients with ventricular tachycardia without clinically apparent heart disease. J Am Coll Cardiol 1989;14(2):372–9.

[5] Oakes DF, Manolis AS, Estes NA 3rd. Limited clinical utility of endomyocardial biopsy in patients presenting with ventricular tachycardia without apparent structural heart disease. Clin Cardiol 1992; 15(1):24–8.

[6] Markowitz SM, Litvak BL, Ramirez de Arellano EA, et al. Adenosine-sensitive ventricular tachycardia: right ventricular abnormalities delineated by magnetic resonance imaging. Circulation 1997; 96(4):1192–200.

[7] Globits S, Kreiner G, Frank H, et al. Significance of morphologic abnormalities detected by MRI in patients undergoing successful ablation of right ventricular outflow tract tachycardia. Circulation 1997;96(8):2633–40.

[8] O'Donnell D, Cox D, Bourke J, et al. Clinical and electrophysiological differences between patients with arrhythmogenic right ventricular dysplasia and right ventricular outflow tract tachycardia. Eur Heart J 2003;24(9):801–10.

[9] Schafers M, Lerch H, Wichter T, et al. Cardiac sympathetic innervation in patients with idiopathic right ventricular outflow tract tachycardia. J Am Coll Cardiol 1998;32(1):181–6.

[10] Schafers M, Wichter T, Lerch H, et al. Cardiac 123I-MIBG uptake in idiopathic ventricular tachycardia and fibrillation. J Nucl Med 1999;40(1):1–5.

[11] Wichter T, Hindricks G, Lerch H, et al. Regional myocardial sympathetic dysinnervation in arrhythmogenic right ventricular cardiomyopathy. An

analysis using 123I-meta-iodobenzylguanidine scintigraphy. Circulation 1994;89(2):667–83.

[12] Gill JS, Hunter GJ, Gane G, et al. Heterogeneity of the human myocardial sympathetic innervation: in vivo demonstration by iodine 123-labeled meta-iodobenzylguanidine scintigraphy. Am Heart J 1993;126(2):390–8.

[13] Nasir K, Rutberg J, Tandri H, et al. Utility of SAECG in arrhythmogenic right ventricle dysplasia. Ann Noninvasive Electrocardiol 2003;8(2):112–20.

[14] Kinoshita O, Fontaine G, Rosas F, et al. Time- and frequency-domain analyses of the signal-averaged ECG in patients with arrhythmogenic right ventricular dysplasia. Circulation 1995;91(3):715–21.

[15] Corrado D, Basso C, Leoni L, et al. Three-dimensional electroanatomical voltage mapping and histologic evaluation of myocardial substrate in right ventricular outflow tract tachycardia. J Am Coll Cardiol 2008;51(7):731–9.

[16] Peters S. Advances in the diagnostic management of arrhythmogenic right ventricular dysplasia-cardiomyopathy. Int J Cardiol 2006;113(1):4–11.

[17] Sticherling C, Zabel M. Arrhythmogenic right ventricular dysplasia presenting as right ventricular outflow tract tachycardia. Europace 2005;7(4):345–7.

[18] Dixit S, Gerstenfeld EP, Lin D, et al. Identification of distinct electrocardiographic patterns from the basal left ventricle: distinguishing medial and lateral sites of origin in patients with idiopathic ventricular tachycardia. Heart Rhythm 2005;2(5):485–91.

[19] Buxton AE, Marchlinski FE, Doherty JU, et al. Repetitive, monomorphic ventricular tachycardia: clinical and electrophysiolgic characteristics in patients with and patients without organic heart disease. Am J Cardiol 1984;54(8):997–1002.

[20] Rahilly GT, Prystowsky EN, Zipes DP, et al. Clinical and electrophysiologic findings in patients with repetitive monomorphic ventricular tachycardia and otherwise normal electrocardiogram. Am J Cardiol 1982;50(3):459–68.

[21] Marchlinski FE, Deely MP, Zado ES. Sex-specific triggers for right ventricular outflow tract tachycardia. Am Heart J 2000;139(6):1009–13.

[22] Lerman BB, Stein K, Engelstein ED, et al. Mechanism of repetitive monomorphic ventricular tachycardia. Circulation 1995;92(3):421–9.

[23] Lerman BB, Belardinelli L, West GA, et al. Adenosine-sensitive ventricular tachycardia: evidence suggesting cyclic AMP-mediated triggered activity. Circulation 1986;74(2):270–80.

[24] Jadonath RL, Schwartzman DS, Preminger MW, et al. Utility of the 12-lead electrocardiogram in localizing the origin of right ventricular outflow tract tachycardia. Am Heart J 1995;130(5):1107–13.

[25] Dixit S, Gerstenfeld EP, Callans DJ, et al. Electrocardiographic patterns of superior right ventricular outflow tract tachycardias: distinguishing septal and free-wall sites of origin. J Cardiovasc Electrophysiol 2003;14(1):1–7.

[26] Iwai S, Cantillon DJ, Kim RJ, et al. Right and left ventricular outflow tract tachycardias: evidence for a common electrophysiologic mechanism. J Cardiovasc Electrophysiol 2006;17(10):1052–8.

[27] Yamawake N, Nishizaki M, Hayashi T, et al. Autonomic and pharmacological responses of idiopathic ventricular tachycardia arising from the left ventricular outflow tract. J Cardiovasc Electrophysiol 2007; 18(11):1161–6.

[28] Callans DJ, Menz V, Schwartzman D, et al. Repetitive monomorphic tachycardia from the left ventricular outflow tract: electrocardiographic patterns consistent with a left ventricular site of origin. J Am Coll Cardiol 1997;29(5):1023–7.

[29] Hachiya H, Aonuma K, Yamauchi Y, et al. Electrocardiographic characteristics of left ventricular outflow tract tachycardia. Pacing Clin Electrophysiol 2000;23(11 Pt 2):1930–4.

[30] Lin D, Ilkhanoff L, Gerstenfeld E, et al. Twelve-lead ECG characteristics of the aortic cusp region guided by intracardiac echo and electroanatomic mapping. Heart Rhythm 2008; doi:10.1016/j.hrthm.2008.

[31] Ouyang F, Fotuhi P, Ho SY, et al. Repetitive monomorphic ventricular tachycardia originating from the aortic sinus cusp: electrocardiographic characterization for guiding catheter ablation. J Am Coll Cardiol 2002;39(3):500–8.

[32] Hachiya H, Aonuma K, Yamauchi Y, et al. How to diagnose, locate, and ablate coronary cusp ventricular tachycardia. J Cardiovasc Electrophysiol 2002; 13(6):551–6.

[33] Daniels DV, Lu YY, Morton JB, et al. Idiopathic epicardial left ventricular tachycardia originating remote from the sinus of Valsalva: electrophysiological characteristics, catheter ablation, and identification from the 12-lead electrocardiogram. Circulation 2006;113(13):1659–66.

[34] Tada H, Nogami A, Naito S, et al. Left ventricular epicardial outflow tract tachycardia: a new distinct subgroup of outflow tract tachycardia. Jpn Circ J 2001;65(8):723–30.

[35] Bazan V, Bala R, Garcia FC, et al. Twelve-lead ECG features to identify ventricular tachycardia arising from the epicardial right ventricle. Heart Rhythm 2006;3(10):1132–9.

[36] Bazan V, Gerstenfeld EP, Garcia FC, et al. Site-specific twelve-lead ECG features to identify an epicardial origin for left ventricular tachycardia in the absence of myocardial infarction. Heart Rhythm 2007;4(11):1403–10.

[37] Ritchie AH, Kerr CR, Qi A, et al. Nonsustained ventricular tachycardia arising from the right ventricular outflow tract. Am J Cardiol 1989;64(10):594–8.

[38] Lemery R, Brugada P, Bella PD, et al. Nonischemic ventricular tachycardia. Clinical course and long-term follow-up in patients without clinically overt heart disease. Circulation 1989;79(5):990–9.

[39] Viskin S, Rosso R, Rogowski O, et al. The "short-coupled" variant of right ventricular outflow tract

tachycardia: a not-so-benign form of benign ventricular tachycardia? J Cardiovasc Electrophysiol 2005; 16(8):912–6.

[40] Noda T, Shimizu W, Taguchi A, et al. Malignant entity of idiopathic ventricular fibrillation and polymorphic ventricular tachycardia initiated by premature extrasystoles originating from the right ventricular outflow tract. J Am Coll Cardiol 2005; 46(7):1288–94.

[41] Kanei Y, Friedman M, Ogawa N, et al. Frequent premature ventricular complexes originating from the right ventricular outflow tract are associated with left ventricular dysfunction. Ann Noninvasive Electrocardiol 2008;13(1):81–5.

[42] Grimm W, Menz V, Hoffmann J, et al. Reversal of tachycardia induced cardiomyopathy following ablation of repetitive monomorphic right ventricular outflow tract tachycardia. Pacing Clin Electrophysiol 2001;24(2):166–71.

[43] Callans DJ. Diagnosing subtle forms of potentially life-threatening diseases. J Am Coll Cardiol 2008; 51(7):740–1.

[44] Corrado D, Basso C, Thiene G. Spectrum of clinicopathologic manifestations of arrhythmogenic right ventricular cardiomyopathy/dysplasia: a multicenter study. J Am Coll Cardiol 1997;30(6):1512–20.

[45] Viskin S, Antzelevitch C. The cardiologists' worst nightmare: sudden death from "benign" ventricular arrhythmias. J Am Coll Cardiol 2005;46(7):1295–7.

[46] Gill JS, Blaszyk K, Ward DE, et al. Verapamil for the suppression of idiopathic ventricular tachycardia of left bundle block-like morphology. Am Heart J 1993;126(5):1126–33.

[47] Mont L, Sexias T, Brugada P, et al. The electrocardiographic, clinical, and electrophysiologic spectrum of idiopathic monomorphic ventricular tachycardia. Am Heart J 1992;124(3):746–53.

[48] Ohe T, Aihara N, Kamakura S. Long-term outcome of verapamil-sensitive sustained left ventricular tachycardia in patients without structural heart disease. J Am Coll Cardiol 1995;25(1):54–8.

[49] Joshi S, Wilbur DJ. Ablation of idiopathic right ventricular outflow tract tachycardia: current perspectives. J Cardiovasc Electrophysiol 2005;16(Suppl 1): S52–8.

[50] Coggins DL, Lee RJ, Sweeney J, et al. Radiofrequence catheter ablation as a cure for idiopathic tachycardia of both left and right ventricular origin. J Am Coll Cardiol 1994;23(6):1333–41.

[51] Klein LS, Miles WM. Ablative therapy for ventricular arrhythmias. Prog Cardiovasc Dis 1995;37(4): 225–42.

[52] Calkins H, Kalbfleisch SJ, el-Atassi R, et al. Relation between efficacy of radiofrequency catheter ablation and site of origin of idiopathic ventricular tachycardia. Am J Cardiol 1993;71(10):827–33.

[53] Gerstenfeld EP, Dixit S, Callans DJ, et al. Quantitative comparison of spontaneous and paced 12-lead electrocardiogram during right ventricular outflow

tract ventricular tachycardia. J Am Coll Cardiol 2003;41(11):2046–53.

[54] Rodriguez LM, Smeets JL, Timmermans C, et al. Predictors for successful ablation of right- and left-sided idiopathic ventricular tachycardia. Am J Cardiol 1997;79(3):309–14.

[55] Wen MS, Taniguchi Y, Yeh SJ, et al. Determinants of tachycardia recurrences after radiofrequency ablation of idiopathic ventricular tachycardia. Am J Cardiol 1998;81(4):500–3.

[56] Obel OA, d'Avila A, Neuzil P, et al. Ablation of left ventricular epicardial outflow tract tachycardia from the distal great cardiac vein. J Am Coll Cardiol 2006; 48(9):1813–7.

[57] Sosa E, Scanavacca M, D'Avila A, et al. Endocardial and epicardial ablation guided by nonsurgical transthoracic epicardial mapping to treat recurrent ventricular tachycardia. J Cardiovasc Electrophysiol 1998;9(3):229–39.

[58] Sosa E, Scanavacca M, D'Avila A. Transthoracic epicardial catheter ablation to treat recurrent ventricular tachycardia. Curr Cardiol Rep 2001;3(6): 451–8.

[59] Friedman PL, Stevenson WG, Bittl JA, et al. Left main coronary artery occlusion during radiofrequency catheter ablation of idiopathic outflow tract ventricular tachycardia (abstr). Pacing Clin Electrophysiol 1997;20(Part II):1184.

[60] Chinushi M, Aizawa Y, Takahashi K, et al. Radiofrequency catheter ablation for idiopathic right ventricular tachycardia with special reference to morphological variation and long-term outcome. Heart 1997;78(3):255–61.

[61] Krittayaphong R, Sriratanasathavorn C, Dumavibhat C, et al. Electrocardiographic predictors of long-term outcomes after radiofrequency ablation in patients with right-ventricular outflow tract tachycardia. Europace 2006;8(8):601–6.

[62] Zipes DP, Foster PR, Troup PJ, et al. Atrial induction of ventricular tachycardia: reentry versus triggered activity. Am J Cardiol 1979;44(1):1–8.

[63] Belhassen B, Rotmensch HH, Laniado S. Response of recurrent sustained ventricular tachycardia to verapamil. Br Heart J 1981;46(6):679–82.

[64] German LD, Packer DL, Bardy GH, et al. Ventricular tachycardia induced by atrial stimulation in patients without symptomatic cardiac disease. Am J Cardiol 1983;52(10):1202–7.

[65] Ward DE, Nathan AW, Camm AJ. Fascicular tachycardia sensitive to calcium antagonists. Eur Heart J 1984;5(11):896–905.

[66] Nakagawa H, Beckman KJ, McClelland JH, et al. Radiofrequency catheter ablation of idiopathic left ventricular tachycardia guided by a Purkinje potential. Circulation 1993;88(6): 2607–17.

[67] Tsuchiya T, Okumura K, Honda T, et al. Significance of late diastolic potential preceding Purkinje potential in verapamil-sensitive idiopathic left

ventricular tachycardia. Circulation 1999;99(18): 2408–13.

[68] Gallagher JJ, Selle JG, Svenson RH, et al. Surgical treatment of arrhythmias. Am J Cardiol 1988; 61(2):27A–44A.

[69] Merliss AD, Seifert MJ, Collins RF, et al. Catheter ablation of idiopathic left ventricular tachycardia associated with a false tendon. Pacing Clin Electrophysiol 1996;19(12 Pt 1):2144–6.

[70] Thakur RK, Klein GJ, Sivaram CA, et al. Anatomic substrate for idiopathic left ventricular tachycardia. Circulation 1996;93(3):497–501.

[71] Lin FC, Wen MS, Wang CC, et al. Left ventricular fibromuscular band is not a specific substrate for idiopathic left ventricular tachycardia. Circulation 1996;93(3):525–8.

[72] Ohe T, Shimomura K, Aihara N, et al. Idiopathic sustained left ventricular tachycardia: clinical and electrophysiologic characteristics. Circulation 1988; 77(3):560–8.

[73] Klein GJ, Millman PJ, Yee R. Recurrent ventricular tachycardia responsive to verapamil. Pacing Clin Electrophysiol 1984;7(6 Pt 1):938–48.

[74] Okumura K, Yamabe H, Tsuchiya T, et al. Characteristics of slow conduction zone demonstrated during entrainment of idiopathic ventricular tachycardia of left ventricular origin. Am J Cardiol 1996;77(5):379–83.

[75] Andrade FR, Eslami M, Elias J, et al. Diagnostic clues from the surface ECG to identify idiopathic (fascicular) ventricular tachycardia: correlation with electrophysiologic findings. J Cardiovasc Electrophysiol 1996;7(1):2–8.

[76] Nogami A, Naito S, Tada H, et al. Verapamil-sensitive left anterior fascicular ventricular tachycardia: results of radiofrequency ablation in six patients. J Cardiovasc Electrophysiol 1998;9(12):1269–78.

[77] Gaita F, Giustetto C, Leclercq JF, et al. Idiopathic verapmil-responsive left ventricular tachycardia: clinical characteristics and long-term follow-up of 33 patients. Eur Heart J 1994;15(9):1252–60.

[78] Wen MS, Yeh SJ, Wang CC, et al. Radiofrequency ablation therapy in idiopathic left ventricular tachycardia with no obvious structural heart disease. Circulation 1994;89(4):1690–6.

[79] Page RL, Shenasa H, Evans JJ, et al. Radiofrequency catheter ablation of idiopathic recurrent ventricular tachycardia with right bundle branch block, left axis morphology. Pacing Clin Electrophysiol 1993;16(2):327–36.

[80] Wen MS, Yeh SJ, Wang CC, et al. Successful radiofrequency ablation of idiopathic left ventricular tachycardia at a site away from the tachycardia exit. J Am Coll Cardiol 1997;30(4):1024–31.

[81] Ouyang F, Cappato R, Ernst S, et al. Electroanatomic substrate of idiopathic left ventricular tachycardia: unidirectional block and macroreentry within the Purkinje network. Circulation 2002; 105(4):462–9.

[82] Lin D, Hsia HH, Gerstenfeld EP, et al. Idiopathic fascicular left ventricular tachycardia: linear ablation lesion strategy for noninducible or nonsustained tachycardia. Heart Rhythm 2005;2(9):934–9.

[83] Sung RJ, Keung EC, Nguyen NX, et al. Effects of beta-adrenergic blockade on verapamil-responsive and verapimil-irresponsive sustained ventricular tachycardias. J Clin Invest 1988;81(3):688–99.

[84] Lerman BB, Stein KM, Markowitz SM, et al. Ventricular arrhythmias in normal hearts. Cardiol Clin 2000;18(2):265–91.

[85] Huang YC, Chang CH, Wang CH, et al. Pheochromocytoma complicated with severe ventricular tachycardia: report of one case. Acta Paediatr Taiwan 2007;48(5):280–4.

ELSEVIER
SAUNDERS

Cardiol Clin 26 (2008) 381–403

CARDIOLOGY
CLINICS

Ventricular Arrhythmias in Heart Failure Patients

Ronald Lo, MD, Henry H. Hsia, MD, FACC*

Division of Cardiovascular Medicine, Stanford University School of Medicine, Cardiac Electrophysiology and Arrhythmia Service, Stanford University Medical Center, 300 Pasteur Drive, H2146, Stanford, CA 94305-5233, USA

Heart failure is a significant major health problem in the United States. An estimated 5 million patients are afflicted by this disease, with an additional 550,000 new cases diagnosed annually. It is a major source of morbidity and mortality and is associated with an increasing number of hospitalizations [1]. Mortality in the heart failure population is primarily by pump failure or by sudden cardiac death (SCD), of which more than 75% is associated with ventricular tachyarrhythmia [2]. There are an estimated 400,000 to 460,000 deaths attributable to SCD in the United States each year, representing an incidence of 0.1% to 0.2% per year in the adult population [3].

Epidemiology

Heart failure can be considered a degradation of systolic or diastolic function. The diagnosis of heart failure is most commonly classified as an ischemic etiology secondary to coronary artery disease and prior myocardial infarction, or as a nonischemic etiology with a variety of causes such as infiltrative, infectious, metabolic, or hemodynamic insults (Box 1) [4]. Ventricular ectopy and nonsustained ventricular tachycardia (VT) are common in patients who have cardiomyopathies and heart failure. It has long been known that the frequency of ventricular ectopy is a risk factor for SCD. Patients who suffered a prior myocardial infarction with frequent premature ventricular complex (PVCs) or nonsustained VT are at a higher risk of SCD irrespective of their ejection fractions. Increasing frequency of PVCs greater than 10 per hour are linked to an even greater SCD risk in patients who have heart disease [5,6]. Despite recent pharmacologic advancements in treatment, mortality remains unacceptably high, with sudden, "unexpected" death occurring in up to 40% to 70% of patients [7,8]. Although the total mortality among patients who have mild heart failure is low, the relative proportion of patients dying suddenly is significant. Patients who have more advanced heart failure have a substantial annual mortality of 40% to 60%; however, the relative proportion of sudden death amounts to less than 30% of all causes of death (Fig. 1) [7,9].

Pathophysiology

Multiple studies have shown that in most patients who have ischemic and nonischemic cardiomyopathies, mechanisms of VT and ventricular fibrillation include myocardial reentry, reentry using the specialized conduction system such as bundle branch reentry (BBR) or intrafascicular reentry, and focal automaticity/triggered activity.

Abnormal automaticity

Ventricular arrhythmias may arise from disturbances in automaticity in myocardial cells. Normal automaticity often originates from cells with "pacemaker activity," which is determined by the rate of phase 4 depolarization of the cardiac action potential. It is a normal property of the sinus node, the atrioventricular node, and the His-Purkinje system. Abnormal automaticity that causes VT has also been demonstrated in subendocardial Purkinje fibers that survive ischemic

---

* Corresponding author.
E-mail address: hhsia@cvmed.stanford.edu
(H.H. Hsia).

Box 1. Etiologies of cardiomyopathy

Ischemia
   Acute and chronic coronary artery
      disease

Infections
   Bacteria
   Spirochetes
   Rickettsia
   Viruses (including HIV)
   Fungi
   Protozoa
   Helminthes

Granulomatous diseases
   Sarcoidosis
   Giant cell myocarditis
   Wegener's granulomatosis

Metabolic disorders
   Beriberi
   Selenium deficiency
   Carnitine deficiency
   Kwashiorkor
   Famililal storage disorders
   Uremia
   Hypokalemia
   Hypomagnesemia
   Hypophosphatemia
   Diabetes mellitus
   Hyperthyroidism
   Hypothyroidism
   Pheochromocytoma
   Acromegaly
   Morbid obesity

Drugs and toxins
   Ethanol
   Cocaine
   Anthracyclines
   Cobalt
   Tricyclic antidepressants
   Phenothiazines
   Catecholamines
   Cyclophosphamide
   Radiation

Other
   Tumors
   Connective tissue disorders
   Familial disorders
   Hereditary neuromuscular and
      neurologic disorders
   Peripartum

---

myocardial injury [10]. Studies in experimental animal models and in failing human hearts have demonstrated abnormal calcium handling. The abnormal calcium metabolism results in decreasing the calcium available to the sarcoplasmic reticulum for release, leading to mechanical dysfunction. Alterations in calcium cycling have also been implicated in the development of arrhythmias by a focal, nonreentrant mechanism in the heart failure population [11]. Pogwizd and colleagues [12,13] studied the role of abnormal calcium handling using three-dimensional mapping of spontaneously occurring VT in human hearts and showed that 100% of VT in nonischemic cardiomyopathy and 50% of VT in ischemic cardiomyopathy may be caused by a focal nonreentrant mechanism.

Triggered arrhythmias

Triggered arrhythmias may occur when there are abnormalities of action potentials that trigger another electrical event by way of abnormal depolarization. The most common abnormality causing triggered arrhythmias are early and late depolarizations, often associated with a prolonged repolarization phase. Early afterdepolarizations (EADs) usually occur in late phase 2 or phase 3 of the action potential. An EAD may occur with an imbalance between the inward and outward currents that favors a net inward current. The EADs may be manifested when there is a decrease in the outward potassium channel or an increase in the inward sodium or calcium currents. EADs may occur when the heart rate is markedly slowed, reducing the outward current from the delayed rectifier potassium channel [14]. EADs are easily inducible in experimental settings with bradycardia or during pauses and are thought to initiate torsades de pointes [15]. Experimental animal models with isochronal mapping have shown that torsades de pointes is consistently initiated first as a focal subendocardial activation, with subsequent beats due to a reentrant mechanism [16].

Delayed afterdepolarizations (DADs) occur in late phase 3 or early phase 4 when the action potential is almost fully repolarized. The development of a DAD is related to conditions that increase intracellular calcium concentrations. With catecholamine stimulation and activation of the beta-adrenergic receptors, an increased intracellular concentration of cAMP results in an increased calcium current and an increased

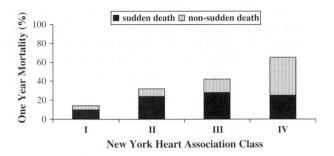

Fig. 1. Annual mortality of heart failure. Prevalence of sudden death and non–sudden death by New York Heart Association functional class and 1-year mortality. (*From* Hsia HH, Jessup ML, Marchlinski FE. Debate: Do all patients with heart failure require implantable defibrillators to prevent sudden death? Curr Control Trials Cardiovasc Med 2000;1(2):98–101.)

calcium release from the sarcoplasmic reticulum. The elevated intracellular calcium subsequently activates the calcium–sodium exchanger, ultimately leading to transient inward sodium current (I_{Ti}) and the DAD (Fig. 2).

Adenosine by way of antiadrenergic effects is able to terminate cAMP-mediated triggered arrhythmias by decreasing the concentrations of intracellular cAMP [17]. Termination of VT by adenosine may be pathognomonic for outflow tract VT caused by cAMP-triggered DADs. In contrast, in other conditions that promote cardiac calcium overload, such as digitalis toxicity, the DADs are mediated by the inhibition of the

sodium potassium ATPase, which secondarily increases intracellular calcium by way of a shift in the equilibrium of the sodium–calcium exchanger. These different mechanisms of DADs may be supported by data showing that adenosine abolishes DADs caused by cAMP stimulation but has no effect on digitalis-induced DADs [18].

Stretch mechanoreceptors may also alter the electrophysiologic properties of the myocardium in heart failure. Stretching or stress in the left ventricle in the normal heart has been shown to shorten the local action potential duration while increasing local spontaneous automaticity and triggered activity [19]. These effects are more

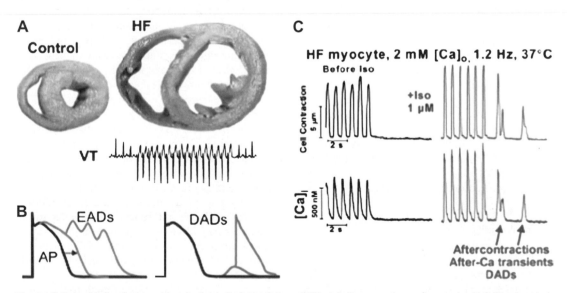

Fig. 2. Cellular basis of triggered arrhythmia in heart failure (HF). (*A*) Cross sections of control and failing hearts in a rabbit HF model. Holter recording of nonsustained VT was seen in 90% of HF versus 0% of control rabbits. (*B*) Diagram of EADs and DADs. AP, action potential. (*C*) Spontaneous aftercontractions (*top*, in μm) and changes in intracellular calcium transients concentration (*bottom*, in nM) in HF myocytes were observed after exposure to isoproterenol (Iso) under 1.2-Hz stimulation (37°C). (*From* Pogwizd SM, Schlotthaurer K, Li L et al. Arrhythmogenesis and contractile dysfunction in heart failure. Circ Res 2001;88:1161; with permission.)

pronounced in structurally abnormal hearts, with greater heterogeneity of action potential durations leading to a wider dispersion in tissue excitability and refractoriness that facilitate unidirectional conduction block [20]. Transient stretch during diastole has been shown to cause local depolarization and trigger action potentials. In dilated canine hearts, stretch mechanoreceptors were reproducibly able to produce spontaneous PVCs [21]. Characterization of stretch-related mechanoreceptors has been located to a nonselective cation channel and related potassium channels [22].

Reentry

Reentrant ventricular arrhythmias represent most of the clinically significant tachycardias. The hallmark of reentrant ventricular arrhythmia is slow conduction, most often due to structural heart disease with scar-based anisotropic conduction abnormalities. Conduction velocity, however, is also mediated by the local cell-to-cell coupling by gap junction proteins such as connexin 43. These connexins are more common along the longitudinal axis than the short axis of the myocytes, leading to a faster conduction velocity along the long axis compared with a slower impulse propagation perpendicular to the cellular syncytium. Disorganization of gap junction distribution and down-regulation of connexins, however, are typical features of myocardial remodeling in hypertrophied or failing hearts, which may play an important role in the development of reentrant arrhythmogenic substrates in human cardiomyopathy [23].

Reentrant VT is characterized by reproducible initiation and termination with programmed stimulation. A stable monomorphic VT can usually be induced from multiple sites in the ventricle. The presence of an excitable gap is a hallmark of stable reentry, with implications that the size and location of the VT circuit is relatively fixed and, at least in part, anatomically defined [24].

Cardiomyopathy

Ischemic

The predominant mechanism of ventricular arrhythmias in patients who have structural heart disease is reentry. Much of what is known about ventricular arrhythmias is based on studies of patients who have coronary artery disease or animal models of myocardial infarction. The pathologic process caused by ischemia or infarct leads to extensive myocyte death and results in aneurysm formation, especially if the infarct is large or transmural [25]. Reentrant arrhythmias typically occur in areas of infarcted myocardium that are adjacent to dense scar. Residual myocardial fibers survive on the endocardium, probably due to perfusion from the ventricular cavity or retrograde perfusion through sinusoidal channels [26]. The surviving myocytes become embedded within regions of fibrosis or scar that constitute substrate for abnormal nonuniform anisotropy, often with conduction block and propagation barrier that promote reentry. Fractionated, long-duration electrograms are commonly recorded from the peri-infarct regions with abnormal, nonuniform anisotropy. Low-level late potentials detected by signal-averaged ECG have been correlated to localized areas of delayed endocardial activation in humans [27–29].

Nonischemic

The anatomic and electrophysiologic substrates for nonischemic cardiomyopathy are less well described. In contrast to ischemic cardiomyopathy in which a distinct scar is present, ventricular myocardium in nonischemic cardiomyopathy often has multiple patchy areas of fibrosis and myofibril disarray with various degrees of myocyte hypertrophy and atrophy [30]. Myocardial dysfunction in nonischemic cardiomyopathy may be secondary to hypertension, diabetes, and metabolic, autoimmune, and infectious causes. Necropsy studies in patients who had idiopathic dilated cardiomyopathy showed that there was a high incidence of endocardial plaque (69%–85%) and myocardial fibrosis (57%) without significant visible scar (14%) [31]. Histologic specimens commonly reveal variable amounts of fibrosis and myofiber disarray that correlate with the degree of nonuniform anisotropic conduction and generation of reentrant wave fronts. In hearts with mild to moderate activation abnormalities, interstitial fibrosis with linear collagen deposition was primarily observed with an overall preserved tissue architecture and cellular alignment. In hearts with severe anisotropy, disturbed activation patterns were observed in areas of dense scar that had muscle bundle disruption similar to the pathologic specimens from patients who had ischemic heart disease and prior myocardial infarction [32].

The mechanism of ventricular arrhythmias in nonischemic cardiomyopathy patients is primarily myocardial scar-based reentry. There is a greater degree of myocardial fibrosis in patients who present with sustained monomorphic VT compared with those presenting with nonsustained arrhythmias [33–35]. Focal initiation of VT, however, may also result from triggered activity with EADs or DADs. Pogwizd and colleagues [13] demonstrated that focal activation can arise in the subendocardium or the subepicardium, with variable interstitial fibrosis. Pathologic findings demonstrated that sites of conduction delay or block consist of areas of extensive interstitial fibrosis with scar formation.

The relationship between inducible arrhythmias and the extent of abnormal endocardial and epicardial substrate in patients who have non-ischemic cardiomyopathy was initially evaluated during surgical epicardial defibrillator patch placement [35]. In patients who had inducible sustained monomorphic VT, a significantly higher incidence of abnormal electrograms was recorded

at epicardial and endocardial layers (47% and 38%, respectively) compared with patients who did not have inducible VT (6% and 18%, respectively). Although a wide individual variation in epicardial electrogram abnormalities predominated in some patients, endocardial abnormalities predominated in others.

Electroanatomic mapping provides a unique insight to the endocardial electrophysiologic substrate for uniform VT in patients who have nonischemic cardiomyopathy. The endocardial substrate is marked by a modest and variable distribution of abnormal low-voltage recordings rarely involving more than 25% of the total endocardial surface area. Furthermore, the predominant distribution of abnormal endocardial electrogram recordings is located at the ventricular base, frequently involving the perivalvular regions (Fig. 3). VTs in these patients typically originate from the basal region of the left

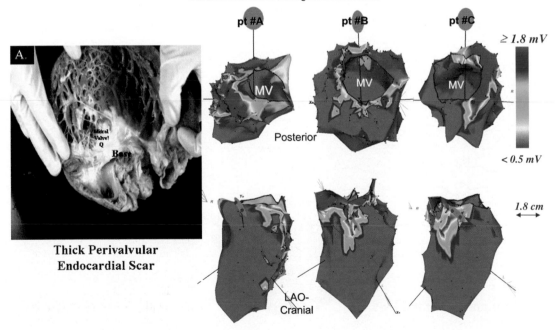

Fig. 3. Endocardial three-dimensional electroanatomic mapping in patients who had nonischemic cardiomyopathy presenting with monomorphic VT. Purple areas represent normal endocardium (amplitude ≥ 1.8 mV), with dense scar depicted in red (amplitude < 0.5 mV). The border zone (amplitude 0.5–1.8 mV) is defined as areas with the color gradient between red and purple. The voltage maps typically demonstrate modest-sized low-voltage endocardial electrogram abnormalities or scar, located near the ventricular base in the perivalvular region. On the left is a pathologic specimen that demonstrates perivalvular scarring at the ventricular base and corresponds to the observed low-voltage areas on the voltage maps. LAO, left anterior oblique; MV, mitral valve. (*Adapted from* Hsia HH, Mofrad PS. Mapping and ablation of ventricular tachycardia in nonischemic cardiomyopathy. In: Wang P, Hsia H, Al-Ahmad A, et al, editors. Ventricular arrhythmias and sudden cardiac death. Oxford (UK): Wiley-Blackwell; 2008; with permission.)

ventricle, corresponding to the locations of the anatomic endocardial substrate (Fig. 4). In comparison to patients who have ischemic cardiomyopathy, the endocardial scar region is significantly smaller in nonischemic cardiomyopathy patients, with a predilection for scar in the base of the heart [34,36,37].

In patients who have dilated cardiomyopathy and fail endocardial ablation, epicardial mapping has demonstrated significant areas of low-voltage scar such that the scar area may be larger on the epicardial surface than on the endocardial surface [38]. In contrast, in patients who have cardiomyopathy due to coronary artery disease, the area of scar has been found to be approximately three times larger in the endocardium compared with the

epicardium. Small islands of viable epicardial myocardium may be observed, located opposite to the corresponding endocardial dense scar region. There is, however, no such relationship between the epicardial and endocardial scars in patients who have nonischemic cardiomyopathy [39].

Ventricular tachycardia related to the His-Purkinje system

BBR is usually seen in patients who have structural heart disease. BBR is a macroreentrant VT involving anterograde conduction by way of the right or left bundle branch, transseptal intramyocardial conduction, and retrograde conduction along the other bundle branch. The

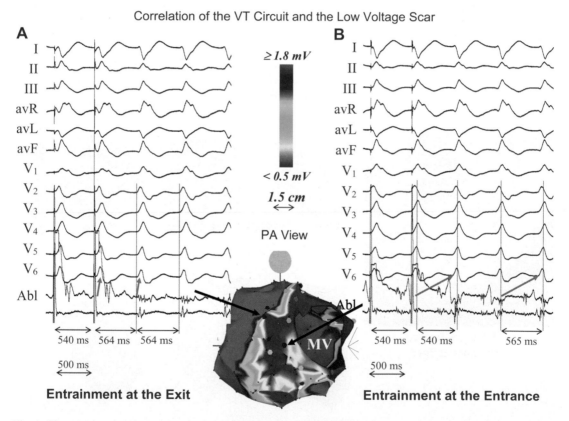

Fig. 4. Electroanatomic voltage map coupled with entrainment mapping for localization of VT circuit. The color gradient corresponds to the left ventricular endocardial bipolar electrogram amplitude as described in Fig. 3. (*A*) Entrainment with minimal surface fusion was observed near the exit site with a short stimulus–QRS interval. (*B*) The entrance site was identified with perfect entrainment and concealed fusion and a long stimulus–QRS interval that matched the electrogram–QRS interval. The VT circuit was located near the left ventricular base, corresponding to the locations of the abnormal endocardial substrate at the perivalvular region defined by the voltage map. MV, mitral valve; PA, posteroanterior. (*From* Hsia HH, Callans DJ, Marchlinski FE. Characterization of endocardial electrophysiological substrate in patients with nonischemic cardiomyopathy and monomorphic ventricular tachycardia. Circulation 2003;108(6):708; with permission.)

prerequisite for BBR VT is conduction delay in the His-Purkinje system, and the average H–V interval in patients who have BBR VT is 80 milliseconds (range, 60–110 milliseconds) [40]. The patients commonly present with a left bundle branch pattern or a nonspecific intraventricular conduction delay on ECG; however, BBR with a right bundle branch block morphology or interfascicular reentry can also be observed [41]. Although BBR is prevalent in patients who have dilated nonischemic cardiomyopathy and present with monomorphic VT, this arrhythmia can occur in cardiomyopathy of any etiology and often coexists with other myocardial reentrant arrhythmias in patients who have structural heart disease [42]. BBR VT accounts for up to 40% of induced sustained arrhythmias in nonischemic cardiomyopathy patients compared with only 6% in patients who have ischemic cardiomyopathy [43]. BBR, however, is also seen with other disorders such as mitral or aortic valve surgery due to close proximity to the His-Purkinje system [44]. Proarrhythmic effects due to conduction delay from flecainide have also been reported to cause BBR [45].

Intrafascicular reentry has been less commonly described (but may be present in patients who have BBR) and typically has a right bundle branch block pattern. A right axis deviation may be observed when there is anterograde conduction down the left anterior fascicle and retrograde conduction up the left posterior fascicle. A left axis deviation may be observed when the reverse path is taken.

The QRS morphology during BBR VT commonly resembles that during sinus rhythm. The diagnosis of BBR is based on carefully detailed electrogram recordings (including recordings from the bundle branches and the His) during the initiation and the sustained reentry. During BBR VT, the onset of the QRS is often preceded by the right bundle potential or the His deflection, with an H–V interval typically equal to or longer than that during sinus rhythm (Fig. 5). Cycle length oscillations of the V–V intervals are preceded by similar changes in the H–H intervals. Entrainment of the bundle branch circuit movement reentry can be achieved by pacing and capturing the right bundle branch or the left fascicle.

Catheter ablation of the right or left bundle branches interrupts the circuit and provides an effective treatment of this arrhythmia [46]; however, a comprehensive electrophysiologic evaluation is essential in patients who have cardiomyopathy because VTs related to the

His-Purkinje system often coexist with other myocardial reentry arrhythmias.

Other cardiomyopathies

Sarcoidosis

Sarcoidosis is a granulomatous disease of unknown etiology. It is characterized by multisystem granulomatous infiltration or discrete fibrosis. Myocardial involvement may be focal or multifocal and the granulomas may become foci for abnormal automaticity and increase the likelihood of reentrant arrhythmias. VT is the most frequently noted arrhythmia in cardiac sarcoid and is the terminal event in 67% of cardiac sarcoid patients [47,48]. Programmed stimulation may induce monomorphic VT, suggesting a reentrant mechanism in patients who have cardiac sarcoid [49]. MRI may also be useful in revealing areas of inflammation in patients who have minimal ventricular dysfunction [50].

Arrhythmogenic right ventricular dysplasia/cardiomyopathy

Arrhythmogenic right ventricular dysplasia/cardiomyopathy (ARVD/C) is a distinct pathologic diagnosis primarily involving fibrosis and fatty infiltration of the right ventricle. Mutations in genes encoding for desmosomal proteins that impair cell adhesion may lead to fibrofatty replacement of myocytes [51]. Additional myocardial mechanical stress may explain the typical phenotypic expressions of ARVD/C that include (1) a strikingly high incidence of the disease in athletic individuals, (2) a latent period for the development of clinical manifestation in early adulthood, and (3) a predilection for the disease to primarily affect certain locations of the right ventricle [52,53].

The extent of right ventricular (RV) involvement may vary from diffuse RV involvement to localized dysplastic regions. Left ventricular or biventricular involvement can also be observed with more recent evidence, suggesting that left ventricular involvement may precede RV involvement [54]. Infiltration of fibrous tissue and fat into regions of normal myocardium, analogous to infarct-related aneurysms in ischemic heart disease, form the arrhythmogenic basis for development of reentrant VT [55]. The extent of RV involvement can vary markedly. Although diffuse RV enlargement and hypokinesis may be present, localized abnormalities consisting of bulging or sacculation of the RV free wall are more characteristic and predominantly involve the

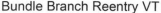

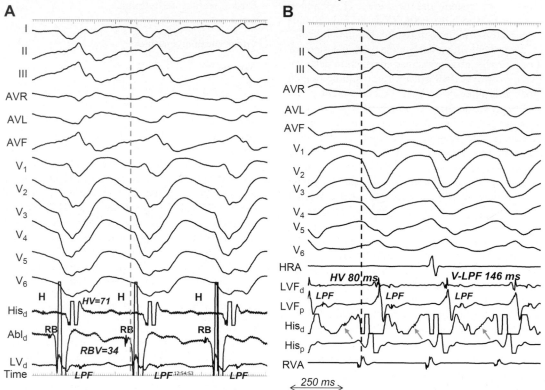

Fig. 5. BBR VT with a left bundle branch block QRS morphology. (*A*) During left bundle branch block VT, His (H) deflections (H–V interval of 71 milliseconds) precedes right bundle (RB) activation (RB–V interval of 34 milliseconds), followed by onset of the QRS. The left posterior fascicle (LPF) potentials followed right ventricular activations, suggesting retrograde penetration up the LPF during a counterclockwise reentry BBR VT. (*B*) Similar observation in a different patient who had nonischemic cardiomyopathy. Presystolic His activation (*arrows*) with an H–V interval of 80 milliseconds, followed by slow transseptal propagation and late retrograde LPF activation with a V–LPF interval of 146 milliseconds. Abld, ablation catheter distal; HRA, high right atrial; LV, left ventricle; LVd, left ventricular mapping catheter distal; RVA, right ventricular apex. (*Adapted from* Hsia HH, Mofrad PS. Mapping and ablation of ventricular tachycardia in nonischemic cardiomyopathy. In: Wang P, Hsia H, Al-Ahmad A, et al, editors. Ventricular arrhythmias and sudden cardiac death. Oxford (UK): Wiley-Blackwell; 2008; with permission.)

infundibular, apical, and subtricuspid-diaphragmatic regions, the so-called "triangle of dysplasia." MRI has been the primary imaging tool for evaluation of ARVD/C, with the ability to determine areas of RV dilatation, aneurysmal outpouching, and fibrofatty infiltration [56].

Chagas' disease

Chagas' disease is a protozoan myocarditis endemic to Central and South America. The vector *Trypanosoma cruzi* is transmitted to human hosts by way of the reduviid bug and may infect up to 4% of the Latin American population. Typically, the patient will develop a nonischemic cardiomyopathy years after the initial infection [57].

The exact etiology of chronic Chagas' cardiomyopathy is unclear and may be due to a cellular-mediated autoimmune reaction with autonomic denervation [58]. The anatomic substrate for VT in Chagas' disease is primarily inferolateral wall motion abnormalities in the left ventricle. Histologic examinations reveal patches of focal and diffuse fibrosis of the myocardium. Recurrent monomorphic VT is common in chronic Chagas' cardiomyopathy; however, the morphologies of VT may vary from patient to patient. Programmed stimulation commonly induces clinical arrhythmia in patients who have Chagas' disease, suggesting that VT resulting from this disease may be due to a reentrant mechanism [59].

Clinical management

Risk stratification

By far, the highest total mortality appears to be in patients who have a depressed ejection fraction and symptoms of heart failure. Sudden, presumably arrhythmic death accounts for a significant proportion of total mortality in patients who have mild symptoms of ventricular dysfunction, whereas progressive hemodynamic deterioration and pump failure are the major causes of death in patients in advanced stage of heart failure (see Fig. 1). A large number of risk factors for arrhythmia recurrence and SCD have been identified in patients who have structural heart disease; however, developing a comprehensive risk stratification strategy remains a challenge.

A depressed ejection fraction remains the most consistent predictor of SCD in patients who have structural heart disease, irrespective of etiology. Patients in the follow-up Multicenter Automatic Defibrillator Implantation Trial (MADIT-II) who had an ejection fraction less than 30% had a rate of SCD of approximately 9.4% at 20 months [60]. In a similar population of patients, however, an ejection fraction greater than 35% and history of myocardial infarction conferred only a 1.8% risk of SCD [61].

The presence of ambient ventricular ectopy also carries prognostic significance. In patients who had prior myocardial infarctions, the presence of frequent PVCs (> 10/h) or nonsustained VT was associated with an increased risk of SCD [62]. In contrast, patients who had prior infarctions but no ventricular ectopy had a less than 1% incidence of SCD [63]. A similar observation was made in patients who had nonischemic dilated cardiomyopathy in the GESICA-GEMA trial. In patients who had heart failure and an average ejection fraction of 19%, the presence of VT was associated with an increased risk of SCD, whereas the absence of VT indicated a lower probability of SCD [64].

Prolongation of the interlead QT interval reflects a dispersion of myocardial repolarization. Such a prolonged vulnerable phase during myocardial recovery and regional heterogeneity has been associated with occurrences of ventricular arrhythmias [65]. The normal QT interval dispersion is around 30 to 70 milliseconds. A measured QT dispersion greater than 80 milliseconds post myocardial infarction was associated with VT with a sensitivity of 73% and a specificity of 86% [66].

T-wave alternans or beat-to-beat variation in the T-wave morphology is believed to be due to regional disturbances in action potential duration leading to dispersion in repolarization and propensity to develop arrhythmias [67]. Microvolt T-wave alternans (MTWA) measures microvolt changes in the T-wave amplitude in alternate beats and has also been found to be a significant predictor of VT events [68]. Abnormal MTWA in patients who have congestive heart failure has been associated with an increased mortality rate [69]. Application of the MTWA test to patients who fit MADIT-II criteria demonstrated that patients who had an abnormal MTWA test had a significantly increased 2-year mortality rate (17.8%) compared with patients who had a normal MTWA (3.8%) [70]. A major limitation of such an MTWA test, however, is the high proportion of indeterminate results.

The autonomic nervous system has also been implicated in causing ventricular arrhythmias. Heart rate variability and baroreflex sensitivity (BRS) are two noninvasive tests used to estimate the function of the autonomic nervous system. Decreased heart rate variability has been shown to be a powerful predictor of mortality and perhaps arrhythmic events in patients who have myocardial infarctions [71,72]. The Autonomic Tone and Reflexes After Myocardial Infarction trial was designed to evaluate the prognostic utility of BRS and heart rate variability in postmyocardial infarction patients. A depressed BRS (defined as < 3 ms/mm Hg) significantly predicted cardiac mortality over an average 21-month follow-up period [73].

The signal-averaged ECG is a high-resolution ECG technique designed to determine the risk of developing VT by measuring the low-amplitude, high-frequency surface ECG signals in the terminal QRS complex that cannot be detected by a standard ECG machine [74]. These late potentials have been correlated to localized areas of delayed endocardial activation in humans, and reflect the substrate for ventricular reentry [27–29]. In patients who have coronary artery disease, signal-averaged ECG has an overall low positive predictive value ranging from 7% to 27%, whereas it has a very high negative predictive value ranging from 96% to 99%. Its utility as a prognostic tool remains controversial in patients who have idiopathic nonischemic cardiomyopathy. An abnormal signal-averaged ECG in patients who have nonischemic cardiomyopathy has been associated with a significantly higher cardiac event rate, with the predominant cause of mortality being sudden death [75].

The diagnostic and prognostic values of an electrophysiology study depend on the underlying pathologic substrate and the spontaneous arrhythmia presentations. The inducibility of monomorphic VT is a powerful marker of risk for SCD, especially in patients who have a history of prior myocardial infarction and reduced ejection fraction or syncope. Programmed electrical stimulation has a sensitivity of about 97% in those who have spontaneous sustained monomorphic VT and a positive predictive value of 65% [76]. In patients who have nonischemic cardiomyopathy, the inducibility of ventricular arrhythmias is much lower. Although the overall sensitivity of programmed stimulation is similar to that in patients who have coronary artery disease, noninducibility in patients who have nonischemic cardiomyopathies does not confer a good prognosis, and patients are still at high risk of SCD [77].

MRI

Advances in MRI have provided unique capabilities to identify morphologic changes in the cardiac chambers in ischemic and nonischemic cardiomyopathies [78]. Applications of gadolinium-enhanced imaging provide detailed characterization of cardiac tissues and identification of areas of scar. Differences between the nonischemic and ischemic subgroups in patients who have ventricular dysfunction and heart failure can be demonstrated on cardiac MRI scans [79,80]. In the studies done by Assomull and colleagues [79] and McCrohon and colleagues [80], all patients who had coronary artery disease had subendocardial or transmural late-gadolinium enhancement, consistent with the typical locations of infarcted myocardium and scars. In contrast, patients who had nonischemic cardiomyopathy had absence of abnormal gadolinium uptake in over half of the population, and patchy or longitudinal striae of midwall enhancement patterns were observed in approximately one third of the patients. The midwall myocardial enhancement in patients who had nonischemic cardiomyopathy was similar to the focal segmental fibrosis found at autopsy. The remaining patients (13%) had a pattern of myocardial enhancement that was indistinguishable from that of ischemic heart disease. These observations were clearly different from the distribution pattern found in patients who had coronary artery disease. Patients who had MRI-documented fibrosis had a significantly greater incidence of SCD and induction of sustained VT by programmed stimulation [81].

Pharmacologic therapy

In addition to their neurohormonal benefits in the management of patients who have heart failure, β-blockers have been shown to be antiarrhythmic and antifibrillatory. Trials using different β-blockers, including atenolol, propranolol, metoprolol, timolol, acebutolol, and carvedilol, have shown consistent reductions in mortality after myocardial infarction [82–86]. The total mortality reduction with these agents is approximately 25% to 40%, with approximately a 32% to 50% reduction in the incidence of SCD. The benefit of reduction of total mortality, cardiovascular mortality, and sudden death risk extends beyond patients who have coronary artery disease to those who have nonischemic cardiomyopathy. It is clear that β-blocker therapy is the cornerstone of heart failure management and is indicated in all patients who have heart failure and no contraindications [87,88].

Angiotensin-converting enzyme (ACE) inhibitors have been well established to decrease the overall mortality in patients after myocardial infarction who have various degrees of systolic heart failure. ACE inhibition has been shown to reduce mortality primarily by inhibiting the progressive architectural changes that lead to inefficient left ventricular function, thus preventing or delaying pump failure. ACE inhibitors, however, were not shown to result in any significant reduction in the incidence of SCD in the Cooperative North Scandinavian Enalapril Survival Study, the Survival And Ventricular Enlargement trial, or the SOLVD trial [89–91], with the exception of the use of ramipril decreasing the incidence of SCD by 30% in post–myocardial infaraction patients who had heart failure [92].

Most trials using antiarrhythmic drug therapy have resulted in worsening outcome in the drug treatment arms. The first of these trials was the Cardiac Arrhythmia Suppression Trial, which demonstrated an increased mortality despite suppression of PVCs using class IC agents, presumably due to proarrhythmia [93]. d-sotalol, a pure I_{Kr} blocker with class III antiarrhythmic effects and little β-blocking activity, also demonstrated a significant mortality increase in patients who had myocardial infarctions and New York Heart

Association (NYHA) class II to III heart failure (Survival With ORal d-sotalol trial) [94]. It was believed that this increase in mortality was due to the lack of β-blocking benefits. Other class III antiarrhythmic agents such as dofetilide appear to be neutral in regard to all-cause mortality and SCD in postmyocardial infarction patients who have heart failure (DIAMOND trial) [95].

Amiodarone, a complex antiarrhythmic drug with multiple pharmacologic actions, is one of the most widely used antiarrhythmic drugs in the heart failure population. Amiodarone does not appear to have any adverse effect on survival or heart failure. In the Survival Trial of Antiarrhythmic Therapy in Congestive Heart Failure, amiodarone had no significant impact on the incidence of SCD or on total mortality [96]; however, multiple smaller studies have shown significant mortality benefits and SCD reduction with the use of this drug [97–99]. Perhaps the largest of

the amiodarone studies are the European Myocardial Infarct Amiodarone Trial and the Canadian Amiodarone Myocardial Infarction Arrhythmia Trial, which focused on patients who had ischemic heart disease and prior myocardial infarction. The results suggested that amiodarone may reduce arrhythmic death, but at the expense of higher mortality from re-infarction and noncardiac mortality [100,101].

Nonpharmacologic therapy (implantable cardioverters-defibrillators)

Initial therapies using implantable cardioverters-defibrillators (ICDs) were targeted at survivors of SCD. Randomized controlled trials involving implantation of ICDs in cardiac arrest survivors demonstrated a significant survival benefit in total mortality and sudden death mortality (Antiarrhythmics Versus Implantable

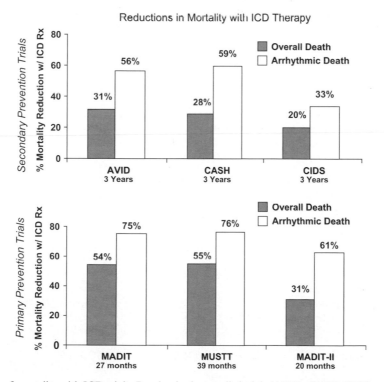

Fig. 6. Reduction of mortality with ICD trials. Randomized controlled trials (AVID, CASH, CIDS; *top*) involving ICD implantation in cardiac arrest survivors demonstrated statistically significant survival benefit in total mortality and sudden death mortality. The relative reduction ranged from 20% to 31% for total mortality and from 33% to 59% for arrhythmic death mortality. Primary prevention trials (MADIT, MUSTT, MADIT-II, *bottom*) with prophylactic ICD implantation in patients who had prior myocardial infarction and ventricular dysfunction demonstrated a relative mortality reduction ranging from 31% to 55% for total mortality and from 61% to 76% for arrhythmic death mortality. The mortality reductions with ICD in primary prevention trials are equal to or greater than those in secondary prevention trials.

Defibrillators trial [AVID] [102], Canadian Implantable Defibrillator Study [CIDS] [103], and Cardiac Arrest Study Hamburg [CASH] [104]). Meta-analysis from the combined secondary prevention trials demonstrated a 57% decrease in the risk of arrhythmic death along with a 30% decrease in all-cause mortality in survivors of SCD (Fig. 6) (Table 1) [105].

With the widespread adoption of ICDs for prevention of SCD in survivors of SCD, the focus was shifted toward prophylactic ICD use for primary prevention in patients who have ventricular dysfunction and are at high risk of sudden death. The MADIT study was the first to evaluate the prophylactic use of ICDs in patients who had prior myocardial infarction, low ejection fraction, and inducible but nonsuppressible ventricular arrhythmias. The use of ICDs in this population was associated with a 54% decrease in all-cause mortality and a 75% decrease in arrhythmia deaths [106]. The MADIT study, however, has been criticized for its small sample size and the low rate of β-blocker usage in the conventional therapy arm.

The utility of electrophysiology study to guide antiarrhythmic therapy in postinfarct patients who have low ejection fraction ($<40\%$) and spontaneous nonsustained VT was subsequently evaluated in the Multicenter UnSustained Tachycardia Trial (MUSTT). The survival benefit associated with electrophysiologically guided therapy was entirely due to the use of defibrillators, not antiarrhythmic drugs. The risk for cardiac arrest or death from arrhythmia among patients who underwent ICD implantation was significantly lower than that among patients who did not have ICD therapy, with a relative risk of 0.24 [107]. A follow-up study, the MADIT-II, was performed in patients who had an ischemic cardiomyopathy and an ejection fraction less than 30%. There was a higher percentage of β-blocker and ACE inhibitor use. With optimized medical treatment, there was a 5.6% absolute mortality benefit and a 30% relative mortality benefit in patients who had defibrillators.

The more recent Sudden Cardiac Death in Heart Failure Trial (SCD-HeFT) included large

Table 1
Defibrillator trials

Trials	Inclusions	Interventions	Results
Primary prevention trials			
AVID	VF, VT/syncope, VT with EF $\leq40\%$	Amiod versus sotalol versus ICD	31% ↓ All-cause mortality in ICD versus drugs in 3 y
CASH	Survivors of VF (no EF requirement)	Metoprolol versus amiod versus propaf versus ICD	37% ↓ All-cause mortality in ICD versus drugs in 2 y 85% ↓ SCD in ICD versus drugs
CIDS	VF, VT/syncope, VT/EF $\leq35\%$, CL <400 ms	Amiod versus ICD	20% ↓ All-cause mortality in ICD versus drugs in 3 y
Secondary prevention trials			
MUSTT	CAD, EF $<40\%$, NSVT	EP versus non–EP-guided Rx, AAD versus ICD	55%–60% ↓ All-cause mortality in ICD versus drugs in 39 mo 73%–76% ↓ SCD in ICD versus drugs
MADIT-I	MI, EF $<35\%$, NSVT, inducible/non-suppressible VA	Conv med versus ICD	Prophylactic ICD ↓ overall mortality (HR: 0.46; $P = .009$), improves survival compared with conv med
MADIT-II	MI, EF $<30\%$	Placebo versus ICD	31% ↓ Overall mortality (HR: 0.69; $P = .016$) 61% ↓ Arrhythmia mortality with ICD
DEFINITE	Nonischemic CM, EF $<36\%$, PVC/NSVT	Placebo versus ICD	↓ SCD (HR: 0.20; $P = .006$) in ICD Insignificant ↓ all-cause mortality in ICD
SCD-HeFT	HF/NYHA II-III, EF $<35\%$	Placebo versus amiod versus ICD	23% ↓ All-cause mortality in ICD versus drugs over 5 y. Amiodarone does not improve survival

Abbreviations: AAD, antiarrhythmic drugs; CAD, coronary artery disease; CL, cycle length; CM, cardiomyopathy; Conv med, conventional medical therapy; EF, ejection fraction; EP, electrophysiology; HF, heart failure; HR, hazard ratio; MI, myocardial infarction; NSVT, nonsustained VT; VA, ventricular arrhythmia; VF ventricular fibrillation. (*From* Heart Rhythm 2006;3(5):page 507.)

cohorts of patients who had ischemic and non-ischemic cardiomyopathies. The enrollment criteria included only symptoms of heart failure and a depressed ejection fraction without arrhythmia indication (ejection fraction <35% and NYHA class II–III heart failure) [108]. Patients were randomized to three arms: optimal medical therapy for heart failure plus placebo, medical therapy plus amiodarone, and medical therapy plus single-lead ICDs. SCD-HeFT demonstrated a 23% mortality benefit in patients implanted with ICDs compared with amiodarone therapy or placebo.

The Defibrillators in Nonischemic Cardiomyopathy Treatment Evaluation trial focused exclusively on patients who had dilated nonischemic cardiomyopathy and ventricular dysfunction. All patients were in NYHA class I to III and received optimal medical therapy (with >85% usage of β-blockers and ACE inhibitors). The implantation of a cardioverter-defibrillator significantly reduced the risk of sudden death from arrhythmia and was associated with a nonsignificant

reduction in the risk of death from any cause in this population [109].

Meta-analysis from the combined secondary prevention trials demonstrated a 57% decrease in the risk of arrhythmic death along with a 30% decrease in all-cause mortality in survivors of SCD [102–105].

Although there is no doubt that the ICD improves survival in high-risk patients, there remains a significant increase in the rate of hospitalization for new or worsening heart failure (Fig. 7) [110]. The development of heart failure is a major determinant of subsequent mortality in heart failure patients despite receiving single-chamber or dual-chamber ICDs. Although the life-prolonging efficacy of ICD therapy is maintained among patients who receive single-chamber devices, there seems to be a significant reduction in ICD benefit after developing heart failure among patients who receive dual-chamber devices. RV pacing with a dual-chamber ICD has been shown to contribute to an increased risk of

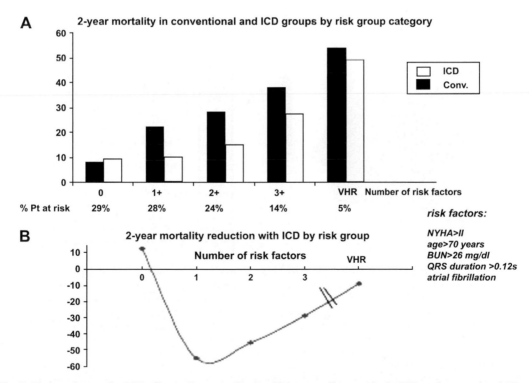

Fig. 7. U-shaped curve for ICD efficacy. Two-year Kaplan-Meier mortality rates in the ICD and conventional (Conv.) therapy groups (*A*), and the corresponding 2-year mortality rate reduction with an ICD, by risk score and in VHR patients (*P* = .05) (*B*). BUN, blood urea nitrogen; VHR, very high risk. (*Modified from* Goldenberg I, Vyas AK, Hall WJ, et al. Risk stratification for primary implantation of a cardioverter-defibrillator in patients with ischemic left ventricular dysfunction. J Am Coll Cardiol 2008;51:294; with permission.)

heart failure after ICD implantation [111,112]. Aggressive heart failure medical management and judicious ICD programming are essential to optimize the benefit of ICD therapy.

Ablative therapy

Prior surgical experiences for treatment of ventricular arrhythmia in patients who have ischemic cardiomyopathy have demonstrated long-term efficacy in preventing arrhythmia

recurrence [113–115]. Catheter ablation also plays an increasing role in the management of patients who have VTs because antiarrhythmic drug therapies are often inadequate to prevent recurrence [116,117]. Catheter ablation techniques, however, usually require identification of the functional components of the reentry circuit and are mostly limited to hemodynamically tolerated monomorphic VTs [118].

The "conventional mapping" strategies for ventricular arrhythmias include activation

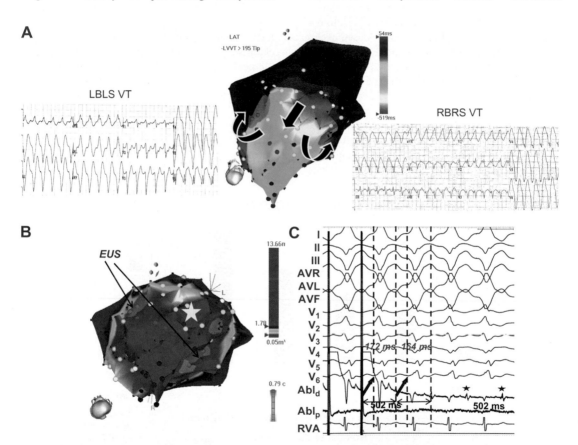

Fig. 8. Electroanatomic mapping in a patient who had a large anterolateral myocardial infarction and sustained monomorphic VT. (*A*) Activation mapping during VT shows a "figure-of-eight" reentry. Temporal isochronal color changes demonstrated an "early-meets-late" activation pattern, with red representing early activation and purple depicting the late area. Two different VTs were induced, with a left bundle branch block–left-superior (LBLS) and a right bundle branch block–right-superior (RBRS) QRS morphology. (*B*) Voltage map shows a large anterolateral scar. The color gradient corresponds to the left ventricular endocardial bipolar electrogram amplitude as described in Fig. 4. Electrical unexcitable scar (EUS) was identified by noncapture with high-output pacing and is depicted by the gray scar (*arrows*). Such dense scar tissues are commonly in proximity to the zone of slow conduction/isthmus of the VT circuit and are often located deep in dense scar (<0.5 mV). (*C*) Entrainment mapping with pacing during VT demonstrated concealed fusion that identified the isthmus site (*stars*), with the electrogram–QRS interval (164 milliseconds) equal to the stimulus–QRS interval of 172 milliseconds. Abld, ablation catheter distal; Ablp, ablation catheter proximal; RVA, right ventricular apical. (*Modified from* Anh D, Hsia H, Callans D. The utility of electroanatomical mapping in catheter ablation of ventricular tachycardias. In: Al-Ahmad A, Callans DJ, Hsia HH, et al, editors. Electroanatomical mapping: an atlas for clinicians. Oxford (UK): Blackwell Publishing; 2008. p. 24; with permission.)

mapping, pace mapping, and entrainment mapping. In addition, the "site-of-origin" of VT can be identified by careful analysis of the QRS morphology on a 12-lead ECG [119,120]. Activation mapping searches for the earliest ventricular depolarization based on the local bipolar electrogram timing, a qS pattern on unipolar recordings as the wave front propagates away from the focus of ventricular activation, or both. Relative timing of recorded signals can be assessed with reference to surface R waves or intracardiac ventricular electrograms. Activation isochrones may be constructed to display the area with the earliest isochronal time as an "early spot" using three-dimensional electroanatomic mapping systems.

Pace mapping for VT localization strives to reproduce the exact QRS morphology compared with that of spontaneous arrhythmias. The method is predicated on the principle that pacing at the exit site of the VT circuit would yield the same surface ECG morphology as the clinical VT, using unipolar pacing or bipolar pacing at low current outputs from a closely spaced bipole [121]. Subtle variations in paced QRS morphology can be observed, however, which may be associated with more than one distinct focus within a limited area [122]. Although previous studies have suggested that pace mapping may be more precise in locating the site of origin compared with activation mapping for focal VTs, a more recent investigation has shown a comparable efficacy between pace mapping and activation mapping with the use of a three-dimensional magnetic electroanatomic mapping system [123].

Entrainment mapping assesses the response of a reentrant arrhythmia to pacing stimulation and is the most reliable method for defining a reentrant VT circuit. Based on the degree of surface ECG fusion, the postpacing interval, and the electrogram-to-QRS timing, one can determine the arbitrarily defined exit, central isthmus, entrance, outer loop, remote, and adjacent bystander sites within a reentrant VT circuit (see Fig. 4; Fig. 8). Entrainment mapping, however, requires that the tachycardia remains hemodynamically stable along with a stable QRS morphology and rate. Pacing during VT may accelerate, terminate, or change to a different arrhythmia, limiting the utility of entrainment mapping.

Substrate mapping

Most induced VTs are often unstable with multiple morphologies and do not permit extensive mapping [124]. Based on the authors' experiences in surgical resection, a recent shift of paradigm has allowed a different approach of VT ablation. This strategy depends on anatomic identification of scar, with infarcted myocardium having different electrogram characteristics than the surrounding tissue. Radiofrequency ablation deployed with reference to anatomic boundaries or myocardial scar may result in successful ablation of VT without ever inducing sustained VT. This substrate-based catheter ablation approach has been shown to be effective in eliminating or controlling scar-based reentrant VTs that were previously considered "unmappable" [125–127].

Electroanatomic mapping couples spatial locations with electrogram recordings and displays a three-dimensional anatomic construct of the cardiac chamber. Such voltage maps depict the location and characteristics of myocardial scar and facilitate mapping of scar-based VTs (see Figs. 4 and 8). The local electrogram amplitude at sites within the VT circuits was recently reported by Hsia and colleagues [128]. Entrance and central isthmus sites are predominantly (84%) located in the "dense scar," with electrogram amplitude less than 0.5 mV. Conversely, exit or outer loop sites are more likely to be located within the border zone (0.5–1.5 mV). Almost all (92%) of the exit sites are located in abnormal myocardium of less than 1.5 mV, with more than half of the exit sites located in the border zone, with voltage between 0.5 and 1.5 mV (Table 2). Careful analysis of the voltage profile helps to identify the approximate location of the VT circuit. Ablation targeted at the scar border zone defined by

Table 2
Local electrogram amplitude for sites within the reentrant circuit

	Entrance	Central isthmus	Exit	Outer loop
Dense scar (<0.5 mV)	17	30	18	6
Border zone (0.5–1.5 mV)	2	7	26	18
Normal (>1.5 mV)	—	—	4	8
Total (136 sites)	19	37	48	32

(*Data from* Hsia HH, Lin D, Sauer WH, et al. Anatomic characterization of endocardial substrate for hemodynamically stable reentrant ventricular tachycardia: identification of endocardial conducting channels. Heart Rhythm 2006;3(5):503–12.)

substrate mapping has been shown to be effective in eliminating VT post myocardial infarction [129]. Furthermore, VT-related conducting channels that correspond to the activation wave front during reentry can be identified (Fig. 9) [128,130]. These VT-related conducting channels may be appropriate targets for ablation. Electrograms with isolated delayed components or late potentials may also serve as surrogates for anisotropic conduction delay. Identification of such late potentials during different rhythms (sinus versus paced) may be an effective adjunct to localize

the arrhythmia substrate for scar-based reentry [131].

A substrate-based ablation strategy targeting the potential VT circuits within the myocardial scar results in successful control of recurrent VT in patients who have cardiomyopathies and heart failure [37]. Multiple linear ablations are typically required, extending from the putative VT exit site at the border zone into the dense scar, often extending up to several centimeters in length [37]. Placement of ablation lines designed to transect the VT-related "conduction channels" in

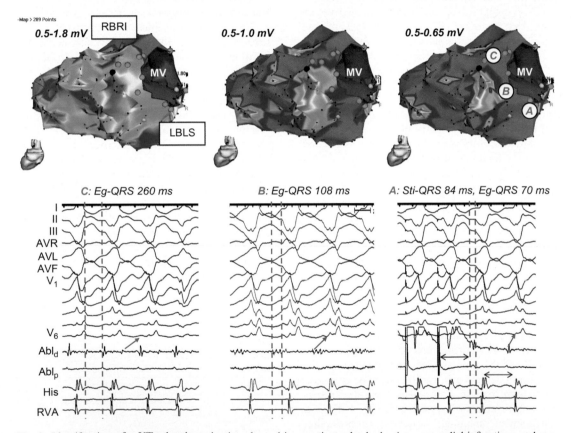

Fig. 9. Identification of a VT-related conducting channel in a patient who had prior myocardial infarctions and presented with sustained VT. Two tachycardias were documented with a right bundle branch block–right-inferior (RBRI) and a left bundle branch block–left-superior (LBLS) QRS morphology. By carefully adjusting the upper and lower color voltage thresholds on the electroanatomic voltage map (0.5–1.8 mV, 0.5–1.0 mV, and 0.5–0.65 mV), a corridor demonstrating a higher voltage amplitude than that of the surrounding areas could be visualized. Entrainment with concealed fusion within the channel was noted at multiple sites (A, B, C), with progressively longer stimulus–QRS (Sti–QRS) intervals equaling electrogram–QRS (Eg–QRS) intervals. This is an example of mitral annular VT with counterclockwise (LBLS) and clockwise (RBRI) reentry VTs around the mitral valve (MV). (*From* Anh D, Hsia H, Callans D. The utility of electroanatomical mapping in catheter ablation of ventricular tachycardias. In: Al-Ahmad A, Callans DJ, Hsia HH, et al, editors. Electroanatomical mapping: an atlas for clinicians. Oxford (UK): Blackwell Publishing; 2008. p. 25; with permission.)

abnormal scar or targeting areas with isolated delayed electrogram recordings may facilitate ablation of multiple stable and unstable VTs, even in the absence of VT induction [128,130–132].

Epicardial mapping

Mapping and ablation of VT still remains a formidable challenge in patients who have scar-based reentrant arrhythmias. The success rate depends on the underlying structural heart disease and the location of VT circuits. The presence of epicardial circuits has been considered one of the main reasons for failure of endocardial ablation. Initial reports from Brazil have demonstrated a high prevalence of epicardial circuits in patients who have Chagas' cardiomyopathy and VT related to old inferior myocardial infarctions [133,134].

In contrast to patients who have coronary artery disease, there is no predilection for subendocardial location of scar and VT circuits in patients who have dilated nonischemic cardiomyopathy. Only modest (approximately one third) endocardial scar is present with a predominant distribution adjacent to valve annuli [36]. Significantly large epicardial scar involvement may be found in selected patients who have nonischemic cardiomyopathy; however, marked individual variations are present [38].

The success of endocardial ablation for VT associated with nonischemic cardiomyopathy appears to be lower than that observed for ischemic VT. This difference may be the result of reentry circuits that are deep to the endocardium or in the epicardial region. Epicardial mapping has led to successful ablation in a significant proportion of these patients after failed endocardial ablation. Approximately one third of patients who have nonischemic cardiomyopathy may require epicardial ablation. The use of a combined epicardial/endocardial approach or a staged approach may improve success rates for ablation of VT [38,39].

Epicardial circuits may be difficult to approach and map using endocardial techniques. The coronary veins can be used for limited access to the epicardium, but the distribution of the coronary venous anatomy places significant constraints on catheter manipulation and placement. The sub-xiphoid transthoracic approach or a surgical approach may be used successfully to gain access to the pericardial and epicardial space to allow for unrestricted access to the epicardial surface of both ventricles [135].

Summary

Ventricular arrhythmia represents a significant cause of mortality and morbidity in patients who have heart failure. The pathophysiologic mechanisms and electroanatomic substrates of ventricular arrhythmia are slowly being elucidated.

Clinical management of ventricular arrhythmia in patients who have heart failure has progressed over the past few decades, with a shift from antiarrhythmic drugs to device therapy. Although implantable defibrillators have a clear impact in reduction of sudden death, optimization of medical neurohormonal therapy and other heart failure management strategies are essential to improve the overall mortality.

Catheter ablation of VT is an effective adjunct in the management of ventricular arrhythmia but remains a significant challenge. Better understanding of the electroanatomic substrates in different cardiomyopathies and identification of other surrogate markers for VT circuits are essential to improve the ablation outcome. Promising advances in robotic and magnetic catheter manipulation may shorten the procedural time and increase safety. Furthermore, incorporation of other imaging technologies such as CT, MRI, or ultrasound with electroanatomic mapping can enhance our ability to efficiently map and ablate ventricular arrhythmia in this patient population.

Future investigations will focus on advancing our understanding of the complex pathophysiology of heart failure. Novel anatomic/physiologic imaging modalities may provide rapid characterization of the substrate for ventricular dysfunction and arrhythmia development and the capacity for serial assessment of disease progression, improving risk stratification.

References

[1] American Heart Association. Heart disease and stroke statistics—2004 update. Dallas (TX): American Heart Association; 2003.

[2] Myerburg RJ, Kessler KM, Zaman L, et al. Survivors of prehospital cardiac arrest. JAMA 1982; 247(10):1485–90.

[3] State-specific mortality from sudden cardiac death—United States, 1999. MMWR Morb Mortal Wkly Rep 2002;51(6):123–6.

[4] Kasper EK, Agema WR, Hutchins GM, et al. The causes of dilated cardiomyopathy: a clinicopathologic review of 673 consecutive patients. J Am Coll Cardiol 1994;23(3):586–90.

[5] Bigger JT, Fleiss JL, Rolnitzky LM. Prevalence, characteristics and significance of ventricular tachycardia detected by 24-hour continuous electrocardiographic recordings in the late hospital phase of acute myocardial infarction. Am J Cardiol 1986;58(13):1151–60.

[6] Bigger JT, Weld FM, Rolnitzky LM. Prevalence, characteristics and significance of ventricular tachycardia (three or more complexes) detected with ambulatory electrocardiographic recording in the late hospital phase of acute myocardial infarction. Am J Cardiol 1981;48(5):815–23.

[7] Kjekshus J. Arrhythmias and mortality in congestive heart failure. Am J Cardiol 1990;65(19): 42I–8I.

[8] Doval HC, Nul DR, Grancelli HO, et al. Randomised trial of low-dose amiodarone in severe congestive heart failure. Grupo de Estudio de la Sobrevida en la Insuficiencia Cardiaca en Argentina (GESICA). Lancet 1994;344(8921):493–8.

[9] Uretsky BF. Implantable defibrillators in patients with coronary artery disease at high risk for ventricular arrhythmia. N Engl J Med 1997;336(23): 1676–7.

[10] Friedman PL, Stewart JR, Wit AL. Spontaneous and induced cardiac arrhythmias in subendocardial Purkinje fibers surviving extensive myocardial infarction in dogs. Circ Res 1973;33(5):612–26.

[11] Pogwizd SM, Bers DM. Calcium cycling in heart failure: the arrhythmia connection. J Cardiovasc Electrophysiol 2002;13(1):88–91.

[12] Pogwizd SM, Hoyt RH, Saffitz JE, et al. Reentrant and focal mechanisms underlying ventricular tachycardia in the human heart. Circulation 1992; 86(6):1872–87.

[13] Pogwizd SM, McKenzie JP, Cain ME. Mechanisms underlying spontaneous and induced ventricular arrhythmias in patients with idiopathic dilated cardiomyopathy. Circulation 1998;98(22):2404–14.

[14] Zeng J, Rudy Y. Early afterdepolarizations in cardiac myocytes: mechanism and rate dependence. Biophys J 1995;68(3):949–64.

[15] January CT, Shorofsky S. Early afterdepolarizations: newer insights into cellular mechanisms. J Cardiovasc Electrophysiol 1990;1(2):161–9.

[16] El-Sherif N, Chinushi M, Caref EB, et al. Electrophysiological mechanism of the characteristic electrocardiographic morphology of torsade de pointes tachyarrhythmias in the long-QT syndrome: detailed analysis of ventricular tridimensional activation patterns. Circulation 1997; 96(12):4392–9.

[17] Farzaneh-Far A, Lerman BB. Idiopathic ventricular outflow tract tachycardia. Heart 2005;91(2): 136–8.

[18] Song Y, Thedford S, Lerman BB, et al. Adenosine-sensitive afterdepolarizations and triggered activity in guinea pig ventricular myocytes. Circ Res 1992; 70(4):743–53.

[19] Dean JW, Lab MJ. Arrhythmia in heart failure: role of mechanically induced changes in electrophysiology. Lancet 1989;1(8650):1309–12.

[20] Antzelevitch C, Fish J. Electrical heterogeneity within the ventricular wall. Basic Res Cardiol 2001;96(6):517–27.

[21] Hansen DE, Craig CS, Hondeghem LM. Stretch-induced arrhythmias in the isolated canine ventricle. Evidence for the importance of mechanoelectrical feedback. Circulation 1990;81(3):1094–105.

[22] Kelly D, Mackenzie L, Hunter P, et al. Gene expression of stretch-activated channels and mechanoelectric feedback in the heart. Clin Exp Pharmacol Physiol 2006;33(7):642–8.

[23] Kostin S, Rieger M, Dammer S, et al. Gap junction remodeling and altered connexin43 expression in the failing human heart. Mol Cell Biochem 2003; 242(1–2):135–44.

[24] Richardson AW, Callans DJ, Josephson ME. Electrophysiology of postinfarction ventricular tachycardia: a paradigm of stable reentry. J Cardiovasc Electrophysiol 1999;10(9):1288–92.

[25] Cabin HS, Roberts WC. True left ventricular aneurysm and healed myocardial infarction. Clinical and necropsy observations including quantification of degrees of coronary arterial narrowing. Am J Cardiol 1980;46(5):754–63.

[26] Friedman PL, Fenoglio JJ, Wit AL. Time course for reversal of electrophysiological and ultrastructural abnormalities in subendocardial Purkinje fibers surviving extensive myocardial infarction in dogs. Circ Res 1975;36(1):127–44.

[27] Marcus NH, Falcone RA, Harken AH, et al. Body surface late potentials: effects of endocardial resection in patients with ventricular tachycardia. Circulation 1984;70(4):632–7.

[28] Simson MB, Untereker WJ, Spielman SR, et al. Relation between late potentials on the body surface and directly recorded fragmented electrograms in patients with ventricular tachycardia. Am J Cardiol 1983;51(1):105–12.

[29] Vassallo JA, Cassidy D, Simson MB, et al. Relation of late potentials to site of origin of ventricular tachycardia associated with coronary heart disease. Am J Cardiol 1985;55(8):985–9.

[30] Nakayama Y, Shimizu G, Hirota Y, et al. Functional and histopathologic correlation in patients with dilated cardiomyopathy: an integrated evaluation by multivariate analysis. J Am Coll Cardiol 1987;10(1):186–92.

[31] Roberts WC, Siegel RJ, McManus BM. Idiopathic dilated cardiomyopathy: analysis of 152 necropsy patients. Am J Cardiol 1987;60(16): 1340–55.

[32] Wu TJ, Ong JJ, Hwang C, et al. Characteristics of wave fronts during ventricular fibrillation in human hearts with dilated cardiomyopathy: role of increased fibrosis in the generation of reentry. J Am Coll Cardiol 1998;32(1):187–96.

[33] Cassidy DM, Vassallo JA, Miller JM, et al. Endocardial catheter mapping in patients in sinus rhythm: relationship to underlying heart disease and ventricular arrhythmias. Circulation 1986; 73(4):645–52.

[34] Hsia HH, Marchlinski FE. Characterization of the electroanatomic substrate for monomorphic ventricular tachycardia in patients with nonischemic cardiomyopathy. Pacing Clin Electrophysiol 2002; 25(7):1114–27.

[35] Perlman RL. Abnormal epicardial and endocardial electrograms in patients with idiopathic dilated cardiomyopathy: relationship to arrhythmias. Circulation 1990;82:I-708.

[36] Hsia HH, Callans DJ, Marchlinski FE. Characterization of endocardial electrophysiological substrate in patients with nonischemic cardiomyopathy and monomorphic ventricular tachycardia. Circulation 2003;108(6):704–10.

[37] Marchlinski FE, Callans DJ, Gottlieb CD, et al. Linear ablation lesions for control of unmappable ventricular tachycardia in patients with ischemic and nonischemic cardiomyopathy. Circulation 2000;101(11):1288–96.

[38] Socjima K, Stevenson WG, Sapp JL, et al. Endocardial and epicardial radiofrequency ablation of ventricular tachycardia associated with dilated cardiomyopathy: the importance of low-voltage scars. J Am Coll Cardiol 2004;43(10):1834–42.

[39] Cesario DA, Vaseghi M, Boyle NG, et al. Value of high-density endocardial and epicardial mapping for catheter ablation of hemodynamically unstable ventricular tachycardia. Heart Rhythm 2006;3(1): 1–10.

[40] Blanck Z, Dhala A, Deshpande S, et al. Bundle branch reentrant ventricular tachycardia: cumulative experience in 48 patients. J Cardiovasc Electrophysiol 1993;4(3):253–62.

[41] Blanck Z, Jazayeri M, Dhala A, et al. Bundle branch reentry: a mechanism of ventricular tachycardia in the absence of myocardial or valvular dysfunction. J Am Coll Cardiol 1993;22(6):1718–22.

[42] Caceres J, Jazayeri M, McKinnie J, et al. Sustained bundle branch reentry as a mechanism of clinical tachycardia. Circulation 1989;79(2):256–70.

[43] Mehdirad AA, Keim S, Rist K, et al. Long-term clinical outcome of right bundle branch radiofrequency catheter ablation for treatment of bundle branch reentrant ventricular tachycardia. Pacing Clin Electrophysiol 1995;18(12 Pt 1):2135–43.

[44] Narasimhan C, Jazayeri MR, Sra J, et al. Ventricular tachycardia in valvular heart disease: facilitation of sustained bundle-branch reentry by valve surgery. Circulation 1997;96(12): 4307–13.

[45] Chalvidan T, Cellarier G, Deharo JC, et al. His-Purkinje system reentry as a proarrhythmic effect of flecainide. Pacing Clin Electrophysiol 2000;23(4 Pt 1):530–3.

[46] Tchou P, Jazayeri M, Denker S, et al. Transcatheter electrical ablation of right bundle branch. A method of treating macroreentrant ventricular tachycardia attributed to bundle branch reentry. Circulation 1988;78(2):246–57.

[47] Roberts WC, McAllister HA, Ferrans VJ. Sarcoidosis of the heart. A clinicopathologic study of 35 necropsy patients and review of 78 previously described necropsy patients. Am J Med 1977;63(1): 86–108.

[48] Sekiguchi M, Hiroe M, Take M, et al. Clinical and histopathological profile of sarcoidosis of the heart and acute idiopathic myocarditis. Concepts through a study employing endomyocardial biopsy. II. Myocarditis. Jpn Circ J 1980;44(4): 264–73.

[49] Winters SL, Cohen M, Greenberg S, et al. Sustained ventricular tachycardia associated with sarcoidosis: assessment of the underlying cardiac anatomy and the prospective utility of programmed ventricular stimulation, drug therapy and an implantable antitachycardia device. J Am Coll Cardiol 1991;18(4):937–43.

[50] Redheuil AB, Paziaud O, Mousseaux E. Ventricular tachycardia and cardiac sarcoidosis: correspondence between MRI and electrophysiology. Eur Heart J 2006;27(12):1430.

[51] Dalal D, Jain R, Tandri H, et al. Long-term efficacy of catheter ablation of ventricular tachycardia in patients with arrhythmogenic right ventricular dysplasia/cardiomyopathy. J Am Coll Cardiol 2007;50(5):432–40.

[52] Kirchhof P, Fabritz L, Zwiener M, et al. Age- and training-dependent development of arrhythmogenic right ventricular cardiomyopathy in heterozygous plakoglobin-deficient mice. Circulation 2006; 114(17):1799–806.

[53] Marcus F, Towbin JA. The mystery of arrhythmogenic right ventricular dysplasia/cardiomyopathy: from observation to mechanistic explanation. Circulation 2006;114(17):1794–5.

[54] Sen-Chowdhry S, Syrris P, Ward D, et al. Clinical and genetic characterization of families with arrhythmogenic right ventricular dysplasia/cardiomyopathy provides novel insights into patterns of disease expression. Circulation 2007;115(13): 1710–20.

[55] Marcus FI, Fontaine GH, Guiraudon G, et al. Right ventricular dysplasia: a report of 24 adult cases. Circulation 1982;65(2):384–98.

[56] Fattori R, Tricoci P, Russo V, et al. Quantification of fatty tissue mass by magnetic resonance imaging in arrhythmogenic right ventricular dysplasia. J Cardiovasc Electrophysiol 2005;16(3): 256–61.

[57] Maguire JH, Hoff R, Sherlock I, et al. Cardiac morbidity and mortality due to Chagas' disease: prospective electrocardiographic study of a Brazilian community. Circulation 1987;75(6):1140–5.

[58] Oliveira JS. A natural human model of intrinsic heart nervous system denervation: Chagas' cardiopathy. Am Heart J 1985;110(5):1092–8.

[59] Scanavacca M, Sosa E. Electrophysiologic study in chronic Chagas' heart disease. Sao Paulo Med J 1995;113(2):841–50.

[60] Moss AJ, Zareba W, Hall WJ, et al. Prophylactic implantation of a defibrillator in patients with myocardial infarction and reduced ejection fraction. N Engl J Med 2002;346(12):877–83.

[61] Makikallio TH, Barthel P, Schneider R, et al. Prediction of sudden cardiac death after acute myocardial infarction: role of Holter monitoring in the modern treatment era. Eur Heart J 2005;26(8): 762–9.

[62] Bigger JT, Fleiss JL, Kleiger R, et al. The relationships among ventricular arrhythmias, left ventricular dysfunction, and mortality in the 2 years after myocardial infarction. Circulation 1984;69(2): 250–8.

[63] Andresen D, Bethge KP, Boissel JP, et al. Importance of quantitative analysis of ventricular arrhythmias for predicting the prognosis in low-risk postmyocardial infarction patients. European Infarction Study Group. Eur Heart J 1990;11(6): 529–36.

[64] Doval HC, Nul DR, Grancelli HO, et al. Nonsustained ventricular tachycardia in severe heart failure. Independent marker of increased mortality due to sudden death. GESICA-GEMA investigators. Circulation 1996;94(12):3198–203.

[65] Kuo CS, Munakata K, Reddy CP, et al. Characteristics and possible mechanism of ventricular arrhythmia dependent on the dispersion of action potential durations. Circulation 1983;67(6): 1356–67.

[66] Puljevic D, Smalcelj A, Durakovic Z, et al. QT dispersion, daily variations, QT interval adaptation and late potentials as risk markers for ventricular tachycardia. Eur Heart J 1997;18(8):1343–9.

[67] Pastore JM, Girouard SD, Laurita KR, et al. Mechanism linking T-wave alternans to the genesis of cardiac fibrillation. Circulation 1999;99(10): 1385–94.

[68] Al-Khatib SM, Sanders GD, Bigger JT, et al. Preventing tomorrow's sudden cardiac death today: part I. Current data on risk stratification for sudden cardiac death. Am Heart J 2007;153(6):941–50.

[69] Klingenheben T, Zabel M, D'Agostino RB, et al. Predictive value of T-wave alternans for arrhythmic events in patients with congestive heart failure. Lancet 2000;356(9230):651–2.

[70] Bloomfield DM, Steinman RC, Namerow PB, et al. Microvolt T-wave alternans distinguishes between patients likely and patients not likely to benefit from implanted cardiac defibrillator therapy: a solution to the Multicenter Automatic Defibrillator Implantation Trial (MADIT) II conundrum. Circulation 2004;110(14):1885–9.

[71] Kleiger RE, Miller JP, Bigger JT, et al. Decreased heart rate variability and its association with increased mortality after acute myocardial infarction. Am J Cardiol 1987;59(4):256–62.

[72] Lown B, Verrier RL. Neural activity and ventricular fibrillation. N Engl J Med 1976;294(21): 1165–70.

[73] La Rovere MT, Bigger JT, Marcus FI, et al. Baroreflex sensitivity and heart-rate variability in prediction of total cardiac mortality after myocardial infarction. ATRAMI (Autonomic Tone and Reflexes After Myocardial Infarction) Investigators. Lancet 1998;351(9101):478–84.

[74] Borggrefe M, Fetsch T, Martinez-Rubio A, et al. Prediction of arrhythmia risk based on signal-averaged ECG in postinfarction patients. Pacing Clin Electrophysiol 1997;20(10 Pt 2):2566–76.

[75] Mancini DM, Wong KL, Simson MB. Prognostic value of an abnormal signal-averaged electrocardiogram in patients with nonischemic congestive cardiomyopathy. Circulation 1993; 87(4):1083–92.

[76] Naccarella F, Lepera G, Rolli A. Arrhythmic risk stratification of post-myocardial infarction patients. Curr Opin Cardiol 2000;15(1):1–6.

[77] Hsia HH, Marchlinski FE. Electrophysiology studies in patients with dilated cardiomyopathies. Card Electrophysiol Rev 2002;6(4):472–81.

[78] White RD. MR and CT assessment for ischemic cardiac disease. J Magn Reson Imaging 2004; 19(6):659–75.

[79] Assomull RG, Pennell DJ, Prasad SK. Cardiovascular magnetic resonance in the evaluation of heart failure. Heart 2007;93(8):985–92.

[80] McCrohon JA, Moon JC, Prasad SK, et al. Differentiation of heart failure related to dilated cardiomyopathy and coronary artery disease using gadolinium-enhanced cardiovascular magnetic resonance. Circulation 2003;108(1):54–9.

[81] Assomull RG, Prasad SK, Lyne J, et al. Cardiovascular magnetic resonance, fibrosis, and prognosis in dilated cardiomyopathy. J Am Coll Cardiol 2006; 48(10):1977–85.

[82] Timolol-induced reduction in mortality and reinfarction in patients surviving acute myocardial infarction. N Engl J Med 1981;304(14):801–7.

[83] A randomized trial of propranolol in patients with acute myocardial infarction. I. Mortality results. JAMA 1982;247(12):1707–14.

[84] Cucherat M, Boissel JP, Leizorovicz A. Persistent reduction of mortality for five years after one year of acebutolol treatment initiated during acute myocardial infarction. The APSI investigators. Acebutolol et Prevention Secondaire de l'Infarctus. Am J Cardiol 1997;79(5):587–9.

[85] Dargie HJ. Effect of carvedilol on outcome after myocardial infarction in patients with left-ventricular dysfunction: the CAPRICORN randomised trial. Lancet 2001;357(9266):1385–90.

[86] Hjalmarson A, Elmfeldt D, Herlitz J, et al. Effect on mortality of metoprolol in acute myocardial infarction. A double-blind randomised trial. Lancet 1981;2(8251):823–7.

[87] MERIT-HF Study Group. Effect of metoprolol CR/XL in chronic heart failure: Metoprolol CR/XL Randomised Intervention Trial in Congestive Heart Failure (MERIT-HF). Lancet 1999; 353(9169):2001–7.

[88] Hjalmarson A, Goldstein S, Fagerberg B, et al. Effects of controlled-release metoprolol on total mortality, hospitalizations, and well-being in patients with heart failure: the Metoprolol CR/XL Randomized Intervention Trial in congestive heart failure (MERIT-HF). MERIT-HF Study Group. JAMA 2000;283(10):1295–302.

[89] The CONSENSUS Trial Study group. Effects of enalapril on mortality in severe congestive heart failure. Results of the Cooperative North Scandinavian Enalapril Survival Study (CONSENSUS). N Engl J Med 1987;316(23):1429–35.

[90] The SOLVD Investigators. Effect of enalapril on survival in patients with reduced left ventricular ejection fractions and congestive heart failure. N Engl J Med 1991;325(5):293–302.

[91] Rutherford JD, Pfeffer MA, Moye LA, et al. Effects of captopril on ischemic events after myocardial infarction. Results of the Survival and Ventricular Enlargement trial. SAVE Investigators. Circulation 1994;90(4):1731–8.

[92] Cleland JG, Erhardt L, Murray G, et al. Effect of ramipril on morbidity and mode of death among survivors of acute myocardial infarction with clinical evidence of heart failure. A report from the AIRE Study Investigators. Eur Heart J 1997; 18(1):41–51.

[93] Echt D, Liebson P, Mitchell L, et al. Mortality and morbidity in patients receiving encainide, flecainide, or placebo. The Cardiac Arrhythmia Suppression Trial N Engl J Med 1991;324(12):781–8.

[94] Waldo AL, Camm AJ, deRuyter H, et al. Effect of d-sotalol on mortality in patients with left ventricular dysfunction after recent and remote myocardial infarction. The SWORD investigators. Survival With Oral d-sotalol. Lancet 1996; 348(9019):7–12.

[95] Kober L, Bloch Thomsen PE, Moller M, et al. Effect of dofetilide in patients with recent myocardial infarction and left-ventricular dysfunction: a randomised trial. Lancet 2000;356(9247):2052–8.

[96] Singh SN, Fletcher RD, Fisher SG, et al. Amiodarone in patients with congestive heart failure and asymptomatic ventricular arrhythmia. Survival Trial of Antiarrhythmic Therapy in Congestive Heart Failure. N Engl J Med 1995;333(2):77–82.

[97] Burkart F, Pfisterer M, Kiowski W, et al. Effect of antiarrhythmic therapy on mortality in survivors of myocardial infarction with asymptomatic complex ventricular arrhythmias: Basel Antiarrhythmic Study of Infarct Survival (BASIS). J Am Coll Cardiol 1990;16(7):1711–8.

[98] Ceremuzynski L, Kleczar E, Krzeminska-Pakula M, et al. Effect of amiodarone on mortality after myocardial infarction: a double-blind, placebo-controlled, pilot study. J Am Coll Cardiol 1992; 20(5):1056–62.

[99] Navarro-Lopez F, Cosin J, Marrugat J, et al. Comparison of the effects of amiodarone versus metoprolol on the frequency of ventricular arrhythmias and on mortality after acute myocardial infarction. SSSD Investigators. Spanish Study on Sudden Death. Am J Cardiol 1993; 72(17):1243–8.

[100] Cairns JA, Connolly SJ, Roberts R, et al. Randomised trial of outcome after myocardial infarction in patients with frequent or repetitive ventricular premature depolarisations: CAMIAT. Canadian Amiodarone Myocardial Infarction Arrhythmia Trial Investigators. Lancet 1997;349(9053): 675–82.

[101] Julian DG, Camm AJ, Frangin G, et al. Randomised trial of effect of amiodarone on mortality in patients with left-ventricular dysfunction after recent myocardial infarction: EMIAT. European Myocardial Infarct Amiodarone Trial Investigators. Lancet 1997;349(9053):667–74.

[102] The Antiarrhythmics Versus Implantable Defibrillators (AVID) investigators. A comparison of antiarrhythmic-drug therapy with implantable defibrillators in patients resuscitated from near-fatal ventricular arrhythmias. The Antiarrhythmics Versus Implantable Defibrillators (AVID) investigators. N Engl J Med 1997;337(22):1576–83.

[103] Connolly SJ, Gent M, Roberts RS, et al. Canadian Implantable Defibrillator Study (CIDS): a randomized trial of the implantable cardioverter defibrillator against amiodarone. Circulation 2000;101(11): 1297–302.

[104] Kuck KH, Cappato R, Siebels J, et al. Randomized comparison of antiarrhythmic drug therapy with implantable defibrillators in patients resuscitated from cardiac arrest: the Cardiac Arrest Study Hamburg (CASH). Circulation 2000;102(7):748–54.

[105] Lee DS, Green LD, Liu PP, et al. Effectiveness of implantable defibrillators for preventing arrhythmic events and death: a meta-analysis. J Am Coll Cardiol 2003;41(9):1573–82.

[106] Moss AJ, Hall WJ, Cannom DS, et al. Improved survival with an implanted defibrillator in patients with coronary disease at high risk for ventricular arrhythmia. Multicenter Automatic Defibrillator Implantation Trial nvestigators. N Engl J Med 1996;335(26):1933–40.

[107] Buxton AE, Lee KL, Fisher JD, et al. A randomized study of the prevention of sudden death in patients with coronary artery disease. Multicenter UnSustained Tachycardia Trial investigators. N Engl J Med 1999;341(25):1882–90.

[108] Bardy GH, Lee KL, Mark DB, et al. Amiodarone or an implantable cardioverter-defibrillator for congestive heart failure. N Engl J Med 2005; 352(3):225–37.

[109] Kadish A, Dyer A, Daubert JP, et al. Prophylactic defibrillator implantation in patients with nonischemic dilated cardiomyopathy. N Engl J Med 2004;350(21):2151–8.

[110] Goldenberg I, Moss AJ, Hall WJ, et al. Causes and consequences of heart failure after prophylactic implantation of a defibrillator in the multicenter automatic defibrillator implantation trial II. Circulation 2006;113(24):2810–7.

[111] Sharma AD, Rizo-Patron C, Hallstrom AP, et al. Percent right ventricular pacing predicts outcomes in the DAVID trial. Heart Rhythm 2005;2(8): 830–4.

[112] Wilkoff BL, Cook JR, Epstein AE, et al. Dual-chamber pacing or ventricular backup pacing in patients with an implantable defibrillator: the Dual Chamber And VVI Implantable Defibrillator (DAVID) trial. JAMA 2002;288(24):3115–23.

[113] Josephson ME, Harken AH, Horowitz LN. Endocardial excision: a new surgical technique for the treatment of recurrent ventricular tachycardia. Circulation 1979;60(7):1430–9.

[114] Krafchek J, Lawrie GM, Roberts R, et al. Surgical ablation of ventricular tachycardia: improved results with a map-directed regional approach. Circulation 1986;73(6):1239–47.

[115] Miller JM, Kienzle MG, Harken AH, et al. Subendocardial resection for ventricular tachycardia: predictors of surgical success. Circulation 1984; 70(4):624–31.

[116] Mason JW. A comparison of electrophysiologic testing with Holter monitoring to predict antiarrhythmic-drug efficacy for ventricular tachyarrhythmias. Electrophysiologic Study versus Electrocardiographic Monitoring Investigators. N Engl J Med 1993;329(7):445–51.

[117] Morady F, Harvey M, Kalbfleisch SJ, et al. Radiofrequency catheter ablation of ventricular tachycardia in patients with coronary artery disease. Circulation 1993;87(2):363–72.

[118] Ellison KE, Stevenson WG, Sweeney MO, et al. Catheter ablation for hemodynamically unstable monomorphic ventricular tachycardia. J Cardiovasc Electrophysiol 2000;11(1):41–4.

[119] Kuchar DL, Ruskin JN, Garan H. Electrocardiographic localization of the site of origin of ventricular tachycardia in patients with prior myocardial infarction. J Am Coll Cardiol 1989; 13(4):893–903.

[120] Miller JM, Marchlinski FE, Buxton AE, et al. Relationship between the 12-lead electrocardiogram during ventricular tachycardia and endocar-

dial site of origin in patients with coronary artery disease. Circulation 1988;77(4):759–66.

[121] Fann JI, Loeb JM, LoCicero J 3rd, et al. Endocardial activation mapping and endocardial pacemapping using a balloon apparatus. Am J Cardiol 1985;55(8):1076–83.

[122] Josephson ME, Waxman HL, Cain ME, et al. Ventricular activation during ventricular endocardial pacing. II. Role of pace-mapping to localize origin of ventricular tachycardia. Am J Cardiol 1982; 50(1):11–22.

[123] Azegami K, Wilber DJ, Arruda M, et al. Spatial resolution of pacemapping and activation mapping in patients with idiopathic right ventricular outflow tract tachycardia. J Cardiovasc Electrophysiol 2005;16(8):823–9.

[124] Soejima K, Suzuki M, Maisel WH, et al. Catheter ablation in patients with multiple and unstable ventricular tachycardias after myocardial infarction: short ablation lines guided by reentry circuit isthmuses and sinus rhythm mapping. Circulation 2001;104(6):664–9.

[125] Rothman SA, Hsia HH, Cossu SF, et al. Radiofrequency catheter ablation of postinfarction ventricular tachycardia: long-term success and the significance of inducible nonclinical arrhythmias. Circulation 1997;96(10):3499–508.

[126] Stevenson WG, Friedman PL, Kocovic D, et al. Radiofrequency catheter ablation of ventricular tachycardia after myocardial infarction. Circulation 1998;98(4):308–14.

[127] Strickberger SA, Man KC, Daoud EG, et al. A prospective evaluation of catheter ablation of ventricular tachycardia as adjuvant therapy in patients with coronary artery disease and an implantable cardioverter-defibrillator. Circulation 1997;96(5): 1525–31.

[128] Hsia HH, Lin D, Sauer WH, et al. Anatomic characterization of endocardial substrate for hemodynamically stable reentrant ventricular tachycardia: identification of endocardial conducting channels. Heart Rhythm 2006;3(5):503–12.

[129] Verma A, Marrouche NF, Schweikert RA, et al. Relationship between successful ablation sites and the scar border zone defined by substrate mapping for ventricular tachycardia post-myocardial infarction. J Cardiovasc Electrophysiol 2005;16(5): 465–71.

[130] Arenal A, del Castillo S, Gonzalez-Torrecilla E, et al. Tachycardia-related channel in the scar tissue in patients with sustained monomorphic ventricular tachycardias: influence of the voltage scar definition. Circulation 2004;110(17):2568–74.

[131] Arenal A, Glez-Torrecilla E, Ortiz M, et al. Ablation of electrograms with an isolated, delayed component as treatment of unmappable

monomorphic ventricular tachycardias in patients with structural heart disease. J Am Coll Cardiol 2003;41(1):81–92.

[132] Hsia HH. Substrate mapping: the historical perspective and current status. J Cardiovasc Electrophysiol 2003;14(5):530–2.

[133] Sosa E, Scanavacca M, d'Avila A, et al. Nonsurgical transthoracic epicardial catheter ablation to treat recurrent ventricular tachycardia occurring late after myocardial infarction. J Am Coll Cardiol 2000;35(6):1442–9.

[134] Sosa E, Scanavacca M, d'Avila A, et al. A new technique to perform epicardial mapping in the electrophysiology laboratory. J Cardiovasc Electrophysiol 1996;7(6):531–6.

[135] Sosa E, Scanavacca M. Epicardial mapping and ablation techniques to control ventricular tachycardia. J Cardiovasc Electrophysiol 2005;16(4):449–52.

ELSEVIER
SAUNDERS

Cardiol Clin 26 (2008) 405–418

CARDIOLOGY
CLINICS

Role of Drug Therapy for Sustained Ventricular Tachyarrhythmias

L. Brent Mitchell, MD, FRCPC

Libin Cardiovascular Institute of Alberta and Department of Cardiac Sciences, Calgary Health Region and University of Calgary Foothills Hospital, 1403 - 29th Street NW Calgary, Alberta T2N 2T9, Canada

Sudden death is responsible for 20% of all deaths in the industrialized world [1]. Most sudden deaths are caused by sustained ventricular tachycardia (VT) or ventricular fibrillation (VF) [2]. Thus, prevention of VT/VF and sudden death has attracted significant attention. Despite the use of implantable cardioverter defibrillators (ICDs), antiarrhythmic drugs still play a dominant role. These therapies, in their broadest sense, include both acute/direct antiarrhythmic drugs (including standard antiarrhythmic agents) and delayed/indirect antiarrhythmic drugs (including agents that modify cardiovascular remodeling processes, thereby reducing the likelihood of future VT/VF and sudden death in patients who have coronary artery disease [CAD], prior myocardial infarction [MI], or congestive heart failure [CHF]). This article examines the current role of pharmacologic therapy for the prevention of VT/VF and sudden death.

Drug therapy for ventricular tachycardia/ventricular fibrillation and sudden death

Randomized, controlled clinical trials (RCTs) show that ICDs are more effective than drugs in preventing sudden death and all-cause mortality. Thus, most patients who have a demonstrated or presumed propensity for VT/VF receive an ICD. Meta-analysis of RCTs of patients who had prior VT/VF (the secondary prevention ICD trials) showed that the use of ICDs reduced all-cause mortality from 27.4% in the control group (most of whom were treated empirically

with amiodarone) to 21.4% (hazard ratio [HR], 0.72; 95% confidence interval [CI], 0.60–0.87) over 2.3 years [3]. Meta-analysis of RCTs of patients who did not have VT/VF (the primary prevention ICD trials) showed that the use of ICDs reduced all-cause mortality from 26.4% in the control group (most of whom received usual care) to 18.5% (HR, 0.75; 95% CI, 0.63–0.91) over the course of 1 year [4]. Nevertheless, most patients use drugs to prevent VT/VF and sudden death, either instead of an ICD when the use of an ICD is inadvisable or, more often, in addition to an ICD to decrease further the risk of sudden death, to decrease VT/VF, to render VT more receptive to ICD treatments, and to treat supraventricular tachyarrhythmias that confuse the ICD.

Class I antiarrhythmic drugs

Class I drugs (sodium-channel blockers) are subdivided further into class Ia drugs that have intermediate onset/offset kinetics and delayed rectifier potassium-channel (I_{Kr}) blockade (quinidine, procainamide, disopyramide), class Ib drugs that have fast kinetics (lidocaine, tocainide, phenytoin, mexiletine), and class Ic drugs that have slow kinetics (propafenone, encainide, flecainide, moricizine).

Effects on ventricular arrhythmias

Class I drugs are the prototypical antiarrhythmic agents. Each has been well demonstrated to suppress spontaneous ventricular premature beats (VPBs) and spontaneous and inducible VT/VF in humans by a large data set that is not reviewed further in this article.

E-mail address: brent.mitchell@calgaryhealthregion.ca

0733-8651/08/$ - see front matter © 2008 Elsevier Inc. All rights reserved.
doi:10.1016/j.ccl.2008.03.004

Effects on sudden death/all-cause mortality

In the Cardiac Arrhythmia Suppression Trials, CAST I [5] and CAST II [6], patients who had prior MI and frequent VPBs participated in a placebo-controlled RCT of encainide, flecainide, or moricizine. Encainide or flecainide increased death/cardiac arrest from 3.5% patients in the placebo group to 8.3% in patients in the treatment group (relative risk [RR], 2.38; 95% CI, 1.59–3.57) over 10 months [5]; moricizine increased death/cardiac arrest from 0.5% in patients in the placebo group to 2.6% in patients in the treatment group (RR, 5.6; 95% CI, 1.7–19.1) within 2 weeks [6]. A meta-analysis of 61 RCTs involving 23,486 patients also showed that class I drugs increased all-cause mortality (odds ratio [OR], 1.13; 95% CI, 1.01–1.27) [7].

Safety

The mortality associated with class I drugs is related in part to ventricular proarrhythmia seen in 1% to 5% of patients [8] and in part to worsening CHF. CAST I [5] showed a statistical trend, and CAST II [6] showed a statistical increase in new/worsened CHF with therapy using class I drugs. Finally, each class I agent also has adverse effects specific to that drug; these effects are especially common with class Ia and Ib drugs.

Inferences

Class I drugs treat and prevent VT/VF but increase sudden death and all-cause mortality. Accordingly, this therapy is reserved for its imperative need when other treatments have failed and the advantages of suppressing VT/VF outweigh the increased risk. In practice, the use of class I agents is limited to short-term therapy of an episode of VT/VF, short-term therapy of an electrical storm of VT/VF, or long-term therapy in patients who have not responded to or are not candidates for any other therapies (including an ICD).

Class II antiarrhythmic drugs

Class II antiarrhythmic drugs have, as their dominant effect, blockade of one or more of the beta subtypes of adrenergic receptors (beta-blockers).

Effects on ventricular arrhythmias

The arrhythmogenic effects of sympathetic stimulation and the antiarrhythmic effects of beta-blockers were reviewed recently [9]. Beta-blockers prevent VT/VF with efficacies comparable to those of class I drugs when used empirically [10] or when their effectiveness is predicted by suppression of either frequent/complex VPBs [11] or inducible VT/VF [12,13]. Ethical concerns, however, precluded the use of placebo controls. Recently, patients who have an ICD have been used to test antiarrhythmic drugs using appropriate ICD therapy as a surrogate for sustained VT/VF. One crossover trial in 11 patients who had sustained VT/VF found the rate of appropriate ICD shocks to be lower with a beta-blocker than without a beta-blocker (0.12 ± 0.24 versus 1.09 ± 1.41 shocks per month; $P = .03$) [13]. The combined results of three RCTs of intravenous beta-blockers in acute MI showed a decrease in sustained VT/VF from 3.1% in the control group to 0.8% in the treatment group (RR, 0.42; 95% CI, 0.32–0.55) [14–16].

Beta-blockers are particularly effective for right ventricular outflow tract VT [17], for rapid polymorphic VT/VF precipitated by sympathetic discharge states [18], and as an adjunct to prevent adrenergic stimulation from reversing the benefits of other antiarrhythmic drugs [19].

Effects on sudden death/all-cause mortality

A meta-analysis of 16 RCTs involving 15,819 patients who had prior MI reported that sudden death was reduced from 5.2% in the control group to 3.6% in the treatment group (OR, 0.68; 95% CI, 0.60–0.80), and a meta-analysis of 24 RCTs involving 20,312 patients who had prior MI reported that all-cause mortality was reduced from 10.0% in the control group to 7.9% in the treatment group (OR, 0.77; 95% CI, 0.70–0.85) after 20 months [20]. Meta-analysis of 17 RCTs involving 3039 patients who had CHF reported that all-cause mortality was reduced from 12.1% in the control group to 7.8% in the treatment group (OR, 0.69; 95% CI, 0.54–0.88) after 9 months, that beta-blockers reduced all-cause mortality in patients who had ischemic cardiomyopathy (OR, 0.69; 95% CI, 0.49–0.98) or nonischemic cardiomyopathy (OR, 0.69; 95% CI, 0.47–0.99), and that the reduction in all-cause mortality with carvedilol (OR, 0.44; 95% CI, 0.28–0.69) was greater than with other beta-blockers (OR, 0.79; 95% CI, 0.56–1.10) [21].

That carvedilol may reduce all-cause mortality more than other beta-blockers was supported by a meta-analysis of 32 RCTs involving 26,580 patients who had prior MI and 28 RCTs involving 15,905 patients who had CHF [22]. Beta-blockers with additional beta$_2$ and/or alpha$_1$ blockade (carvedilol, timolol, propranolol) reduced all-cause mortality (post-MI: OR, 0.69; 95% CI, 0.61–0.79; CHF: OR, 0.58; 95% CI, 0.48–0.71) more than selective beta$_1$-blockers (metoprolol, bisoprolol, atenolol); (post-MI: OR, 0.79; 95% CI, 0.66–0.95); (HF: OR, 0.67; 95% CI, 0.58–0.77) which in turn reduced all-cause mortality, more than beta-blockers with intrinsic sympathomimetic activity (oxprenolol, bucindolol, xamoterol, practolol, alprenolol, acebutolol, pindolol) (post-MI: OR, 0.85; 95% CI, 0.74–0.99; CHF: OR, 0.90; 95% CI, 0.77–1.06). In the Carvedilol or Metoprolol European Trial, 3029 patients who had CHF were assigned randomly to carvedilol or metoprolol [23]. Carvedilol reduced the rate of sudden death from 17% in patients treated with metoprolol to 14% (OR, 0.81; 95% CI, 0.68–0.97) and reduced all-cause mortality from 40% in patients treated with metoprolol to 34% (OR, 0.83; 95% CI, 0.74–0.93) over 58 months [24].

Carvedilol is a beta$_1$-, beta$_2$-, and alpha$_1$-blocker; does not cause beta$_1$-receptor up-regulation; blocks the rapidly activating component of the I_{Kr}; and, at higher dosages, blocks L-type calcium channels ($I_{Ca,L}$), the transient outward potassium current (I_{to}), and the slowly activating component of the delayed rectifier (I_{Ks}) [22,25]. Thus, there is biologic rationale for the contention that carvedilol has greater antiarrhythmic activity than other beta-blockers.

The Carvedilol Prospective Randomized Cumulative Survival (COPERNICUS) and Carvedilol Post-infarct Survival Control in Left Ventricular Dysfunction (CAPRICORN) trials tested carvedilol against VT/VF [26,27]. In COPERNICUS, in 2289 patients who had class III-IV CHF and a left ventricular ejection fraction (LVEF) below 0.25, VT decreased from 2.3% in the placebo group to 1.0% in the carvedilol group (RR, 0.62; 95% CI, 0.15–0.55), and VF decreased from 2.0% in the placebo group to 1.0% in the carvedilol group (RR, 0.68; 95% CI, 0.48–0.94; $P < .05$) over 10.4 months. In the CAPRICORN trial in 1959 patients who had a prior MI and an LVEF of 0.40 or lower, VT/VF decreased from

3.9% in the placebo group to 0.9% in the carvedilol group (HR, 0.24; 95% CI, 0.11–0.49) over 1.3 years.

Safety

The antiarrhythmic benefits of beta-blockers are achieved at very low risk. The only expressions of proarrhythmia with beta-blockers are sinus bradycardia and atrioventricular (AV) block. The latter has been estimated to occur in less than 1% of patients [20].

Inferences

Beta-blockers treat and prevent VT/VF and reduce sudden death and all-cause mortality. Given the safety of beta-blockers, nearly all patients who have a propensity to VT/VF should receive this therapy. Exceptions include patients unable to tolerate beta-blockers and patients who do not have structural heart disease who have an idiopathic VT that responds to other therapy. In this regard, it is possible that carvedilol has advantages over other beta-blockers.

Class III antiarrhythmic drugs

Class III drugs (potassium-channel blockers) include d,l-sotalol, d-sotalol, dofetilide, azimilide, and amiodarone.

Effects on ventricular arrhythmias

Reviews documenting the antiarrhythmic efficacy of d,l-sotalol [28], d-sotalol [29], dofetilide [30], azimilide [31], and amiodarone [32] have been published.

D,l-sotalol was superior to placebo [33] and beta-blockers [34] for suppression of VPBs, was comparable to class Ia drugs for suppression of VPBs [35], and was effective for prevention of VT/VF [36]. The Electrophysiologic Study Versus Electrocardiographic Monitoring trial tested seven randomized antiarrhythmic drugs in 486 patients who had VT/VF [37]. D,l-sotalol, compared with imipramine, mexiletine, pirmenol, procainamide, propafenone, and quinidine, suppressed inducible VT/VF more than class I drugs (25% versus 16%; $P < .001$), had fewer adverse events than class I drugs (23% versus 47%; $P < .001$), and had a lower 1-year probability of VT/VF recurrence on predicted effective therapy (0.20 ± 0.04) than class I drugs (range, 0.38–0.60) [36].

Empiric d,l-sotalol was evaluated in a placebo-controlled RCT involving 302 patients who had prior VT/VF and an ICD [38]. D,l-sotalol reduced the probability of death or appropriate ICD therapy from 0.42 in the placebo group (most of whom were not treated with beta-blockers) to 0.27 in the d,l-sotalol group (RR, 0.56; 95% CI, 0.36–0.85) after 1 year. D,l-sotalol was compared with standard beta-blockers in three RCTs. In one trial, d,l-sotalol increased the 1-year probability of both VT and fast VT/VF (0.43 and 0.46, respectively) compared with metoprolol (0.17 and 0.12, respectively; $P = .02$) [39]; in the other two trials there was no difference in VT/VF between the patients treated with d,l-sotalol and those treated with standard beta-blockers [40,41].

D-sotalol, a relatively pure I_{Kr} blocker, was superior to placebo for suppression of VPBs [42], was superior to class Ia drugs for suppression of inducible sustained VT/VF [43], and was effective for long-term prevention of VT/VF [44].

Dofetilide, another relatively pure I_{Kr} blocker, was superior to placebo for suppression of inducible VT/VF [45] and for time to first appropriate ICD therapy in patients who had prior sustained VT/VF [46]. Dofetilide was equivalent to d,l-sotalol for suppression of inducible VT [47,48].

Azimilide blocks both components of delayed rectifier (I_{Kr} and I_{Ks}), is a weak blocker of the $I_{Ca,L}$, and has weak alpha- and beta-blocking effects [31,49]. These actions should increase antiarrhythmic potency by lessening reverse use dependence and should reduce the probability of torsade de pointes. In an animal model of torsade de pointes, azimilide was less proarrhythmic than dofetilide or d,l-sotalol [50]. Azimilide is effective for suppression of both VPBs and inducible VT/VF [49]. Two RCTs tested azimilide for prevention of VT/VF in patients who had spontaneous or inducible VT/VF and who had an ICD. In a dose-ranging study in 172 patients, Singer and colleagues [51] reported the annual incidence of appropriate ICD therapy was reduced from 36% in patients who received placebo to 10%, 12%, and 9%, respectively, in patients who received 35 mg, 75 mg, and 125 mg azimilide daily (all comparisons, $P < .0001$). In the Shock Inhibition Evaluation with Azimilide trial, 633 patients who had prior VT/VF and an ICD were assigned randomly to placebo, to azimilide, 75 mg/d, or to azimilide, 125 mg/d [52]. The annual number of appropriate ICD therapies decreased from 25.1 in the placebo group to 17.1 in patients who received azimilide, 75 mg/d ($P = .02$) and to 9.6 in patients who received azimilide, 125 mg/d (all comparisons, $P < .05$).

Amiodarone expresses class I, II, III, and IV antiarrhythmic effects, is the most potent antiarrhythmic drug, has a low risk of torsade de pointes ($<1\%$), has very slow pharmacokinetics, and has frequent and unusual long-term adverse effects [32]. In the Cardiac Arrest in Seattle: Conventional Versus Amiodarone Drug Evaluation trial, 228 patients resuscitated from VT/VF were assigned randomly to empiric amiodarone or to a class I drug predicted to be effective by its suppression of frequent and complex VPBs or inducible VT/VF [53]. Amiodarone reduced the 2-year probability of cardiac death or sustained VT/VF from approximately 0.48 in patients taking the class I drug to approximately 0.23 ($P < .001$). In the Optimal Pharmacologic Therapy in Cardioverter Defibrillator Patients trial, standard beta-blockers, d,l-sotalol, and amiodarone plus a standard beta-blocker were compared for the prevention of appropriate ICD therapy in patients who had spontaneous or inducible VT/VF [41]. The use of amiodarone plus a standard beta-blocker reduced the annual VT/VF rate from 0.45 in patients receiving standard beta-blockers and from 0.39 in patients receiving d,l-sotalol to 0.19 ($P < .001$).

Effects on sudden death/all-cause mortality

Julian and colleagues [54] randomly assigned 1456 patients who had prior MI to d,l-sotalol or placebo. They found no difference in sudden death between the patients receiving placebo and patients receiving d,l-sotalol (2.4% versus 2.9%; RR, 1.07; 95% CI, 0.82–1.39). They similarly found no difference in all-cause mortality between patients receiving placebo and patients receiving d,l-sotalol (8.9% versus 7.3%; RR, 0.81; 95% CI, 0.55–1.19) after 1 year.

The Survival with Oral D-sotalol (SWORD) investigators randomly assigned 3121 patients who had prior MI and who had an LVEF of 0.40 or lower to d-sotalol or placebo [55]. After 5 months, d-sotalol increased the rate of death from presumed arrhythmic causes from 2.0% in patients receiving placebo to 3.6% (RR, 1.77; 95% CI, 1.15–2.74) and increased all-cause mortality from 3.1% in patients receiving placebo to 5.1% (RR, 01.65; 95% CI, 1.15–2.36).

The Danish Investigations of Arrhythmia and Mortality on Dofetilide (DIAMOND) group randomly assigned 1518 patients who had CHF to dofetilide or placebo with mandated drug initiation in hospital (DIAMOND-CHF) [56].

After 18 months, there were no differences between the patients receiving dofetilide or placebo in death ascribed to arrhythmia (20% and 20%, respectively) or in all-cause mortality (41% and 42%, respectively). These investigators also randomly assigned 1510 patients who had prior MI with an LVEF of 0.35 or lower to dofetilide or placebo with mandated drug initiation in hospital (DIAMOND-MI) [57]. After 15 months, there were no differences between patients treated with dofetilide or placebo in death assumed to be caused by arrhythmia (17% and 18%, respectively) or in all-cause mortality (31% and 32%, respectively).

In the Azimilide Post-infarct Survival Evaluation (ALIVE) trial, 3381 patients who had prior MI and an LVEF of 0.15 to 0.35 were assigned randomly to azimilide or placebo [58]. After 1 year, there were no significant differences between the patients treated with azimilide and patients who received placebo in death attributed to arrhythmia (6.7% and 5.4%, respectively) or in all-cause mortality (12% and 12%, respectively).

Meta-analysis of eight RCTs involving 5101 patients who had prior MI and of five RCTs involving 1452 patients who had CHF reported that amiodarone reduced the rate of sudden death from 5.7% in patients in the control group to 4.0% (HR, 0.71; 95% CI, 0.59–0.85) and reduced all-cause mortality from 12.3% in patients in the control group to 10.9% (HR, 0.87; 95% CI, 0.78–0.99) without affecting New York Heart Association (NYHA) status [59]. In the Sudden Cardiac Death in Heart Failure Trial, 2521 patients who had CHF with an LVEF of 0.35 (stratified by NYHA class) were assigned randomly to placebo, amiodarone, or an ICD [60]. There was no difference in all-cause mortality between patients treated with amiodarone and patients receiving placebo (HR, 1.06; 97.5% CI, 0.86–1.30), although there was an increase in all-cause mortality in patients who had NYHA class III disease taking amiodarone (HR, 1.44; 95% CI, 1.05–1.97).

Safety

The use of a class III drug carries a risk of torsade de pointes: 1% to 5% with d,l-sotalol, 1% to 2% with d-sotalol, 1% to 3% with dofetilide, less than 1% with azimilide, and less than 1% with amiodarone [29,61].

In RCTs, adverse events (particularly dizziness, depression, and nausea [54]) caused d,l-sotalol to be discontinued more often than placebo (27% versus 12%; RR, 1.54; 95% CI, 1.15–2.04) [38]. In the SWORD trial, there were no differences in serious adverse effects, including recognized torsade de pointes, between d-sotalol and placebo [55]. In the DIAMOND-CHF and DIAMOND-MI trials the dofetilide dosage initially was fixed [56,57]. Later, the dofetilide dosage was individualized based on creatinine clearance and QT interval. In the patients treated with dofetilide, torsade de pointes occurred in 4.8% of patients who had CHF before the dosing change and in 2.9% of these patients after the dosing change and in 3.0% of patients who had prior MI before the dosing change and in 0.6% of these patients after the dosing change. Seventy-six percent of the torsade de points episodes in the DIAMOND-CHF trial and 71% of the torsade de pointes episodes in DIAMOND-MI occurred during the 3-day drug-initiation hospitalization. Other adverse events occurred equally in patients treated with dofetilide and patients receiving placebo. One comparison of dofetilide and d,l-sotalol reported that withdrawals for adverse events were equal (19% and 26%, respectively) and that the risks of ventricular proarrhythmia were equal during acute titration (4.5% and 3.1%, respectively) and during follow-up (4.9% and 7.7%, respectively) [51]. Three RCTs found adverse events to occur equally with azimilide and placebo [51,52,58] except for severe neutropenia (0.9% versus 0.2%, respectively; $P = .01$) [58]. In the ALIVE trial, torsade de pointes occurred in 0.3% of patients treated with azimilide and in 0.1% of patients receiving placebo [58]. The Amiodarone Trials Meta-Analysis investigators found amiodarone to have more adverse events than placebo: hypothyroidism (7.0% and 1.1%, respectively), hyperthyroidism (1.4% and 0.5%, respectively), peripheral neuropathy (0.5% and 0.2%, respectively), lung infiltrates (1.6% and 0.5%, respectively), bradycardia (2.4% and 0.8%, respectively), and liver abnormalities (1.0% and 0.4%, respectively) [59].

Inferences

Class III drugs treat and prevent VT/VF. D,l-sotalol, d-sotalol, and dofetilide have a significant risk of torsade de pointes. Azimilide has a smaller risk of torsade de pointes. In patients who have structural heart disease, d,l-sotalol, dofetilide, and azimilide have no effect on sudden death or all-cause mortality; d-sotalol increases sudden death and all-cause mortality. Amiodarone has a lesser risk of torsade de pointes, has a greater adverse effect profile, and decreases sudden death and all-cause mortality in patients who have structural heart disease. In general, class III drugs are more effective and better tolerated than class I drugs. Accordingly, class III drugs are used only when other treatments have failed and the advantages of suppressing VT/VF outweigh the risk of torsade de pointes and, with some drugs, the increase in all-cause mortality. In practice, class III agents are used for short-term therapy of an episode of VT/VF, for short-term therapy of an electrical storm of VT/VF, or for long-term therapy in patients who have not responded to or are not candidates for other therapies (excluding class I drugs). In these settings, amiodarone is preferred. Nevertheless, if time permits, amiodarone may be preceded by a trial of other class III agents (traditionally d,l-sotalol, but dofetilide or azimilide also are appropriate).

Class IV antiarrhythmic drugs

Class IV drugs (the nondihydropyridine calcium-channel blockers verapamil and diltiazem) have as their dominant electrophysiologic effect inhibition the $I_{Ca,L}$.

Effects on ventricular arrhythmias

Class IV drugs have minimal effects on re-entrant ventricular arrhythmias [62] but are effective for ventricular arrhythmias based on triggered activity. Thus, class IV drugs are useful for Belhassen VT (left septal or verapamil-sensitive VT) [63], for right ventricular outflow tract VT [64], for catecholaminergic polymorphic VT [65], and for some VTs related to acute myocardial ischemia, particularly those associated with coronary artery spasm [66].

Effects on sudden death/all-cause mortality

A meta-analysis of RCTs of class IV drugs included 26 trials of 21,644 patients who had prior MI and reported that class IV drugs had no effect on all-cause mortality (OR, 1.03; 95% CI, 0.94–1.13) [7].

Safety

Class IV drugs have an excellent safety profile in patients without structural heart disease. Withdrawal for adverse effects is uncommon and is comparable to placebo (4%–8%). Serious adverse effects, such AV block or rash, occur in less than 2% of patients [67]. Nevertheless, in patients who have depressed left ventricular function, class IV drugs may hasten the progression of CHF [68].

Inferences

The use of class IV drugs for VT/VF is limited to niche indications. They are first-line therapies for Belhassen VT and for VT/VF related to coronary artery spasm. They also are used for right ventricular outflow tract VT or catecholaminergic polymorphic VT for patients who cannot take or who have not responded to beta-blocker therapy. Most such patients are not at risk for progression of CHF.

Statins

Hydroxymethylglutaryl coenzyme-A reductase inhibitors (statins) have many effects other than cholesterol lowering. These pleiotropic effects include those on signaling pathways for inflammation, endothelial nitric oxide synthesis, plasminogen, endothelin-1, platelet activation, angiotensin II receptor regulation, sympathetic nerve activity, oxidative stress, left ventricular mass regression, left ventricular reverse remodeling, and antiarrhythmic effects [69]. The last includes changes in properties of the sarcolemmal membrane with resultant alterations in ion-channel function.

Effects on ventricular arrhythmias

A meta-analysis of three nonrandomized studies in patients who had CAD with prior VT/VF and an ICD reported that lipid-lowering drugs reduced appropriate ICD therapy from 58% in 457 patients not taking taking lipid-lowering drugs to 38% in 264 patients taking lipid-lowering drugs (89% of which were statins) (RR, 0.60; 95% CI, 0.49–0.73) after 16 months [70–72]. The Cholesterol Lowering and Arrhythmia Recurrences after Internal Defibrillator Implantation trial randomly assigned 106 patients who had CAD and prior VT/VF and an ICD to atorvastatin or placebo [73]. By intention-to-treat, atorvastatin had a nonsignificant effect, reducing appropriate ICD therapy from 36% in the placebo group to 21% in the atorvastatin group (HR, 0.58; $P = .07$). By treatment received, atorvastatin significantly reduced appropriate ICD therapy from 40% in the placebo group to 16% in the atorvastatin group (HR, 0.39; $P = .02$).

A nonrandomized substudy of the Multicenter Automatic Defibrillator Implantation II Trial reported that patients who had CAD, depressed LVEF, and a primary-prevention ICD who took a statin had a lower 2-year probability of first appropriate ICD therapy than patients who did not take a statin (0.26 versus 0.35; HR, 0.72; 95% CI, 0.52–0.99) after 17 months [74]. The Defibrillators in Non-Ischemic Cardiomyopathy Treatment Evaluation reported that patients who had nonischemic cardiomyopathy who had a primary-prevention ICD and who took a statin had a nonsignificant reduction in first appropriate ICD shock compared with patients who did not take a statin (12.5% versus 15.6%; HR, 0.80; 95% CI, 0.35–1.84) after 29 months [75].

Effects on sudden death/all-cause mortality

Meta-analysis of 10 RCTs involving 22,275 patients who had CAD reported that statins reduced the rate of sudden death from 3.8% in the control group to 3.0% in patients treated with statin (HR, 0.81; 95% CI, 0.71–0.93) after 4.4 years [76]. Another meta-analysis of 14 RCTs involving 90,056 patients who had CAD reported that statins reduced all-cause mortality from 9.7% in the control group to 8.5% in patients treated with statin (HR, 0.87; 95% CI, 0.84–0.91) after 5 years [77]. Patients who had CHF were excluded from most statin RCTs because of safety concerns [78]. Recently, the Controlled Rosuvastatin Multinational heart failure trial randomly assigned 5011 patients aged 60 years and older who had CHF and a depressed LVEF to rosuvastatin or placebo and reported equivalent risks of all-cause mortality (29.0% and 30.4%, respectively; HR, 0.95; 95% CI, 0.86–1.05) after 33 months [79].

Safety

The Cholesterol Treatment Trialists' collaborators meta-analysis of statin trials reported a nonsignificant 5-year excess risk of rhabdomyolysis with statins of 0.01% ($P = .4$) [77].

Inferences

Statins prevent VT/VF, sudden cardiac death, and all-cause mortality in patients who have CAD (and perhaps in patients who have idiopathic dilated cardiomyopathy or advanced CHF) with a very low risk of therapy. Statins should be used in patients who have CAD and may be considered in patients who have idiopathic congestive cardiomyopathy or advanced CHF if VT/VF management is problematic.

Renin-angiotensin-aldosterone system inhibitors

Activation of the renin-angiotensin-aldosterone system (RAAS) results in dysregulation of many cardiovascular processes causing vascular and myocardial inflammation, vascular smooth muscle proliferation, myocyte hypertrophy, endothelial dysfunction, myocardial fibrosis, thrombotic cascade activation, platelet activation, oxidative pathway activation, interstitial matrix remodeling, coronary plaque destabilization, hypokalemia, and hypomagnesemia [80,81]. The RAAS may be suppressed by inhibiting angiotensin-converting enzyme (ACE) hydrolysis of inactive angiotensin I to active angiotensin II with an ACE inhibitor, by blocking the AT_1 receptor through which many deleterious effects of angiotensin II are mediated with an angiotensin receptor blocker (ARB), or by blocking the effects of aldosterone with an aldosterone blocker.

Effects on ventricular arrhythmias

Other than by correction of hypokalemia or hypomagnesemia, suppression of the RAAS would not be expected to be acutely antiarrhythmic. Some studies report that ACE inhibitors decrease VPB frequency and complexity; others do not. In general, the positive studies were longer-term trials in patients who had CHF associated with increases in serum potassium or decreases in autonomic sympathetic tone [82–84]. In one trial in patients who had inducible VT, captopril treatment had no significant effect on the inducibility of VT [85]. Few studies have examined the antiarrhythmic effects of ARBs in humans. One study found that losartan had no significant effects on the frequency or complexity of spontaneous VPBs in hypertensive men who had preserved left ventricular systolic function [86]. Three RCTs of spironolactone in patients who had CHF reported a decrease in the frequency and complexity of VPBs [87–89]. Again, these were longer-term trials, and efficacy was correlated inversely with plasma or erythrocyte magnesium levels.

Effects on sudden death/all-cause mortality

Meta-analyses of ACE inhibitor RCTs consider patients in three groups: patients who have CHF of any cause (mostly CAD), patients who have had a recent MI (often with CHF or depressed LVEF), and patients who have demonstrated or possible CAD without CHF or left ventricular dysfunction. In patients who have CHF, a meta-analysis of 32 RCTs involving 7105 patients reported that treatment with an ACE inhibitor reduced the rate of sudden death nonsignificantly from 5.6% in the control group to 4.7% (OR, 0.91; 95% CI, 0.73–1.12) while reducing all-cause mortality from 21.9% in the control group to 15.8% (OR, 0.77; 95% CI, 0.67–0.88) [90]. A meta-analysis of 15 RCTs involving 15,104 patients who had a recent MI reported that treatment with ACE inhibitors reduced the rate of sudden death from 6.6% in the control group to 5.3% (OR, 0.80; 95% CI, 0.70–0.92) and reduced all-cause mortality from 16.8% in the control group to 14.4% (OR, 0.83; 95% CI, 0.71–0.97) [91]. In patients who had documented or possible CAD and preserved left ventricular function, meta-analysis of six RCTs involving 33,500 patients reported that treatment with ACE inhibitors reduced all-cause mortality from 8.3% in the control group to 7.2% (OR, 0.87; 95% CI, 0.81–0.94) over 4.4 years [92]. A substudy in the Heart Outcome Prevention Evaluation trial in patients who had or were at high risk of developing CAD without overt CHF reported that treatment with ramipril reduced the rate of sudden death/documented arrhythmic death/resuscitated cardiac arrest from 4.2% in the control group to 3.3% (OR, 0.79; 95% CI, 0.64–0.98) over 4.5 years [93].

A meta-analysis of nine RCTs involving 4623 patients who had CHF who were not receiving ACE inhibitors reported that treatment with ARBs decreased all-cause mortality from 17.7% in the control group to 10.6% (OR, 0.83; 95% CI, 0.60–1.00) after 18 months [94]. In eight RCTs evaluating ARBs against ACE inhibitors in 5201 patients who had CHF, all-cause mortality in patients receiving ARBs was no different from that in patients receiving an ACE inhibitor (11.5% versus 12.8%; OR, 1.06; 95% CI, 0.90–1.13) over 14 months. In seven RCTs evaluating ARBs added to ACE inhibitors in 8260 patients who had CHF, all-cause mortality in patients receiving an ARB plus an ACE inhibitor was no different from that in patients receiving only an ACE inhibitor (21.2% versus 22.6%; OR, 0.97; 95% CI, 0.87–1.08) over 27 months. Two RCTs found no difference in all-cause mortality between patients who had high-risk acute MI and depressed LVEF treated with an ARB and an ACE inhibitor and those treated with an ACE inhibitor alone [95,96].

The Randomized Aldactone Evaluation Study (RALES) randomly assigned 1663 patients who had class III-IV CHF treated with ACE inhibitors to receive spironolactone or placebo [97]. Treatment with spironolactone reduced the rate of sudden death from 13.1% in the control group to 10.0% (RR, 0.71; 95% CI, 0.54–0.95) and reduced all-cause mortality from 46% in the control group to 35% (RR, 0.70; 95% CI, 0.60–0.82) after 24 months. Similarly, the Eplerenone Post-acute Myocardial Infarction Heart Failure Efficacy and Survival Study (EPHESUS) randomly assigned 6642 patients who had recent MI and an LVEF of 0.40 or less and (except for patients who had diabetes) symptomatic CHF on optimal CHF therapy to eplerenone or placebo [98]. Treatment with eplerenone reduced the rate of sudden death from 6.1% in the control group to 4.9% (RR, 0.79; 95% CI, 0.64–0.97) and reduced all-cause mortality from 16.7% in the control group to 14.4% (RR, 0.85; 95% CI, 0.75–0.96) after 16 months.

Safety

A meta-analysis of 36 RCTs involving 18,234 patients reported that therapy was withdrawn more often from patients receiving an ACE inhibitor than from control patients because of cough (2.0% versus 1.1%; RR, 3.19; 95% CI, 2.22–4.57), hypotension (1.6% versus 0.8%; RR, 1.95; 95% CI, 1.39–2.74), renal dysfunction (0.9% versus 0.5%; RR, 1.84; 95% CI, 1.20–2.81), and hyperkalemia (0.4% versus 0.03%; RR, 7.11; 95% CI, 2.11–3.94) [99].

In the Candesartan in Heart Failure: Assessment of Reduction in Mortality and Morbidity–Alternative study, the ARB was withdrawn more frequently than placebo for hypotension (3.7% versus 0.9%; RR, 1.63; 95% CI, 1.22–2.19), renal dysfunction (6.1% versus 2.7%; RR, 1.42; 95% CI, 1.15–1.76), and hyperkalemia (1.9% versus 0.3%; RR, 1.74; 95% CI, 1.14–2.66) [100]. Meta-analysis of RCTs involving 17,337 patients who had CHF or high-risk patients who had prior MI reported that the combination of ARB and ACE inhibitor was withdrawn more often than the ACE inhibitor alone because of adverse effects (11.5% versus 9.0%; RR, 1.28; 95% CI, 1.17–1.40) [101]. The most common reasons for withdrawal were hypotension (11.1% versus 7.5%; RR, 1.48; 95% CI, 1.34–1.62), renal dysfunction

(4.1% versus 2.4%; RR, 1.76; 95% CI, 1.49–2.09), and hyperkalemia (1.6% versus 0.8%; RR, 2.46; 95% CI, 0.68–8.87) [101].

In the RALES trial, therapy was discontinued for adverse events more often in patients receiving spironolactone (8%) than in patients receiving placebo (5%) [97]. The most common adverse effect was gynecomastia or breast pain in men (10% versus 1%). In EPHESUS, this adverse effect was rare. The major adverse effect was serious hyperkalemia in 5.5% of patients taking eplerenone, compared with 3.9% of patients taking placebo ($P = .002$) [98]. This finding was offset by serious hypokalemia in 8.4% of patients taking eplerenone compared with 13.1% of patients taking placebo ($P < .001$).

Inferences

ACE inhibitors, ARBs, and aldosterone blockers have antiarrhythmic effects by increasing potassium and magnesium concentrations and by decreasing sympathetic tone in patients who have CHF. In long-term use they also prevent the development of VT/VF and sudden death in patients who have significant structural heart disease. Thus, an ACE inhibitor or, when an ACE inhibitor is poorly tolerated, an ARB should be used in patients who have structural heart disease. Aldosterone blockers should be used in patients who have class III-IV CHF and for other patients with demonstrated or presumed VT/VF propensity when potassium and/or magnesium conservation is desired.

Digoxin

The dominant actions of digoxin are an inhibition of sodium-potassium ATPase, thereby augmenting transmembrane sodium–calcium exchange resulting in increased intracellular calcium, a reduction of sympathetic tone, and an augmentation of parasympathetic tone [102]. Digoxin also may inhibit the RAAS. In therapeutic concentrations, digoxin has no direct ventricular electrophysiologic effects [103]. In toxic concentrations, myocyte calcium loading causes delayed afterdepolarizations and VT [104]. Unfortunately, the window between therapeutic and toxic dosages of digoxin is small.

Effects on ventricular arrhythmias

Two placebo-controlled RCTs in patients who had CHF found digoxin to have no effect on the frequency or complexity of VPBs [105,106]. A crossover trial suggested that 0.375 mg/d of digoxin reduced the frequency but not the complexity of VPB, perhaps through its sympatholytic effects [107].

Effects on sudden death/all-cause mortality

The Digitalis Investigator Group (DIG) trial randomly assigned 6800 patients who had class II-IV CHF in sinus rhythm with an LVEF of 0.45 or less to digoxin or placebo [108]. After a follow-up of 37 months, there was no significant difference between the digoxin and the placebo groups in all-cause mortality (34.8% and 35.1%, respectively; RR, 0.99; 95% CI, 0.91–1.07) or in cardiac mortality (29.9% and 29.5%, respectively; RR, 1.01; 95% CI, 0.93–1.10). Treatment with digoxin, however, trended to reduce CHF deaths, from 13.2% in the placebo group to 11.6% (RR, 0.88; 95% CI, 0.77–1.01; $P = .06$). Although the incidence of sudden death was not reported, if cardiac mortality was unaffected and CHF mortality was reduced, sudden death must have increased. In this regard, the incidence of VT/VF was higher in the digoxin group than in the placebo group (1.1% versus 0.8%; RR, 1.40; 95% CI, 0.84–2.3; $P = .20$).

A post hoc analysis of DIG trial data examined the effects of digoxin on CHF death and all-cause mortality in male participants who survived 1 month as a function of trough serum digoxin concentration at 1 month [109]. Compared with 1171 men in the placebo group who survived 1 month, patients who had digoxin concentrations of 0.5 to 0.8 ng/mL (n = 572) had an absolute 6.3% lower rate of all-cause mortality (95% CI, 2.1%–10.5%), a 3.7% lower rate of cardiovascular mortality (95% CI, 0.4% 7.7%), and a 4.7% lower rate of CHF mortality (95% CI, 2.1%–7.3%). Comparable reductions in cardiac and CHF mortality suggest a similar reduction in sudden death. In men who had digoxin concentrations of 0.9 to 1.1 ng/mL (n = 322), the rates of all-cause mortality, cardiovascular mortality, and heart failure mortality were similar to those in the placebo group. Those who had digoxin concentrations of 1.2 ng/mL or higher (n = 277) had an absolute higher rate of all-cause mortality (11.8%; 95% CI, 5.7%–18.0%) and a higher rate of cardiovascular mortality (11.5%; 95% CI, 5.4%–17.5%) but an equivalent rate of CHF mortality (1.9%; 95% CI, −2.6%–6.3%). The increase in cardiac mortality but not in CHF mortality suggests an increase in the rate of sudden death.

Safety

In addition to the possible increase in sudden death, other safety issues with digoxin are frequent drug–drug interactions [102] and digoxin intoxication [102,108]. In the DIG trial suspected digoxin intoxication was more common in patients receiving active treatment (11.9%) than in patients receiving placebo (7.9%) and included supraventricular tachyarrhythmias in 2.5% of patients receiving digoxin and 1.2% of patients receiving placebo (RR, 2.10; 95% CI, 1.45–3.07) and second- or third-degree AV block in 1.2% of patients receiving digoxin and 0.4% of patients receiving placebo (RR, 2.87; 95% CI, 1.56–5.28) [108].

Inferences

Digoxin has no role in the treatment of VT/VF and may increase the rate of sudden death. Patients who have difficult-to-control VT/VF who are receiving digoxin therapy may be helped by ensuring that the serum digoxin concentration is less than 0.9 ng/mL.

Summary

Class I, III, and IV drugs have immediate/direct antiarrhythmic effects. Class I drugs treat and prevent VT/VF at the expense of an increase in sudden death and all-cause mortality. Class III drugs treat and prevent VT/VF with a variable effect on sudden death and all-cause mortality. Class IV drugs treat and prevent certain forms of VT with no effect on sudden death or all-cause mortality. Accordingly, class I and III agents are used for short-term therapy of an episode or storm of VT/VF or for long-term therapy in patients who have not responded to or are not candidates for all other therapies (including the ICD). In these settings, class III agents that do not have a detrimental effect on sudden death (d,l-sotalol, amiodarone) are preferred. Class IV drugs are used in niche applications: as first-line treatment for Belhassen VT or coronary artery spasm VT/VF and after beta-blockers for right ventricular outflow tract VT or catecholaminergic polymorphic VT.

Beta-blockers have both immediate/direct and delayed/indirect antiarrhythmic effects. They treat and prevent VT/VF and decrease sudden death and all-cause mortality in patients who have structural heart disease. Most patients who have a propensity to VT/VF should receive a beta-blocker. Carvedilol may have advantages over other beta-blockers in this setting.

Statins, ACE inhibitors, ARBs, and aldosterone blockers have delayed/indirect antiarrhythmic effects that are expressed dominantly by a decrease in the rate of sudden death and all-cause mortality in patients who have structural heart disease. Statins should be used in patients who have CAD and may be considered in patients who have idiopathic congestive cardiomyopathy or advanced CHF if VT/VF management is problematic. An ACE inhibitor or, when an ACE-inhibitor is poorly tolerated, an ARB should be used in patients who have structural heart disease. Aldosterone blockers should be used in patients who have class III-IV CHF and for other patients who have a propensity to VT/VF when potassium and/or magnesium conservation is desired.

Digoxin has no role in the treatment or prevention of VT/VF and may increase the rate of sudden death. Patients who have difficult-to-control VT/VF who are receiving digoxin therapy may be helped by ensuring that the serum digoxin concentration is less than 0.9 ng/mL.

References

[1] Zheng ZJ, Croft JB, Giles WH, et al. Sudden cardiac death in the United States, 1989 to 1998. Circulation 2001;104(18):2158–63.

[2] Bayes de Luna AB, Coumel P, Leclercq JF. Curriculum in cardiology: ambulatory sudden cardiac death; mechanisms of production of fatal arrhythmia on the basis of data from 157 cases. Am Heart J 1989;117(1):151–9.

[3] Connolly SJ, Hallstrom AP, Cappato R, et al. Meta-analysis of the implantable cardioverter defibrillator secondary prevention trials. Eur Heart J 2000;21(24):2071–8.

[4] Nanthakumar K, Epstein AE, Kay GN, et al. Prophylactic implantable cardioverter-defibrillator therapy in patients with left ventricular systolic dysfunction: a pooled analysis of 10 primary prevention trials. J Am Coll Cardiol 2004;44(11):2166–72.

[5] Echt DS, Liebson PR, Mitchell LB, et al. Mortality and morbidity in patients receiving encainide, flecainide, or placebo. N Engl J Med 1991; 324(12):781–8.

[6] Cardiac Arrhythmia Suppression Trial II Investigators. Effect of the antiarrhythmic agent moricizine on survival after myocardial infarction. N Engl J Med 1992;327(4):227–33.

[7] McAlister FA, Teo KK. Antiarrhythmic therapies for the prevention of sudden cardiac death. Drugs 1997;54(2):235–52.

[8] Friedman PL, Stevenson WG. Proarrhythmia. Am J Cardiol 1998;82(7 Suppl 1):50N–8N.

[9] Dorian P. Antiarrhythmic action of ß-blockers: potential mechanisms. J Cardiovasc Pharmacol Ther 2005;10(Suppl 1):S15–22.

[10] Steinbeck G, Andresen D, Bach P, et al. A comparison of electrophysiologically guided antiarrhythmic drug therapy with beta-blocker therapy in patients with symptomatic, sustained ventricular tachyarrhythmias. N Engl J Med 1992;327(14): 987–92.

[11] Lown B, Graboys TB. Management of patients with malignant ventricular arrhythmias. Am J Cardiol 1977;39(6):910–8.

[12] Duff HJ, Mitchell LB, Wyse DG. Antiarrhythmic efficacy of propranolol: comparison of low and high serum concentrations. J Am Coll Cardiol 1986;8(4):959–65.

[13] Leclercq JF, Leenhardt A, Coumel P, et al. Efficacy of beta-blocking agents in reducing the number of shocks in patients implanted with first-generation automatic defibrillators. Eur Heart J 1992;13(9): 1180–4.

[14] Yusuf S, Sleight P, Rossi PRF, et al. Reduction in infarct size, arrhythmias, chest pain, and morbidity by early intravenous beta-blockade in suspected acute myocardial infarction. Circulation 1983; 67(6 Pt 2):I32–41.

[15] Rydén L, Arniego R, Arnmar K, et al. A double-blind trial of metoprolol in acute myocardial infarction: effects on ventricular tachycardia. N Engl J Med 1983;308(11):614–8.

[16] Norris RM, Brown MA, Clarke ED, et al. Prevention of ventricular fibrillation during acute myocardial infarction by intravenous propranolol. Lancet 1984;324(8408):883–6.

[17] Lerman BB, Belardinelli L, West GA, et al. Adenosine-sensitive ventricular tachycardia: evidence suggesting cyclic AMP-mediated triggered activity. Circulation 1986;74(2):270–80.

[18] Sung RJ, Shen EN, Morady F, et al. Electrophysiologic mechanisms of exercise-induced sustained ventricular tachycardia. Am J Cardiol 1983;51(3): 525–30.

[19] Reiter MJ, Reiffel JA. Importance of beta blockade in the therapy of serious ventricular arrhythmias. Am J Cardiol 1998;82(4 Suppl 1):9I–19I.

[20] Yusuf S, Peto R, Lewis J, et al. Beta blockade during and after myocardial infarction: an overview of the randomized trials. Prog Cardiovasc Dis 1985;27(5):335–71.

[21] Heidenreich PA, Lee TT, Massie BM. Effect of beta-blockade on mortality in patients with heart failure: a meta-analysis of randomized clinical trials. J Am Coll Cardiol 1997;30(1): 27–34.

[22] Packer M. Do ß-blockers prolong survival in heart failure only by inhibiting the ß1-receptor? A perspective on the results of the COMET trial. J Card Fail 2003;9(6):429–43.

[23] Poole-Wilson PA, Swedberg K, Cleland JG, et al. Comparison of carvedilol and metoprolol outcomes in patients with chronic heart failure in the Carvedilol or Metoprolol European Trial (COMET): randomized controlled trial. Lancet 2003;362(9377):7–13.

[24] Torp-Pedersen C, Poole-Wilson PA, Swedberg K, et al. Effects of metoprolol and carvedilol on cause-specific mortality and morbidity in patients with chronic heart failure (COMET). Am Heart J 2005;149(2):370–6.

[25] El-Sharif N, Turitto G. Electrophysiologic effects of carvedilol: is carvedilol an antiarrhythmic agent? Pacing Clin Electrophysiol 2005;28(9):985–90.

[26] Packer M, Fowler MB, Roecker EB, et al. Effect of carvedilol on the morbidity of patients with severe chronic heart failure. Results of the Carvedilol Prospective Randomized Cumulative Survival (COPERNICUS) study. Circulation 2002;106(17): 2194–9.

[27] McMurray J, Køber L, Robertson M, et al. Antiarrhythmic effect of carvedilol after acute myocardial infarction: results of the Carvedilol Post-Infarct Survival Control in Left Ventricular Dysfunction (CAPRICORN) trial. J Am Coll Cardiol 2005; 45(4):525–30.

[28] Anderson JL, Prystowski EN. Sotalol: an important new antiarrhythmic. Am Heart J 1999;137(3): 388–409.

[29] Advani SV, Singh BN. Pharmacodynamic, pharmacokinetic and antiarrhythmic properties of d-sotalol, the dextro-isomer of sotalol. Drugs 1995;49(5):664–79.

[30] Mounsey JP, DiMarco JP. Dofetilide. Circulation 2000;102(21):2665–70.

[31] Clemett D, Markham A. Azimilide. Drugs 2000; 59(2):271–7.

[32] Vassallo P, Trohman RG. Prescribing amiodarone: an evidence-based review of clinical indications. JAMA 2007;298(11):1312–22.

[33] Anatasiou-Nana MI, Gilbert EM, Miller RH, et al. Usefulness of d,l sotalol for suppression of chronic ventricular arrhythmias. Am J Cardiol 1991;67(6): 511–6.

[34] Deedwania PC. Suppressant effects of conventional beta blockers and sotalol on complex and repetitive ventricular premature beats. Am J Cardiol 1990; 65(2):43A–50A.

[35] Lidell C, Rehnquist N, Sjögren A, et al. Comparative efficacy of oral sotalol and procainamide in patients with chronic ventricular arrhythmias: a multicenter study. Am Heart J 1985;109(5 Pt 1): 970–5.

[36] Mason JW, ESVEM Investigators. A comparison of seven antiarrhythmic drugs in patients with

ventricular tachyarrhythmias. N Engl J Med 1993; 329(7):452–8.

[37] Mason JW, ESVEM Investigators. A comparison of electrophysiologic testing with Holter monitoring to predict antiarrhythmic-drug efficacy for ventricular tachyarrhythmias. N Engl J Med 1993;329(7):445–51.

[38] Pacifico A, Hohnloser SH, Williams JH, et al. Prevention of implantable-defibrillator shocks by treatment with sotalol. N Engl J Med 1999; 340(24):1855–62.

[39] Seidl K, Hauer B, Schwick NG, et al. Comparison of metoprolol and sotalol in preventing ventricular tachyarrhythmias after the implantation of a cardioverter/defibrillator. Am J Cardiol 1998; 82(6):744–8.

[40] Kettering K, Mewis C, Dörnberger V, et al. Efficacy of metoprolol and sotalol in the prevention of recurrences of sustained ventricular tachyarrhythmias in patients with an implantable cardioverter defibrillator. Pacing Clin Electrophysiol 2002;25(11):1571–6.

[41] Connolly SJ, Dorian P, Roberts RS, et al. Comparison of ß-blockers, amiodarone plus ß-blockers, or sotalol for prevention of shocks from implantable cardioverter defibrillators: the OPTIC study: a randomized trial. JAMA 2006; 295(2):165–71.

[42] Barbey JT, Echt DS, Thompson KA, et al. Effect of d-sotalol on ventricular arrhythmias in man. Circulation 1985;72(4 Pt 2):170–5.

[43] Schwartz J, Crocker K, Wynn J, et al. The antiarrhythmic effects of d-sotalol. Am Heart J 1987; 114(3):539–44.

[44] Brachmann J, Schols W, Beyer T, et al. Acute and chronic antiarrhythmic efficacy of d-sotalol in patients with sustained ventricular tachyarrhythmias. Eur Heart J 1993;14(Suppl H):85–7.

[45] Echt DS, Lee JT, Murray KT, et al. A randomized, double-blind, placebo-controlled, dose-ranging study of dofetilide in patients with inducible sustained ventricular tachyarrhythmias. J Cardiovasc Electrophysiol 1995;6(9):687–99.

[46] O'Toole M, O'Neill G, Kluger J, et al. Efficacy and safety of oral dofetilide in patients with an implanted defibrillator: multicenter study [abstract]. Circulation 1999;100(18):I–794.

[47] Boriani G, Biffi M, De Simone N, et al. Repolarization changes in a double-blind crossover study of dofetilide versus sotalol in the treatment of ventricular tachycardia. Pacing Clin Electrophysiol 2000; 23(11 Pt 2):1935–8.

[48] Boriani G, Lubinski A, Capucci A, et al. A multicentre double-blind randomized crossover comparative study on the efficacy and safety of dofetilide vs sotalol in patients with inducible sustained ventricular tachycardia and ischaemic heart disease. Eur Heart J 2001; 22(23):2180–91.

[49] Karam R, Marcello S, Brooks RR, et al. Azimilide dihydrochloride, a novel antiarrhythmic agent. Am J Cardiol 1998;81(6 Suppl 1):40D–6D.

[50] Brooks RR, Drexler AP, Maynard AE, et al. Proarrhythmia of azimilide and other class III antiarrhythmic agents in the adrenergically stimulated rabbit. Proc Soc Exp Biol Med 2000;223(2):183–9.

[51] Singer I, Al-Khalidi H, Niazi I, et al. Azimilide decreases recurrent ventricular tachyarrhythmias in patients with implantable cardioverter defibrillators. J Am Coll Cardiol 2004;43(1):39–43.

[52] Dorian P, Borggrefe M, Al-Khalidi HR, et al. Placebo-controlled, randomized clinical trial of azimilide for prevention of ventricular tachyarrhythmias in patients with an implantable cardioverter defibrillator. Circulation 2004;110(24): 3646–54.

[53] CASCADE Investigators. Randomized antiarrhythmic drug therapy in survivors of cardiac arrest (the CASCADE study). Am J Cardiol 1993;72(3): 280–7.

[54] Julian DG, Prescott RJ, Jackson FS, et al. Controlled trial of sotalol for one year after myocardial infarction. Lancet 1982;319(8282):1142–7.

[55] Waldo AL, Camm AJ, deRuyter H, et al. Effect of d-sotalol on mortality in patients with left ventricular dysfunction after recent and remote myocardial infarction. Lancet 1996;348(9019):7–12.

[56] Torp-Pedersen C, Møller M, Bloch-Thomsen PE, et al. Dofetilide in patients with congestive heart failure and left ventricular dysfunction. N Engl J Med 1999;341(12):857–65.

[57] Køber L, Bloch Thomsen PE, Møller M, et al. Effect of dofetilide in patients with recent myocardial infarction and left-ventricular dysfunction: a randomised trial. Lancet 2000;356(9247):2052–8.

[58] Camm AJ, Pratt CM, Schwartz PJ, et al. Mortality in patients after a recent myocardial infarction: a randomized placebo-controlled trial of azimilide using heart rate variability for risk stratification. Circulation 2004;109(8):990 6.

[59] Amiodarone Trials Meta-Analysis (ATMA) Investigators. Effect of prophylactic amiodarone on mortality after acute myocardial infarction and in congestive heart failure: meta-analysis of individual data from 6500 patients in randomized trials. Lancet 1997;350(9089):1417–24.

[60] Bardy GH, Lee KL, Mark DB, et al. Amiodarone or an implantable cardioverter defibrillator for congestive heart failure. N Engl J Med 2005;352(3): 225–37.

[61] Brendorp B, Pedersen OD, Torp-Pedersen C, et al. A benefit-risk assessment of class III antiarrhythmic agents. Drug Saf 2002;25(12):847–65.

[62] Mason JW, Swerdlow CD, Mitchell LB. Efficacy of verapamil in chronic, recurrent ventricular tachycardia. Am J Cardiol 1983;51(10):1614–7.

[63] Belhassen B, Shapira I, Pelleg A, et al. Idiopathic recurrent sustained ventricular tachycardia

responsive to verapamil: an ECG-electrophysiologic entity. Am Heart J 1984;108(4 Pt 1):1034–7.

[64] Iwai S, Cantillon DJ, Kim RJ, et al. Right and left ventricular outflow tract tachycardias: evidence for a common electrophysiologic mechanism. J Cardiovasc Electrophysiol 2006;17(10):1052–8.

[65] Sumitomo N, Harada K, Nagashima M, et al. Catecholaminergic polymorphic ventricular tachycardia: electrocardiographic characteristics and optimal therapeutic strategies to prevent sudden death. Heart 2003;89(1):66–70.

[66] Grenadier E, Alpan G, Maor N, et al. Polymorphous ventricular tachycardia in acute myocardial infarction. Am J Cardiol 1984;53(9):1280–3.

[67] Russell RP. Side effects of calcium channel blockers. Hypertension 1988;11(3 Pt 2):II42–4.

[68] Goldstein RE, Boccuzzi SJ, Cruess D, et al. Diltiazem increases late-onset congestive heart failure in postinfarction patients with early reduction in ejection fraction. Circulation 1991;83(1):52–60.

[69] Shanes JG, Minadeo KN, Moret A, et al. Statin therapy in heart failure: prognostic effects and potential mechanism. Am Heart J 2007;154(4): 617–23.

[70] De Sutter J, Tavernier R, De Buyzere M, et al. Lipid-lowering drugs and recurrences of life-threatening ventricular arrhythmias in high-risk patients. J Am Coll Cardiol 2000;36(3):766–72.

[71] Mitchell LB, Powell JL, Gillis AM, et al. Are lipid-lowering drugs also antiarrhythmic drugs? An analysis of the antiarrhythmics versus implantable defibrillators (AVID) trial. J Am Coll Cardiol 2003;42(1):81–7.

[72] Chiu JH, Abdelhadi RH, Chung MK, et al. Effect of statin therapy on risk of ventricular arrhythmia among patients with coronary artery disease and an implantable cardioverter-defibrillator. Am J Cardiol 2005;95(4):490–1.

[73] Cholesterol lowering and arrhythmia recurrences after internal defibrillator implantation: the CLARIDI Trial. Available at: www.clinicalstudy results.org/documents/company-study_578_0.pdf. Accessed January 8, 2008.

[74] Vyas AK, Guo H, Moss AJ, et al. Reductions in ventricular tachyarrhythmias with statins in the multicenter automatic defibrillator implantation trial (MADIT)-II. J Am Coll Cardiol 2006;47(4): 769–73.

[75] Goldberger JJ, Subacius H, Schaechter A, et al. Effects of statin therapy on arrhythmic events and survival in patients with nonischemic dilated cardiomyopathy. J Am Coll Cardiol 2006;48(6): 1228–33.

[76] Levantesi G, Scarano M, Marfisi R, et al. Meta-analysis of effects of statin treatment on risk of sudden death. Am J Cardiol 2007;100(11):1644–50.

[77] Cholesterol Treatment Trialists' (CTT) Collaborators. Efficacy and safety of cholesterol-lowering treatment: prospective meta-analysis of data from 90 056 participants in 14 randomised trials of statins. Lancet 2005;366(9493):1267–78.

[78] Rauchhaus M, Clark AL, Doehner W, et al. The relationship between cholesterol and survival in patients with chronic heart failure. J Am Coll Cardiol 2003;42(11):1933–40.

[79] Kjekshus J, Apetrei E, Barrios V, et al. Rosuvastatin in older patients with systolic heart failure. N Engl J Med 2007;357(22):2248–61.

[80] Altas SA. The renin-angiotensin aldosterone system: pathophysiological role and pharmacologic inhibition. J Manag Care Pharm 2007;13(8 Suppl S-b):S9–20.

[81] Maisel WH, Stevenson WG. Sudden death and the electrophysiological effects of angiotensin-converting enzyme inhibitors. J Card Fail 2000;6(2):80–2.

[82] Cleland JG, Dargie HJ, Hodsman GP, et al. Captopril in heart failure: a double-blind controlled trial. Br Heart J 1984;52(5):530–5.

[83] Webster MWI, Fitzpatrick A, Nicholls G, et al. Effect of enalapril on ventricular arrhythmias in congestive heart failure. Am J Cardiol 1985;56(8): 566–9.

[84] Hattori Y, Atsushi S, Hiroaki F, et al. Effects of captopril on ventricular arrhythmias in patients with congestive heart failure. Clin Ther 1997; 19(3):481–6.

[85] Bashir Y, Sneddon JF, O'Nunain S, et al. Comparative electrophysiological effects of captopril or hydralazine combined with nitrate in patients with left ventricular dysfunction and inducible ventricular tachycardia. Br Heart J 1992;67(5):355–60.

[86] Zakynthinos E, Pierrutsakos Ch, Daniil Z, et al. Losartan controlled blood pressure and reduced left ventricular hypertrophy but did not alter arrhythmias in hypertensive men with preserved systolic function. Angiology 2005;56(4):439–49.

[87] Barr CS, Lang CC, Hanson J, et al. Effects of adding spironolactone to angiotensin-converting enzyme inhibitor in chronic congestive heart failure secondary to coronary artery disease. Am J Cardiol 1995;76(17):1259–65.

[88] Ramires FJ, Mansur A, Coelho O, et al. Effect of spironolactone on ventricular arrhythmias in congestive heart failure secondary to idiopathic or to ischemic cardiomyopathy. Am J Cardiol 2000; 85(10):1207–11.

[89] Gao X, Peng L, Adhikari CM, et al. Spironolactone reduced arrhythmias and maintained magnesium homeostasis in patients with congestive heart failure. J Card Fail 2007;13(3):170–7.

[90] Garg R, Yusuf S, Collaborative Group on ACE Inhibitor Trials. Overview of randomized trials of angiotensin-converting enzyme inhibitors on mortality and morbidity in patients with heart failure. JAMA 1995;273(18):1450–6.

[91] Domanski MJ, Exner DV, Borkowf CB, et al. Effect of angiotensin converting enzyme inhibition on sudden cardiac death in patients following acute

myocardial infarction: a meta-analysis of randomized clinical trials. J Am Coll Cardiol 1999;33(3): 598–604.

[92] Al-Mallah MH, Tleyjeh IM, Abdel-Latif AA, et al. Angiotensin-converting enzyme inhibitors in coronary artery disease and preserved left ventricular systolic function. J Am Coll Cardiol 2006;47(8): 1576–83.

[93] Teo KK, Mitchell LB, Pogue J, et al. Effect of ramipril in reducing sudden deaths and nonfatal cardiac arrests in high-risk individuals without heart failure or left ventricular dysfunction. Circulation 2004;110(11):1413–7.

[94] Lee VC, Rhew DC, Dylan M, et al. Meta-analysis: angiotensin-receptor blockers in chronic heart failure and high-risk acute myocardial infarction. Ann Intern Med 2004;141(9):693–704.

[95] Pfeffer MA, McMurray JJ, Velazquez EJ, et al. Valsartan, captopril, or both in myocardial infarction complicated by heart failure, left ventricular dysfunction, or both. N Engl J Med 2003;349(13): 1893–906.

[96] Dickstein K, Kjekshus J. Effects of losartan and captopril on mortality and morbidity in high-risk patients after acute myocardial infarction: the OPTIMAAL randomized trial. Optimal trial in myocardial infarction with angiotensin II antagonist losartan. Lancet 2002;360(9335):752–60.

[97] Pitt B, Zannad F, Remme WJ, et al. The effect of spironolactone on morbidity and mortality in patients with severe heart failure. N Engl J Med 1999;341(10):709–17.

[98] Pitt B, Remme W, Zannad F, et al. Eplerenone, a selective aldosterone blocker, in patients with left ventricular dysfunction after myocardial infarction. N Engl J Med 2003;348(14):1309–21.

[99] Agustí A, Bonet S, Arnau JM, et al. Adverse effects of ACE inhibitors in patients with chronic heart failure and/or ventricular dysfunction. Drug Saf 2003;26(12):895–908.

[100] Granger CB, McMurray JJV, Yusuf A, et al. Effects of candesartan in patients with chronic heart failure and reduced left-ventricular systolic function intolerant to angiotensin-converting-enzyme inhibitors: the CHARM-Alternative trial. Lancet 2003;362(9386):772–6.

[101] Phillips CO, Kashani A, Ko DK, et al. Adverse effects of combination angiotensin II receptor blockers plus angiotensin-converting enzyme inhibitors for left ventricular dysfunction: a quantitative review of data from randomized clinical trials. Arch Intern Med 2007;167(18):1930–6.

[102] Eichhorn EJ, Gheorghiade M. Digoxin. Prog Cardiovasc Dis 2002;44(4):251–66.

[103] Ruch SR, Nishio M, Wasserstrom JA. Effect of cardiac glycosides on action potential characteristics and contractility in cat ventricular myocytes: role of calcium overload. J Pharmacol Exp Ther 2003;307(1):419–28.

[104] Rocchetti M, Besana A, Mostacciuolo G, et al. Diverse toxicity associated with cardiac $Na+/K+$ pump inhibition: evaluation of electrophysiological mechanisms. J Pharmacol Exp Ther 2003;305(2): 765–71.

[105] Captopril-Digoxin Multicenter Research Group. Comparative effects of therapy with captopril and digoxin in patients with mild to moderate heart failure. JAMA 1988;259(4):539–44.

[106] DiBianco R, Shabetai R, Kostuk W, et al. A comparison of oral milrinone, digoxin, and their combination in the treatment of patients with chronic heart failure. N Engl J Med 1989;320(11): 677–83.

[107] Gradman AH, Cunningham M, Harbison MA, et al. Effects of oral digoxin on ventricular ectopy in relation to left ventricular function. Am J Cardiol 1983;51(5):765–9.

[108] Digitalis Investigator Group. The effect of digoxin on mortality and morbidity in patients with heart failure. N Engl J Med 1997;336(8):525–33.

[109] Rathore SS, Curtis JP, Wang Y, et al. Association of serum digoxin concentration and outcomes in patients with heart failure. JAMA 2003;289(7): 871–8.

Use of Traditional and Biventricular Implantable Cardiac Devices for Primary and Secondary Prevention of Sudden Death

Matthew H. Klein, MD, Michael R. Gold, MD, PhD*

Division of Cardiology, Medical University of South Carolina, 25 Courtenay Drive, Room 7031 ART, MSC 592, Charleston, SC 29425, USA

Sudden cardiac death (SCD) accounts for 450,000 deaths yearly in the United States and remains a major public health problem [1]. There is a dismal survival rate following such an event [2–4], with only 3% to 28% of patients who experience SCD surviving to hospital discharge [5]. Therapy for survivors of SCD and sustained ventricular tachycardia (VT) focused initially on types 1 and 3 antiarrhythmic drugs. The results of these trials were disappointing, which led to the development of the implantable cardioverter defibrillator (ICD). Multiple randomized clinical trials have shown a significant mortality benefit of defibrillator therapy compared with antiarrhythmic drug therapy for secondary prevention of SCD [6–10], and ICDs long have been considered the standard of care in this group. Furthermore, clinical trials of antiarrhythmic drugs for the primary prevention of sudden death have failed to show consistent benefit [11]. Paradoxically, other drug classes, such as β-blockers, angiotensin-converting enzyme (ACE) inhibitors, aldosterone antagonists, and statins appear to have moderate efficacy for preventing SCD in high-risk cohorts. Multiple trials completed over the past decade have documented the effectiveness of the ICD for primary prevention to reduce the risk of SCD and overall mortality in patients at high risk for lethal arrhythmias [12]. Because ventricular tachyarrhythmias are considered the underlying cause of SCD in most subjects, most cardiac rhythm device studies designed to reduce mortality have focused on ICD technology with or without pacing.

Cardiac resynchronization therapy (CRT) using biventricular pacing has emerged as an important adjunctive therapy for patients who have systolic heart failure and intraventricular conduction delay. Several large multicenter trials of CRT have shown an improvement in exercise capacity and quality of life with a reduction in hospitalizations among subjects who have advanced heart failure, QRS prolongation and a reduced left ventricular ejection fraction (LVEF). A reduction of sudden death and all-cause mortality also has been demonstrated with CRT, with or without ICD backup. In addition, bradycardia initiates some sudden death episodes, and pacing may be effective to reduce sudden death by preventing asystole or affecting repolarization. This article reviews the clinical trials evaluating the effects of ICD and pacing therapy on SCD.

Secondary prevention implantable cardioverter defibrillator trials

Several prospective, randomized trials evaluated the role of the ICD in secondary prevention of SCD [6–10], defined as those patients who previously experienced an episode of sustained ventricular tachyarrhythmia. The first and largest published study was the Antiarrhythmics versus Implantable Defibrillators (AVID) trial in 1997, which enrolled 1016 patients who had survived one or more episodes of ventricular fibrillation

* Corresponding author.
E-mail address: goldmr@musc.edu (M.R. Gold).

0733-8651/08/$ - see front matter © 2008 Elsevier Inc. All rights reserved.
doi:10.1016/j.ccl.2008.03.006

(VF) or had symptomatic, sustained VT and a reduced LVEF [6]. The study patients were randomized to either ICD or antiarrhythmic drug therapy, which was primarily amiodarone. Patients assigned to the defibrillator group were found to have a 31% relative reduction in mortality, leading the data safety monitoring board to terminate the trial prematurely. This translated into an average improvement in life expectancy of 2.7 months, although this is likely an underestimate of the benefit of this therapy, because median follow-up was only 18 months. Additionally, the AVID investigators performed a prospective cost-effectiveness analysis and found that the cost of an ICD compared with antiarrhythmic therapy was approximately $67,000 per year of life saved [13].

The Canadian Implantable Defibrillator Study (CIDS) [7] reported on 659 patients who had a history of cardiac arrest, sustained VT, or syncope with a depressed ejection fraction (EF) and inducible sustained ventricular arrhythmia. Subjects were randomized to treatment with an ICD or amiodarone. A 20% relative decrease in mortality from all causes was observed in the defibrillator group, which did not reach statistical significance.

The Cardiac Arrest Study Hamburg (CASH) [8] included 346 patients who survived a cardiac arrest and randomly were assigned to receive an ICD or antiarrhythmic drug therapy (amiodarone, metoprolol, or propafenone). Relative to the patients in AVID and CIDS, the subjects enrolled in CASH were healthier, with a higher mean LVEF. The propafenone arm had a 61% excess total mortality during the first year of

follow-up and was stopped early. The final analysis included the 288 remaining patients, and compared the defibrillator group versus the metoprolol and amiodarone groups at 57 months mean follow-up. As with CIDS, CASH showed a trend toward decreased total mortality in the ICD group (23% relative risk reduction), which did not reach statistical significance.

Connolly and colleagues [14] performed a meta-analysis of the AVID, CIDS, and CASH trials and found that ICD therapy, compared with amiodarone, resulted in significant relative reductions in total mortality (28%) and arrhythmic death (50%) (Fig. 1). The mean survival benefit of an ICD, as compared with drug therapy, was estimated to be 4.4 months over a follow-up period of 6 years. Furthermore, defibrillator therapy improved mortality outcomes regardless of the presence of structural heart disease, use of β-blockers, prior surgical revascularization, or presenting arrhythmia (VT or VF). This analysis also showed that patients who had LVEF greater than 35% derived significantly less benefit from ICD therapy than those who had more significant LV dysfunction. A second meta-analysis, which separately compared the effectiveness of ICD therapy versus medical therapy for both primary and secondary prevention of arrhythmic events, found a significant decrease in all-cause mortality in the ICD group in the secondary prevention trials [15].

Both the AVID and CIDS investigators performed subgroup analyses to determine the benefit of ICD therapy based on LVEF [16,17]. In the AVID trial, patients who had LVEF less than

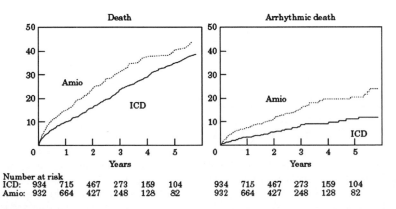

Fig. 1. Cumulative risk of total mortality and arrhythmic death with implantable cardioverter–defibrillator (ICD) versus amiodarone from secondary prevention trials (*Reproduced from* Connolly SJ, Hallstrom AP, Cappato R, et al. Meta-analysis of the implantable cardioverter defibrillator secondary prevention trials: AVID, CASH, and CIDS studies. Eur Heart J 2000;21(24):2074; with permission.)

35% showed a 40% relative mortality reduction with an ICD versus drug therapy, whereas those who had an LVEF greater than 35% did not benefit significantly [16]. Likewise, the subgroup analysis from CIDS found that patients who had more severe LV dysfunction (LVEF less than 35%) gained a greater mortality benefit from defibrillator therapy than those who had a more preserved LVEF [17]. A separate investigation from the AVID population compared survival rates across different quintiles of LVEF. In the antiarrhythmic drug group but not the ICD group, survival was associated strongly with left ventricular (LV) systolic function. The authors concluded that this effect likely was related to the superiority of the ICD in treating malignant ventricular arrhythmias [18].

Substudies from the CIDS and AVID trials were designed to uncover additional baseline characteristics that would predict benefit of ICD therapy. In the CIDS trial, high-risk patients (defined by two or more of the following: LVEF less than or equal to 35%, age greater than or equal to 70, and New York Heart Association class 3 or 4), were found to have a 50% relative risk reduction for total mortality, whereas patients who had one or no risk factors derived no benefit [17]. In separate substudies that included patients in the other secondary prevention trials, however, LVEF remained the only risk factor predictive of ICD efficacy [15,19]. A retrospective substudy from AVID sought to identify baseline variables that were predictive of low arrhythmia recurrence based on a review of stored ICD event data [20]. Factors that significantly predicted low arrhythmia recurrence rate were VF as the index arrhythmia, no history of cerebrovascular disease, higher LVEF, no tachyarrhythmia history, and need for revascularization [20]. Raitt and colleagues [21] examined spontaneous arrhythmias occurring in AVID patients randomized to an ICD. Those patients who had VT as their index arrhythmia were significantly more likely to have appropriate therapy than those who presented initially with VF. These findings suggest that there are important differences in the electrophysiologic characteristics between these two patient populations [21].

Another substudy from the AVID registry involved patients with life-threatening ventricular arrhythmias thought to be secondary to a reversible cause, a group that was not eligible for randomization [22]. Compared with patients who had a primary ventricular arrhythmia (no

reversible cause identified), mortality for patients who had a transient or identifiable cause was equally high [23]. It was also noteworthy that patients who had hemodynamically stable VT had a similar prognosis as those who had unstable VT [24]. These results call into question the previously held beliefs that patients who have stable VT and those who have a potentially reversible cause have a good prognosis and are not candidates for an ICD. Rather, it may be that other nonarrhythmic clinical characteristics, such as ischemia, heart failure, or LV dysfunction, may be more important for determining sudden and all-cause mortality. This finding has led to an increase in the practice of ICD implantation for patients who have documented sustained ventricular arrhythmias and concurrent electrolyte abnormalities, heart failure exacerbations, or ischemia (in the absence of an ST elevation myocardial infarction).

One criticism of the AVID results was related to an imbalance between β-blocker usage observed between the study groups (40% of patients received β-blockers in the ICD arm versus 11% in the antiarrhythmic drug arm of the trial), which could modify the observed benefits of ICD therapy [6,25]. An AVID substudy evaluated the effects of β-blockade in both the randomized and nonrandomized populations followed in the trial [25]. In patients treated with either an ICD or amiodarone, β-blocker use did not alter survival. AVID-eligible patients who were not randomized to either amiodarone or ICD therapy, however, experienced a 53% mortality reduction with β-blockers compared with those who did not receive β-blockers. The authors postulated that β-blocker use led to a reduction in SCD, but this survival benefit was no longer prominent when patients also were receiving specific antiarrhythmic therapy with amiodarone or a defibrillator [25].

An AVID substudy collected quality of life data on 800 trial participants surviving to at least 1 year of follow-up [26]. Similar alterations in self-perceived quality of life were observed among participants treated with antiarrhythmic drugs and those treated with ICDs. The development of sporadic shocks was associated with a reduction in physical functioning and mental well-being among ICD recipients. Among patients treated with antiarrhythmic drugs, a similar reduction in both physical functioning and mental well-being occurred in those who developed adverse symptoms related to therapy [26]. Quality-of-life outcomes from the CIDS trial were somewhat different from those observed in AVID. In a post-hoc analysis, emotional and physical health scores improved significantly in the ICD group and were either unchanged or deteriorated in the amiodarone group. The investigators noted, however, that quality of life did not improve in the subgroup of ICD patients who received five or more shocks from their device during the 12-month follow-up period [27].

Brodsky and colleagues [28] investigated the utility of electrophysiologic (EP) studies in AVID patients following VT, VT with syncope, or sustained VT in the setting of LV dysfunction. In this setting, the EP study did not predict death or recurrent arrhythmias accurately during follow-up. Another potential predictor evaluated by the AVID group was electrical storm, defined as multiple temporally related episodes of VT or VF. Electrical storm was found to be a significant risk factor for overall mortality within the 3 months following its occurrence, and to a lesser extent beyond that time [29].

Although the aforementioned secondary prevention trials generally followed patients for a limited time, long-term outcomes were assessed in a subset of VT/VF survivors from the CIDS trial. Patients were followed for a mean duration of 5.6 years. The all-cause annual mortality rate in the amiodarone group was found to be 5.5% versus 2.8% in the ICD group [30]. Although the initial CIDS trial only showed a modest mortality advantage of ICD therapy over amiodarone, the CIDS long-term substudy investigators found a progressive increase in the benefits of defibrillator therapy over time [31]. In addition, 82% of patients receiving amiodarone experienced drug-related adverse effects, and 50% of patients on amiodarone required dose reduction or discontinuation [30]. This highlights some of the problems interpreting the relatively short-term follow-up of most ICD trials. The efficacy of ICDs does not appear to wane over time, whereas drug therapy may become less effective or lead to increased intolerance as the cardiac substrate changes or systemic accumulation progresses. Therefore, the benefit of ICD therapy compared with antiarrhythmic drugs may continue to increase with longer follow-up. Moreover, the duration of median follow-up is much shorter than battery longevity, so the cost of ICD therapy likely is overestimated, and the prolongation of life likely is underestimated.

Primary prevention trials

Clinical trials of antiarrhythmic drug therapy for the primary prevention of sudden death had variable results, showing harm, no effect, or an inconsistent benefit [11]. Given the high morality rate associated with an out-of-hospital cardiac arrest and the disappointing results of antiarrhythmic drugs, multiple trials were undertaken to examine the efficacy of defibrillator therapy in high-risk cohorts (Table 1). The first of these trials to be published was the Multicenter Automatic Defibrillator Implantation Trial (MADIT-I) [32], which enrolled 196 patients who had coronary artery disease (CAD), spontaneous nonsustained ventricular tachycardia (NSVT), LVEF less than or equal to 35%, and inducible VT that was not suppressed with the use of intravenous procainamide. The investigators found a 54% relative reduction in all-cause mortality over a mean follow-up period of 27 months in the defibrillator group compared with the group assigned to conventional medical therapy. This mortality reduction translated into a number needed-to-treat (NNT) of 3 over 36 months. The cost of ICD therapy compared with conventional care was $27,000 per life-year gained in MADIT, which compares favorably with other cardiac interventions [33].

The Multicenter Unsustained Tachycardia Trial (MUSTT) [34] was a randomized trial that enrolled a similar population to that of MADIT-I. Patients who had a history of myocardial infarction (MI), LVEF less than or equal to 40%, and spontaneous NSVT underwent an EP study. Those patients who had inducible VT (n = 704) were assigned randomly to either no therapy or antiarrhythmic therapy, while patients who did not have inducible VT were followed in a registry. The patients who randomly were assigned to EP-guided therapy underwent serial drug testing followed by random assignment of an antiarrhythmic drug. The most common drugs prescribed were class 1 antiarrhythmics (26%), followed by amiodarone (10%) and sotalol (9%). ICD therapy could be used only after failure of at least one antiarrhythmic drug. Although MUSTT frequently has been considered to be a defibrillator trial, it may be described better as a test of an EP-guided treatment strategy in which an ICD could be prescribed at an investigator's discretion [35]. Of note, the frequency of defibrillator prescription varied among the trial centers and over time. Despite these limitations, the 5-year all-cause mortality among the 161 patients

Table 1
Selected clinical trials of implantable cardioverter defibrillator therapy for primary prevention of sudden cardiac death

Trial	Number of patients	Inclusion criteria	Mean follow-up (months)	Control therapy	Relative risk reduction (%)	Absolute risk reduction (%)	P value
MADIT-I [32]	196	Nonrecent MI (>3 wks) or CABG (>3 mos), EF ≤35%, spontaneous NSVT, and inducible VT	27	Medical therapy	54	22.8	0.009
MUSTT [34]	704	Nonrecent MI (≥4 days), EF ≤40%, spontaneous NSVT, and inducible VT	39	Medical therapy	51	23	<.001 (ICD versus medical therapy)
MADIT-II [40]	1232	EF ≤30%, remote MI (>1 mo)	20	Medical therapy	31	5.4	0.02
AMIOVIRT [51]	103	EF ≤35%, NICM, NSVT	24	Medical therapy	13	1.7	0.8
Cardiomyopathy Trial (CAT) [52]	104	NYHA II-III, EF ≤30%, NICM, recent-onset heart failure (≤9 mos)	23	Medical therapy	17	5.4	0.6
DEFINITE [53]	458	NICM, EF <35%, NSVT, or ≥10 PVCs/hr	29	Medical therapy	35	5.2	0.08
SCD-HeFT [54]	1676	NYHA II-III, nonrecent MI or revascularization (>30 days), nonrecent heart failure onset (>3 mos)	46	Placebo	23	6.8	<0.01

Abbreviations: CABG, coronary artery bypass graft surgery; EF, ejection fraction; LVEF, left ventricular ejection fraction; MI, myocardial infarction; NICM, nonischemic cardiomyopathy; NSVT, nonsustained ventricular tachycardia; NYHA, New York Heart Association functional class; PVC, premature ventricular complex; VT, ventricular tachycardia.

who received ICD therapy during the initial hospitalization was 24%, which was significantly lower than the 171 patients treated with antiarrhythmic drugs (55% mortality) and the 353 patients who received no therapy (48% mortality). This translated into a 49% relative risk reduction for defibrillators as compared with drug therapy. Antiarrhythmic therapy was associated with a nonsignificant worsening of survival compared with standard medical therapy.

The MUSTT investigators also examined the prognostic significance of inducible VT during EP testing by comparing the long-term outcomes of patients who did not receive therapy [36]. Over a 5-year follow-up period, patients in whom sustained VT could not be induced had a significantly lower risk of sudden death or cardiac arrest than similar patients who had inducible VT. The overall mortality was also significantly lower in patients without inducible VT; however, the absolute difference in mortality between the patients

who were inducible at the time of study and those who were noninducible was only 4% (48% versus 44%, respectively). These data suggest that the group of noninducible patients also might benefit from a primary prevention strategy, and that an EP study may be an inadequate risk stratification tool [37].

Multiple substudies from MUSTT sought to identify clinical risk factors that would predict increased risk of SCD. For the patients enrolled in MUSTT who did not receive antiarrhythmic therapy, the risk of total mortality and arrhythmic death was significantly greater among patients who had LVEF less than 30%, compared with patients who had LVEF 30% to 40% [38]. A recently published multivariate analysis from MUSTT, however, showed that EF alone may not be an adequate assessment of risk. Multiple other clinical factors, including functional class, history of heart failure, NSVT not related to bypass surgery, age, LV conduction abnormalities, and atrial fibrillation, were found to influence total mortality and arrhythmic death. In addition, patients who have LVEF greater than 30% and other risk factors may be at higher risk for events than patients who have LVEF less than or equal to 30% but no other risk factors [12].

A MUSTT substudy compared the outcomes of enrolled patients based on race, and found multiple differences between blacks and whites [39]. These differences included a higher ICD implantation rate in whites versus blacks (50% versus 28%, respectively) and higher probability of inducible sustained VT on serial EP testing in whites, making whites more likely to be eligible for ICD implantation. Whites assigned to EP-guided therapy had a lower risk of arrhythmic death and overall mortality compared with blacks. Beyond the discrepancy in ICD implantation, there may be differences in arrhythmic substrates and proarrhythmic responses to antiarrhythmic drugs between the two races that partially explain these outcomes [39].

The second Multicenter Automatic Defibrillator Implantation Trial (MADIT II) [40] evaluated patients who had CAD, a history of MI, and LVEF less than or equal to 30%, and compared ICD therapy with standard medical care. This allowed for a larger segment of the population at risk for SCD to be included compared with MADIT (subsequently referred to as MADIT I), as patients were not required to have spontaneous or inducible arrhythmias. Patients treated with an ICD had a 31% relative reduction in mortality compared with standard medical therapy (14.2% versus 19.8%, respectively) during an average follow-up of 20 months. Antiarrhythmic drugs (primarily amiodarone) were used in less than 20% of subjects in both groups.

The MADIT-II investigators performed a subsequent analysis of defibrillator benefit as a function of time from MI to enrollment [41]. A mortality benefit was found among patients who had a remote MI (18 months or greater), but not in patients who had a more recent MI (less than 18 months). Furthermore, the mortality risk increased as a function of time from MI, and remained substantial for up to 15 years. This is contrary to older data suggesting that the highest risk period for SCD after MI was in the first year. This likely reflects a change in the management of these patients with aggressive use of reperfusion strategies and medical therapy to block neurohormonal activation, including β-blockers, ACE inhibitors and aldosterone

antagonists. ICD benefit also was analyzed retrospectively based on time from last coronary revascularization [42]. Patients implanted more than 6 months after coronary revascularization received significant benefit from an ICD, whereas patients implanted less than 6 months following revascularization showed no benefit. This difference may be because of a relatively low risk for SCD in the early period following revascularization [42].

The benefit of ICD therapy in patients who were enrolled in MADIT-II was evaluated based on various clinical risk factors. In subjects randomized to treatment with a defibrillator, there was no significant difference in outcomes across New York Heart Association class or across varying degrees of LV dysfunction [43]. In a separate post-hoc analysis, all-cause mortality and SCD were increased across progressive degrees of renal dysfunction. Patients who had severe renal dysfunction, however, had no mortality benefit from ICD therapy, whereas patients who had no renal disease or mild to moderate disease had a significant survival benefit [44]. The MADIT-II investigators also assessed obesity as a risk factor for arrhythmic events [45]. In obese patients, there was a 64% increase in the risk of appropriate ICD therapy compared with nonobese patients over a follow-up period of 2 years.

Another intriguing analysis from the MADIT-II database examined the clinical course and subsequent mortality risk to patients following successful termination of a ventricular tachyarrhythmia by an ICD [46]. Patients who received successful appropriate ICD therapy had an 80% 1-year survival rate. Compared with MADIT-II patients not receiving therapy, patients receiving successful ICD therapy were at higher risk for heart failure and nonsudden cardiac death, suggesting that this group may require special attention during follow-up. A further evaluation examined factors that predict increased risk of ICD-appropriate therapy or death. In a multivariate analysis, interim hospitalizations for heart failure and coronary events subsequently were associated with an increased risk of ICD therapy for ventricular tachyarrhythmias and death [47].

Outcomes and effectiveness data were gathered based on race and gender differences in two separate MADIT-II substudies [48,49]. ICD therapy was associated with a reduction in mortality and SCD in whites; in contrast, there was no significant outcomes benefit for blacks [48]. Women enrolled in MADIT-II had similar mortality and

ICD effectiveness, but fewer episodes of ventricular arrhythmias, compared with men [49].

A cost-effectiveness analysis also was performed based on the results of MADIT-II [50]. The estimated cost per life-year saved was $235,000 for the 3.5-year follow-up, a relatively high value. Projections out to 12 years follow-up, however, were substantially lower, ranging from $78,600 to $114,000 per year-of-life saved.

Several randomized primary prevention trials have been published comparing antiarrhythmic drugs with ICD therapy in patients with nonischemic cardiomyopathy (NICM). The Amiodarone versus Implantable Cardioverter–Defibrillator Trial (AMIOVIRT) [51] was a small study (n=103) of patients who had nonischemic LV dysfunction and asymptomatic NSVT. To be included in the trial, patients had to have a chronic (longer than 6 months) diagnosis of LV dysfunction. Over a 2-year average follow-up period, there was no statistically significant mortality difference between the group treated with an ICD versus the group treated with amiodarone.

The Cardiomyopathy Trial (CAT) [52] evaluated 104 patients who had NICM and LVEF less than 30% with recent onset heart failure (less than or equal to 9 months from enrollment). The trial compared ICD implantation with standard medical therapy. At a mean follow-up of 5.5 years, survival was not significantly different between the two groups.

The next trial to evaluate ICD therapy in this patient population was the Defibrillators in Non-Ischemic Cardiomyopathy Treatment Evaluation (DEFINITE) [53]. There were 488 patients who had NICM, LVEF less than or equal to 35%, and frequent premature ventricular beats or NSVT randomized to standard medical care or standard care plus an ICD. There was a trend toward improved overall mortality, the primary endpoint, at 2-year follow-up in the ICD group (14.1% versus 7.9%), but this did not reach statistical significance ($P = .08$). For sudden death, a secondary endpoint of the trial, a significant reduction in the ICD group was observed (3 in the ICD group versus 14 in the standard care group, $P = .006$).

These relatively small studies showed at best a trend for mortality reduction among patients who have NICM. This is in contrast to the large benefit noted in most studies involving patients with known ischemic heart disease. Many of these studies were underpowered to address the issue of mortality benefit in this population. To help

evaluate this issue more definitively, the National Institutes of Health (NIH) helped sponsor a large landmark trial. The Sudden Cardiac Death–Heart Failure Trial (SCD-HeFT) [54] evaluated 2521 patients who had ischemic and nonischemic cardiomyopathy, symptomatic heart failure, and LVEF less than or equal to 35%. The cohort included 70% who had NYHA class 2 functional status and 30% who had class 3. There were three arms to the trial: ICD therapy, amiodarone, and placebo. The defibrillators used in this trial were simple single-lead, programmed as shock-only devices. Medical management of heart failure patients in SCD-HeFT was exceptional, with 96% of patients on an ACE inhibitor or angiotensin receptor blocker at baseline, and 69% of patients on β-blockers. The primary end-point was all-cause mortality. At 5 years follow-up, patients randomly assigned to receive an ICD had a 23% relative risk reduction in mortality (7% absolute risk reduction) compared with placebo, and this benefit was similar in patients who had both ischemic and non-ischemic cardiomyopathy. Amiodarone therapy had a similar risk of death compared with placebo.

Mark and colleagues [55] published a cost-effectiveness analysis from SCD-HeFT. For an assumed pulse generator longevity of 5 years, there was a calculated cost-effectiveness of $33,192 per life-year saved for ICD therapy compared with amiodarone. This number compares favorably with the cost-effectiveness data presented from MADIT-II and AVID, perhaps because of the longer duration of follow-up in the SCD-HeFT trial. Similar cost-effectiveness data from SCD-HeFT were projected between etiologies of heart failure, whether ischemic or nonischemic in origin.

A recent substudy from SCD-HeFT specifically evaluated the population enrolled in the trial with atrial fibrillation (AF). In those randomized to ICD therapy, patients who had AF on baseline electrocardiogram were more likely to receive both appropriate and inappropriate shocks than patients in sinus rhythm at baseline. Total mortality rates were found to be similar between the two groups [56].

Nanthakumar and colleagues [57] performed a pooled analysis of treatment with and without ICDs in 10 trials for primary prevention of SCD, and included results of the AMIOVIRT, CAT, MADIT-I, MADIT-II, Comparison of Medical Therapy, Pacing, and Defibrillation in Heart Failure (COMPANION), DEFINITE, and SCD-HeFT trials (Fig. 2). ICD therapy provided between a 5.8% and 7.9% absolute mortality reduction ($P = .003$) compared with optimal medical management in patients who had LV systolic dysfunction, regardless of etiology. This translates into an NNT of 13 to 17 for ICD therapy over a period of approximately 34 months, depending on which trials were included in the analysis. This finding remains statistically significant regardless of the exclusion of any one trial.

Several older trials evaluated the efficacy of prophylactic ICD therapy in specific circumstances. The Coronary Artery Bypass Graft Patch (CABG Patch) trial compared treatment with an ICD versus standard care in 900 patients undergoing elective coronary bypass surgery with EF less than or equal to 35% and abnormal signal-averaged electrocardiograms (SAECG) [58]. Over a mean follow-up period of 32 months, there was no statistical difference in all-cause mortality between the two groups (hazard ratio for ICD group 1.07, $P = .64$). One plausible explanation for the lack of benefit observed with ICD therapy in this trial is the independent reduction in mortality associated with coronary bypass surgery alone. A subgroup analysis from the Studies of Left Ventricular Dysfunction (SOLVD) trials evaluated outcomes of patients who had prior history of coronary artery bypass surgery [59]. Prior coronary artery bypass surgery was associated with a 25% reduction in risk of death and a 46% reduction in risk of SCD compared with patients not undergoing surgery, both statistically

significant. Thus, the prophylactic benefit of ICD implantation may not exist in this relatively protected population. Alternatively, the use of older thoracotomy ICD systems, the limited value of SAECG for risk stratification, or an improvement in systolic function following bypass surgery may have contributed to the lack of benefit of ICD therapy in this cohort.

The Defibrillators in Acute Myocardial Infarction Trial (DINAMIT) was a primary prevention trial enrolling patients who had recent MI (within 6 to 40 days of enrollment) [60]. Additional inclusion criteria included LV systolic dysfunction (EF less than or equal to 35%) and impaired cardiac autonomic function, as manifested by low heart rate variability or high 24-hour resting heart rate. There was no statistical benefit in all-cause mortality for the ICD group at a mean follow-up of 30 months (hazard ratio for ICD group 1.08, $P = .66$). Although ICD therapy was associated with a significant reduction in death from arrhythmic causes, this was offset by an increase risk of death from nonarrhythmic causes in this group. As previously discussed in a subgroup analysis from MADIT-II, this lack of benefit may be related to improved medical therapies and more aggressive reperfusion strategies after MI in the present era. [41] Additionally, although impaired heart rate variability likely identifies a group of patients at high risk for arrhythmic death following MI, this marker also identifies patients who have LV dysfunction at high risk for progressive pump failure [61], which

Comparison: 01 ICD vs. Control (Overall)
Outcome: 01 All-Cause Mortality

Study or sub-category	Treatment n/N	Control n/N	RR (random) 95% CI	Weight %	RR (random) 95% CI
AMIOVIRT	6/51	7/52		2.76	0.87 [0.32, 2.42]
CABG Patch	101/446	95/454		12.79	1.08 [0.84, 1.39]
CAT	13/50	17/54		5.93	0.83 [0.45, 1.52]
COMPANION	105/595	131/617		13.19	0.83 [0.66, 1.05]
DEFINITE	28/229	40/229		8.46	0.70 [0.45, 1.09]
DINAMIT	62/332	58/342		11.00	1.10 [0.80, 1.52]
MADIT 1	15/95	39/101		7.12	0.41 [0.24, 0.69]
MADIT 2	105/742	97/490		12.71	0.71 [0.56, 0.92]
MUSTT	35/161	255/537		11.42	0.46 [0.34, 0.62]
SCD HeFT	182/829	244/847		14.62	0.76 [0.65, 0.90]
Total (95% CI)	3530	3723		100.00	0.75 [0.63, 0.91]

Total events: 652 (Treatment), 983 (Control)
Test for heterogeneity: Chi² = 29.67, df = 9 (P = 0.0005), I² = 69.7%
Test for overall effect: Z = 3.00 (P = 0.003)

0.1 0.2 0.5 1 2 5 10
Favours treatment   Favours control

Fig. 2. Summary of implantable cardioverter–defibrillator (ICD) primary prevention trials (*Reproduced from* Nanthakumar K, Epstein AE, Kay GN, et al. Prophylactic implantable cardioverter–defibrillator therapy in patients with left ventricular systolic dysfunction: a pooled analysis of 10 primary prevention trials. J Am Coll Cardiol 2004;44(11):2170; with permission.)

defibrillators are incapable of treating. Finally, there may be a higher competing risk of fatal heart failure and recurrent ischemic events early post-MI that precludes demonstration of ICD benefit.

Pacemaker trials

Bradycardia and asystole represent additional mechanisms by which SCD may occur. Although intracardiac pacing is clearly efficacious for treating bradyarrhythmias, the mortality benefit in prevention of SCD is difficult to establish or quantify. There is little doubt that pacing prevents mortality in the setting of acquired complete heart block, although this observation never was subjected to prospective study. Multiple randomized trials have evaluated atrial-based (dual-chamber or atrial) pacing versus ventricular pacing in bradycardic patients; none of these trials have shown a reduction in mortality [62]. Additionally, a recent meta-analysis by Healey and colleagues, [62] while finding a reduction in the incidence of AF with atrial-based pacing, found no improvement in mortality, heart failure outcomes, or cardiovascular death compared with ventricular pacing.

Cardiac resynchronization therapy

The two large long-term randomized trials that have assessed the role of cardiac resynchronization therapy (CRT) on mortality are the COMPANION [63] and the Effect of Cardiac Resynchronization on Morbidity and Mortality in Heart Failure (CARE-HF) [64] trials. The COMPANION study, comprised of 1520 patients who had NYHA class 3 or 4 symptoms and QRS duration greater than 120 milliseconds, had three treatment arms: CRT with ICD, CRT alone, and optimal medical therapy. Patients who had LV dysfunction from both ischemic and nonischemic causes were included. The composite primary endpoint was death or hospitalization from any cause. There was a 40% relative risk reduction ($P < .001$) in the composite primary endpoint for the CRT with ICD group and a 34% relative risk reduction ($P < .002$) in the CRT alone group compared with medical therapy. With respect to all-cause mortality, a prespecified secondary endpoint, there was a 36% relative risk reduction ($P = .003$) in the CRT with ICD group and a 24% relative risk reduction ($P = .059$) in the CRT alone group compared with medical therapy.

This translates into a NNT of only approximately 14 patients for the CRT with ICD group to prevent one death over a 1-year period, a large mortality reduction. This benefit remained consistent across multiple clinical and demographic variables including patient age, gender, QRS duration, cause of LV dysfunction, LVEF, blood pressure, and medication use.

CARE-HF was the second large randomized trial (n = 813) to evaluate the role of CRT in patients who had advanced heart failure (NYHA Class III-IV), cardiomyopathy, and LV dyssynchrony. Patients were randomly assigned to CRT (without ICD function) or medical therapy. The primary endpoint was death from any cause or unplanned cardiovascular hospitalization. Over a mean follow-up of 29 months, there was a 16% absolute risk reduction in the primary endpoint ($P < .001$) and a 10% absolute risk reduction ($P < .002$) in the secondary endpoint of all-cause mortality. There was also a significant benefit in multiple hemodynamic and echocardiographic parameters with CRT including improvement in LVEF and reductions in interventricular mechanical delay, end–systolic volume index, and area of the mitral regurgitant jet. CRT also provided better quality of life and symptomatic outcomes compared with medical therapy alone ($P < .01$).

A recent meta-analysis reviewed the outcomes from COMPANION, CARE-HF, and several smaller randomized trials of CRT versus medical therapy only [65–71]. All patients enrolled in the studies were characterized by symptomatic heart failure, LV systolic dysfunction, and cardiac dyssynchrony. Overall mortality (fixed effects odds ratio 0.72, 95% CI 0.59 to 0.88) and heart failure hospitalizations (fixed effects odds ratio 0.55, 95% CI 0.44 to 0.68) were reduced markedly with CRT (Fig. 3).

Summary

Over the past two decades, the indications for ICD use have broadened based on a series of landmark clinical trials. The ICD consistently has shown a reduction in SCD and overall mortality in the treatment of patients with prior symptomatic ventricular arrhythmias. A series of primary prevention trials demonstrated a significant benefit of prophylactic ICD therapy versus antiarrhythmic drugs for the treatment of high-risk ischemic and nonischemic cardiomyopathy patients. Currently, LVEF remains the best

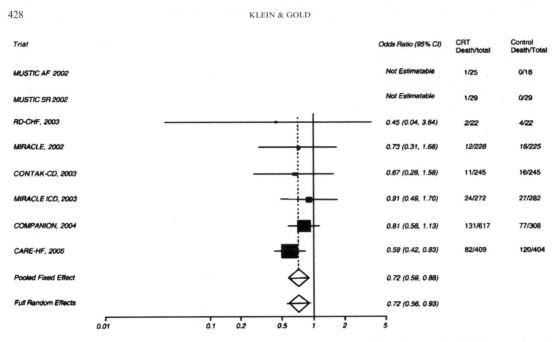

Fig. 3. Summary of cardiac resynchronization trials on mortality (*Reproduced from* Freemantle N, Tharmanathan P, Calvert MJ, et al. Cardiac resynchronisation for patients with heart failure due to left ventricular systolic dysfunction—a systematic review and meta-analysis. Eur J Heart Fail 2006;8(4):438; with permission.)

predictor of benefit in these populations. Recent clinical trials also provide evidence for the morbidity and mortality benefit of CRT using biventricular pacing in advanced heart failure patients who have a prolonged QRS duration.

Despite the aforementioned primary prevention trials that defined a subset of patients at high risk for SCD, most patients who present with SCD would not meet present criteria for prophylactic ICD implantation before their sudden death event. Thus, there remains a large cohort of patients at risk for SCD presently not well identified. Conversely, most patients who receive ICDs based on current guidelines do not require device therapy for ventricular tachyarrhythmias over the first 3 to 5 years of follow-up. Thus, further studies to improve risk stratification are needed.

References

[1] Zheng ZJ, Croft JB, Giles WH, et al. Sudden cardiac death in the United States, 1989 to 1998. Circulation 2001;104(18):2158–63.

[2] Bigger JT. Expanding indications for implantable cardiac defibrillators. N Engl J Med 2002;346(12): 931–3.

[3] de Vreede-Swagemakers JJ, Gorgels AP, Dubois-Arbouw WI, et al. Out-of-hospital cardiac arrest in the 1990s: a population-based study in the Maastricht area on incidence, characteristics, and survival. J Am Coll Cardiol 1997;30(6):1500–5.

[4] Weaver WD, Hill D, Fahrenbruch CE, et al. Use of the automatic external defibrillator in the management of out-of-hospital cardiac arrest. N Engl J Med 1988;319(11):661–6.

[5] Merit-HF Study Group. Effect of metoprolol CR/XL in chronic heart failure: the Metoprolol CR/Xl Randomized Intervention Trial In Congestive Heart Failure (MERIT-HF). Lancet 1999;353(9169): 2001–7.

[6] A comparison of antiarrhythmic drug therapy with implantable defibrillators in patients resuscitated from near-fatal ventricular arrhythmias. The Antiarrhythmic Versus Implantable Defibrillators (AVID) Investigators. N Engl J Med 1997;337(22):1576–83.

[7] Connolly SJ, Gent M, Roberts RS, et al. Canadian Implantable Defibrillator Study (CIDS): a randomized trial of the implantable cardioverter defibrillator against amiodarone. Circulation 2000;101(11): 1297–302.

[8] Kuck KH, Cappato R, Siebels J, et al. Randomized comparison of antiarrhythmic drug therapy with implantable defibrillators in patients resuscitated from cardiac arrest: the Cardiac Arrest Study Hamburg (CASH). Circulation 2000;102(7):748–54.

[9] Nademanee K, Veerakul G, Mower M, et al. Defibrillator versus beta-blockers for unexplained death in Thailand (DEBUT): a randomized clinical trial. Circulation 2003;107(17):2221–6.

[10] Lau EW, Griffith MJ, Pathmanathan RK, et al. The Midlands Trial Of Empirical Amiodarone Versus

Electrophysiology-guided Interventions and Implantable Cardioverter-Defibrillators (MAVERIC): a multicentre prospective randomized clinical trial on the secondary prevention of sudden cardiac death. Europace 2004;6(4):257–66.

[11] Naccarelli GV, Wolbrette DL, Dell'Orfano JT, et al. A decade of clinical trial developments in postmyocardial infarction, congestive heart failure, and sustained ventricular tachyarrhythmia patients: from CAST to AVID and beyond. J Cardiovasc Electrophysiol 1998;9(8):864–91.

[12] Buxton AE, Lee KL, Hafley GE, et al. Limitations of ejection fraction for prediction of sudden death risk in patients with coronary artery disease: lessons from the MUSTT study. J Am Coll Cardiol 2007; 50(12):1150–7.

[13] Larsen G, Hallstrom A, McAnulty J, et al. Cost-effectiveness of the implantable cardioverter–defibrillator versus antiarrhythmic drugs in survivors of serious ventricular tachyarrhythmias: results of the Antiarrhythmics Versus Implantable Defibrillators (AVID) economic analysis substudy. Circulation 2002;105(17):2049–57.

[14] Connolly SJ, Hallstrom AP, Cappato R, et al. Meta-analysis of the implantable cardioverter defibrillator secondary prevention trials: AVID, CASH, and CIDS studies. Eur Heart J 2000;21(24): 2071–8.

[15] Lee D, Green L, Liu P, et al. Effectiveness of implantable defibrillators for preventing arrhythmic events and death: a meta-analysis. J Am Coll Cardiol 2003;41(9):1573–82.

[16] Domanski MJ, Sakseena S, Epstein AE, et al. Relative effectiveness of the implantable cardioverter defibrillator and antiarrhythmic drugs in patients with varying degrees of left ventricular dysfunction who have survived malignant ventricular arrhythmias. AVID Investigators. Antiarrhythmics Versus Implantable Defibrillators. J Am Coll Cardiol 1999;34(4):1090–5.

[17] Sheldon R, Connolly S, Krahn A, et al. Identification of patients most likely to benefit from implantable cardioverter defibrillator therapy. The Canadian Implantable Defibrillator Study. Circulation 2000;101(14):1660–4.

[18] Domanski MJ, Epstein A, Hallstrom A, et al. Survival of antiarrhythmic or implantable cardioverter defibrillator-treated patients with varying degrees of left ventricular dysfunction who survived malignant ventricular arrhythmias. J Cardiovasc Electrophysiol 2002;13(6):580–3.

[19] Exner DV, Sheldon RS, Pinski SL, et al. Do baseline characteristics accurately discriminate between patients likely versus unlikely to benefit from implantable defibrillator therapy? Evaluation of the Canadian implantable defibrillator study implantable cardioverter defibrillator efficacy score in the antiarrhythmics versus implantable defibrillators trial. Am Heart J 2001;141(1):99–104.

[20] Hallstrom AP, McAnulty JH, Wilkoff BL, et al. Patients at lower risk of arrhythmia recurrence: a subgroup in whom implantable defibrillators may not offer benefit. Antiarrhythmics Versus Implantable Defibrillator (AVID) trial investigators. J Am Coll Cardiol 2001;37(4):1093–9.

[21] Raitt M, Klein R, Wyse G, et al. Comparison of arrhythmia recurrence in patients presenting with ventricular fibrillation versus ventricular tachycardia in the Antiarrhythmics Versus Implantable Defibrillators (AVID) trial. Am J Cardiol 2003; 91(7):812–6.

[22] Wyse DG, Friedman PL, Brodsky MA, et al. Life-threatening ventricular arrhythmias due to transient or correctable causes: high risk for death in follow-up. J Am Coll Cardiol 2001;38(6):1718–24.

[23] Anderson JL, Hallstrom AP, Cappato R, et al. Design and results of the Antiarrhythmics vs Implantable Defibrillators (AVID) registry. AVID investigators. Circulation 1999;99(13):1692–9.

[24] Raitt MH, Renfroe EG, Epstein AE, et al. Stable ventricular tachycardia is not a benign rhythm: insights from the Antiarrhythmics Versus Implantable Defibrillators (AVID) registry. Circulation 2001; 103(2):244–52.

[25] Exner DV, Reiffel JA, Epstein AE, et al. Beta-blocker use and survival in patients with ventricular fibrillation or symptomatic ventricular tachycardia: the Antiarrhythmics Versus Implantable Defibrillators (AVID) trial. J Am Coll Cardiol 1999;34(2): 325–33.

[26] Schron EB, Exner DV, Yao Q, et al. Quality of life in the antiarrhythmics versus implantable defibrillators trial: impact of therapy and influence of adverse symptoms and defibrillator shocks. Circulation 2002;105(5):589–94.

[27] Irvine J, Dorian P, Baker B, et al. Quality of life in the Canadian Implantable Defibrillator Study (CIDS). Am Heart J 2002;144(2):282–9.

[28] Brodsky MA, Mitchell LB, Halperin BD, et al. Prognostic value of baseline electrophysiologic studies in patients with sustained ventricular tachyarrhythmia: the Antiarrhythmics Versus Implantable Defibrillators (AVID) trial. Am Heart J 2002;144(3):478–84.

[29] Exner DV, Pinski SL, Wyse DG, et al. Electrical storm presages nonsudden death: the Antiarrhythmics Versus Implantable Defibrillators (AVID) trial. Circulation 2001;103(16):2066–71.

[30] Bokhari F, Newman D, Greene M, et al. Long-term comparison of the implantable cardioverter defibrillator versus amiodarone: eleven-year follow-up of a subset of patients in the Canadian Implantable Defibrillator Study (CIDS). Circulation 2004; 110(2):112–6.

[31] Prystowsky EN. Prevention of sudden cardiac death. Clin Cardiol 2005;28(11 Suppl 1):I12–8.

[32] Moss AJ, Hall WJ, Cannom DS, et al. Improved survival with an implanted defibrillator in patients with coronary disease at high risk for ventricular

arrhythmia. Multicenter Automatic Defibrillator Implantation Trial Investigators. N Engl J Med 1996;335(26):1933–40.

[33] Mushlin AI, Hall WJ, Zwanziger J, et al. The cost-effectiveness of automatic implantable cardiac defibrillators: results from MADIT. Multicenter Automatic Defibrillator Implantation Trial. Circulation 1998;97(21):2129–35.

[34] Buxton AE, Lee KL, Fisher JD, et al. A randomized study of the prevention of sudden death in patients with coronary artery disease. Multicenter Unsustained Tachycardia Trial Investigators. N Engl J Med 1999;341(25):1882–90 [Erratum, N Engl J Med 2000;342(17): 1300].

[35] DiMarco JP. Implantable cardioverter defibrillators. N Engl J Med 2003;349(19):1836–47.

[36] Buxton AE, Lee KL, Dicarlo L, et al. Electrophysiologic testing to identify patients with coronary artery disease who are at risk for sudden death. N Engl J Med 2000;342(26):1937–45.

[37] Goldberger Z, Lampert R. Implantable cardioverter defibrillators: expanding indications and technologies. JAMA 2006;295(7):809–18.

[38] Buxton AE, Lee KL, Hafley GE, et al. Relation of ejection fraction and inducible ventricular tachycardia to mode of death in patients with coronary artery disease. An analysis of patients enrolled in the multicenter unsustained tachycardia trial. Circulation 2002;106(19):2466–72.

[39] Russo AM, Hafley GE, Lee KL, et al. Racial differences in outcome in the multicenter unsustained tachycardia trial (MUSTT): a comparison of whites versus blacks. Circulation 2003;108(1): 67–72.

[40] Moss AJ, Zareba W, Hall WJ, et al. Prophylactic implantation of a defibrillator in patients with myocardial infarction and reduced ejection fraction. N Engl J Med 2002;346(12):877–83.

[41] Wilber DJ, Zareba W, Hall WJ, et al. Time dependence of mortality risk and defibrillator benefit after myocardial infarction. Circulation 2004;109(9): 1082–4.

[42] Goldenberg I, Moss AJ, McNitt S, et al. Time dependence of defibrillator benefit after coronary revascularization in the Multicenter Automatic Defibrillator Implantation Trial (MADIT)-II. J Am Coll Cardiol 2006;47(9):1811–7.

[43] Zareba W, Piotrowicz K, McNitt S, et al. Implantable cardioverter–defibrillator efficacy in patients with heart failure and left ventricular dysfunction (from the MADIT II population). Am J Cardiol 2005;95(12):1487–91.

[44] Goldenberg I, Moss AJ, McNitt S, et al. Relations among renal function, risk of sudden cardiac death, and benefit of the implanted cardiac defibrillator in patients with ischemic left ventricular dysfunction. Am J Cardiol 2006;98(4):485–90.

[45] Pietrasik G, Goldenberg I, McNitt S, et al. Obesity as a risk factor for sustained ventricular tachyarrhythmias in MADIT II patients. J Cardiovasc Electrophysiol 2007;18(2):181–4.

[46] Moss AJ, Greenberg H, Case RB, et al. Long-term clinical course of patients after termination of ventricular tachyarrhythmia by an implanted defibrillator. Circulation 2004;110(25):3760–5.

[47] Singh JP, Hall WJ, McNitt S, et al. Factors influencing appropriate firing of the implanted defibrillator for ventricular tachycardia/fibrillation. J Am Coll Cardiol 2005;46(9):1712–20.

[48] Vorobiof G, Goldenberg I, Moss AJ, et al. Effectiveness of the implantable cardioverter defibrillator in blacks versus whites (from MADIT-II). Am J Cardiol 2006;98(10):1383–6.

[49] Zareba W, Moss AJ, Jackson Hall W, et al. Clinical course of implantable cardioverter defibrillator therapy in postinfarction women with severe left ventricular dysfunction. J Cardiovasc Electrophysiol 2005;16(12):1265–70.

[50] Zwanziger J, Hall WJ, Dick AW, et al. The cost-effectiveness of implantable defibrillators: results from the Multicenter Automatic Defibrillator Implantation Trial (MADIT)-II. J Am Coll Cardiol 2006;47(11):2310–8.

[51] Strickberger SA, Hummel JD, Bartlett TG, et al. Amiodarone versus implantable cardioverter–defibrillator: randomized trial in patients with nonischemic dilated cardiomyopathy and asymptomatic nonsustained ventricular tachycardia-AMIOVIRT. J Am Coll Cardiol 2003;41(10):1707–12.

[52] Bänsch D, Antz M, Boczor S, et al. Primary prevention of sudden death in idiopathic dilated cardiomyopathy: the Cardiomyopathy Trial (CAT). Circulation 2002;105(12):1453–8.

[53] Kadish A, Schaechter A, Subacius H, et al. Prophylactic defibrillator implantation in patients with nonischemic dilated cardiomyopathy. N Engl J Med 2004;350(21):2151–8.

[54] Bardy GH, Lee KL, Mark DB, et al. Amiodarone or an implantable cardioverter–defibrillator for congestive heart failure. N Engl J Med 2005;352(3):225–37.

[55] Mark DB, Nelson CL, Anstrom KJ, et al. Cost-effectiveness of defibrillator therapy or amiodarone in chronic stable heart failure: results from the Sudden Cardiac Death in Heart Failure Trial (SCD-HeFT). Circulation 2006;114(2):135–42.

[56] Singh SN, Poole J, Anderson J, et al. Role of amiodarone or implantable cardioverter defibrillator in patients with atrial fibrillation and heart failure. Am Heart J 2006;152(5):974 e7–11.

[57] Nanthakumar K, Epstein AE, Kay GN, et al. Prophylactic implantable cardioverter defibrillator therapy in patients with left ventricular systolic dysfunction: a pooled analysis of 10 primary prevention trials. J Am Coll Cardiol 2004;44(11):2166–72.

[58] Bigger JT Jr. Prophylactic use of implanted cardiac defibrillators in patients at high risk for ventricular arrhythmias after coronary artery bypass graft surgery. Coronary Artery Bypass Graft (CABG) Patch

Trial Investigators. N Engl J Med 1997;337(22): 1569–75.

[59] Veenhuyzen GD, Singh SN, McAreavey D, et al. Prior coronary artery bypass surgery and risk of death among patients with ischemic left ventricular dysfunction. Circulation 2001;104(13):1489–93.

[60] Hohnloser SH, Kuck KH, Dorian P, et al. Prophylactic use of an implantable cardioverter–defibrillator after acute myocardial infarction. N Engl J Med 2004;351(24):2481–8.

[61] Nolan J, Batin PD, Andrews R, et al. Prospective study of heart rate variability and mortality in chronic heart failure: results of the United Kingdom heart failure evaluation and assessment of risk trial (UK-heart). Circulation 1998;98(15):1510–6.

[62] Healey JS, Toff WD, Lamas GA, et al. Cardiovascular outcomes with atrial-based pacing compared with ventricular pacing: meta-analysis of randomized trials, using individual pacing data. Circulation 2006;114(1):3–5.

[63] Bristow MR, Saxon LA, Boehmer J, et al. Cardiac resynchronization in chronic heart failure. N Engl J Med 2004;350(21):2140–50.

[64] Cleland JG, Daubert JC, Erdmann E, et al. The effect of cardiac resynchronization on morbidity and mortality in heart failure. N Engl J Med 2005; 352(15):1539–49.

[65] Freemantle N, Tharmanathan P, Calvert MJ, et al. Cardiac resynchronisation for patients with heart failure due to left ventricular systolic dysfunction—a systematic review and meta-analysis. Eur J Heart Fail 2006;8(4):433–40.

[66] Higgins SL, Hummel JD, Niazi IK, et al. Cardiac resynchronization therapy for the treatment of heart failure in patients with intraventricular conduction delay and malignant ventricular tachyarrhythmias. J Am Coll Cardiol 2003;42(8):1454–9.

[67] Young JB, Abraham WT, Smith AL, et al. Combined cardiac resynchronization and implantable cardioversion defibrillation in advanced heart failure. The MIRACLE ICD trial. JAMA 2003; 289(20):2685–94.

[68] Cazeau S, Leclercq C, Lavergne T, et al. Effects of multisite biventricular pacing in patients with heart failure and intraventricular conduction delay. N Engl J Med 2001;344(12):873–80.

[69] Leclercq C, Walker S, Linde C, et al. Comparative effects of permanent biventricular and right univentricular pacing in heart failure patients with chronic atrial fibrillation. Eur Heart J 2002; 23(22):1780–7.

[70] Leclercq C, Cazeau S, Lellouche D, et al. Upgrading from right ventricular pacing to biventricular pacing in previously paced patients with advanced heart failure: a randomized controlled study. Pacing Clin Electrophysiol 2007;30(Suppl 1)):S23–30.

[71] Abraham WT, Fisher WG, Smith AL, et al. Cardiac resynchronization therapy with or without an implantable defibrillator in advanced chronic heart failure. N Engl J Med 2002;346(24):1845–53.

ELSEVIER
SAUNDERS

Cardiol Clin 26 (2008) 433–439

CARDIOLOGY
CLINICS

Unresolved Issues in Implantable Cardioverter-Defibrillator Therapy

Pamela K. Mason, MD*, John P. DiMarco, MD, PhD

*Department of Internal Medicine, Cardiovascular Division, PO Box 800158, University of Virginia Health System,
Charlottesville, VA 22908, USA*

Over the last 15 years, a series of well-designed randomized clinical trials has clearly demonstrated that implantable cardioverter-defibrillator (ICD) therapy reduces mortality in select high-risk populations [1,2]. The initial key studies were secondary prevention trials that showed that ICD therapy was superior to antiarrhythmic drug therapy in patients who had survived an episode of sustained ventricular tachycardia or cardiac arrest. Such patients were known to have a high risk for recurrence, and ICD therapy reduced total mortality by 25% to 37%. Subsequently, primary prevention trials that included patients who had ischemic or nonischemic cardiomyopathies showed that ICD implantation lowered mortality by a similar percentage in high-risk patients who did not have a prior history of a sustained arrhythmia. In early 2005, the Centers for Medical and Medicaid Services issued guidelines for ICD implantation [3] that included secondary and primary indications. Well over 140,000 ICDs are now being implanted each year in the United States alone. Despite the widespread acceptance of ICD therapy, many questions related to its optimal use remain (Box 1). This article discusses several key issues now confronting clinicians.

Epidemiology

Although multiple investigators have estimated that there are about 350,000 sudden cardiac deaths in the United States each year, this number may not accurately describe the population that could benefit from ICD therapy because not all these deaths are out-of-hospital deaths that might be prevented by an ICD. According to 1999 data from the Centers for Disease Control and Prevention [4], only about 64% of all cardiac deaths occur out-of-hospital or in a hospital emergency department (Fig. 1). Slightly more than one third of cardiac deaths occur among hospitalized patients. Presumably, many of the patients who died during a hospital stay were being effectively monitored and their deaths were not sudden or unexpected. More recently, the American Heart Association (AHA) estimated that the true incidence of out-of-hospital cardiac arrest is about 0.55/1000 population or 165,000 events annually in the United States [5]. The same AHA statistical report also estimated that about two thirds of unexpected sudden cardiac deaths occur in subjects who do not have prior recognized heart disease. This latter group of victims is an unlikely potential target for an expensive and invasive therapy like an ICD.

Studies have also shown that the age of sudden death victims is increasing and that the proportion of out-of-hospital cardiac arrest victims who have ventricular fibrillation documented by emergency medical teams has decreased significantly [5,6]. Asystole and pulseless electrical activity are now the initial rhythms most commonly recorded. Elderly patients account for a large fraction of the cardiac deaths that occur outside the hospital. In the 1999 data cited previously, over 40% of all emergency room or out-of-hospital cardiac deaths occurred in individuals older than 75 years, with 24% of those older than 85 years (Fig. 2). Although these deaths may be classified as sudden, they may not be unexpected or preventable. These observations suggest that the strategies for increased ICD utilization that are targeted at

---

* Corresponding author.
E-mail address: pkm5f@virginia.edu (P.K. Mason).

individuals identified as being at high or very high
risk will have a relatively small impact from a public health perspective.

Subgroup analysis

Randomized trials are designed to test a hypothesis involving a single or a composite primary
end point that applies to the entire study group.
After the trial has been completed, however, it is
common to examine subgroups to see whether
results from the entire population hold for patients
who have certain clinical characteristics. Subgroup
analysis may be useful for formulating new hy-
potheses that can be tested in future trials, but the
results of such analyses must be interpreted and
applied to individual patients by clinicians with
great caution. Attempts to guide therapy based on
analysis of subgroups from the Sudden Cardiac
Death in Heart Failure Trial (SCD-HeFT) [7] il-
lustrate this problem. The main conclusion of the
SCD-HeFT was that ICD therapy was superior
to placebo and amiodarone for reducing total
mortality in patients who had ischemic or nonischemic cardiomyopathies, class II or class III
heart failure symptoms, and a left ventricular ejection fraction of 0.35 or less. Subgroup analysis,
however, showed that the hazard ratio was not significantly reduced among women, in those who
had an ejection fraction of 0.30 or higher, and in
diabetics. Excluding individuals in these groups
from ICD therapy would be difficult for clinicians
in light of current published guidelines [3]. Subgroup analysis may also give discordant results
when different trials are examined. For example,
in SCD-HeFT, ICD therapy was beneficial in patients who had class II but not class III heart failure symptoms, whereas in the Defibrillators in
Nonischemic Cardiomyopathy Treatment Evaluation trial [8], most of the benefit with ICD therapy
observed was in the class III subgroup. Women did
not benefit in SCD-HeFT but did in the Multicenter Defibrillator Implantation Trial II (MADIT-
II) [9]. Most studies are statistically designed to
have adequate power to test the primary hypothesis only in the entire study group. Observations
made in subgroups may be thought provoking
but are rarely convincing enough to warrant clinical decisions contrary to the overall result.

Antiarrhythmic drug therapy

Some argue that antiarrhythmic drug therapy
should not be used in the era of ICD therapy. The
major secondary and primary intervention trials
compared ICD therapy to antiarrhythmic drug
therapy or to no therapy. In the secondary prevention trials, patients in whom antiarrhythmic
drugs were believed necessary to control frequent
or recurrent arrhythmias were excluded. In clinical
practice, however, antiarrhythmic drugs are frequently required. Several studies have now shown
that the use of antiarrhythmic drugs decreases
ICD shock frequency and may thus make long-
term ICD therapy more acceptable [10–12]. An example can be seen in the Optimal Pharmacological
Therapy in Cardioverter Defibrillator Patients
trial [10], in which therapy with sotalol and amiodarone plus a β-blocker produced significant reductions in ICD shocks. Similar data have been

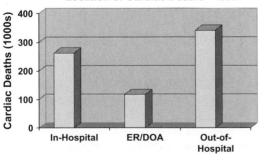

Fig. 1. Cardiac deaths in the United States during 1999
by location as compiled by the Centers for Disease Control and Prevention. ER/DOA, death in or on arrival to
the emergency room. (*Data from* Center for Disease
Control and Prevention. State-specific mortality from
sudden cardiac death—United States, 1999. MMWR
Morb Mortal Wkly Rep 2002;51(6);123–6.)

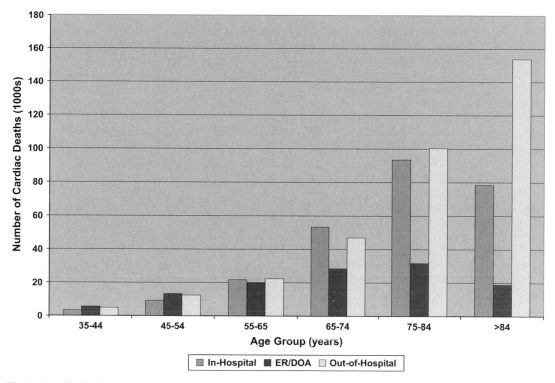

Fig. 2. Age distribution of cardiac deaths in the United States during 1999 as compiled by the Centers for Disease Control and Prevention. ER/DOA, death in or on arrival to the emergency room. (*Data from* Center for Disease Control and Prevention. State-specific mortality from sudden cardiac death—United States, 1999. MMWR Morb Mortal Wkly Rep 2002;51(6);123–6.)

reported for sotalol [11] and azimilide [12]. Thus, many patients, particularly those who receive an ICD for secondary prevention or who require ICD therapy for ventricular tachycardia or ventricular fibrillation after an implant for a primary prevention indication, would benefit from the careful prescription of an antiarrhythmic drug.

Comorbidities

Patients entered in clinical trials are not always representative of the patients encountered by clinicians, of whom many have multiple coexisting diseases [13]. The presence of coexisting disease is rarely mentioned in ICD clinical guidelines [14] beyond a general admonition not to implant unless the patient has a "reasonable expectation of survival with a good functional status for more than 1 year." Some studies specifically exclude patients who have certain high-risk characteristics. For example, the MADIT-II [9] excluded all patients who had moderately severe renal insufficiency. Studies are also often affected by "pre-enrollment" bias because investigators select patients who they

think will be "good" and reliable candidates for the study. These patients tend to be healthier and less complicated than many patients seen in everyday clinical practice who might be difficult to follow according to a strict trial protocol.

Advanced age is perhaps the most important factor that is not taken into consideration by published guidelines. In the published primary and secondary ICD prevention trials, the mean age for enrollees was between 58 and 64 years [1,2,14]. Although they were not specifically excluded, relatively few patients older than 80 years were enrolled. In contrast, recent data from the ICD Registry compiled by the National Cardiovascular Data Registry show that 15% of all ICD recipients are older than 80 years, and an additional 16% are between 75 and 79 years old [15]. Other studies have shown that the ratio of sudden to non–sudden deaths declines steeply as the age range of subjects increases [16,17]. This finding limits any potential benefit of an ICD in this age range despite the fact that even very elderly patients would still be considered candidates by guideline criteria.

Other groups have begun to study the impact of comorbidities on the value of ICD therapy. Parkash and colleagues [18] reviewed survival data from a large ICD database from a single institution. These investigators devised a scoring system that included the following risk factors: age 80 years or older (2 points), ejection fraction less than 0.30, atrial fibrillation, creatinine greater than 1.8 mg/dL, and class III or IV heart failure symptoms. Patients who had risk scores of 1 or 2 had low mortality with ICD therapy but patients who had risk scores of 3 or greater had high 6-month and 1-year death rates. In a retrospective analysis of all ICD recipients in Ontario, Canada, Lee and colleagues [19] showed that age, heart failure, peripheral vascular disease, pulmonary disease, diabetes with complications, renal disease, and malignancy all independently had an adverse effect on survival in ICD recipients. In an analysis of the MADIT-II database, Goldenberg and colleagues [20] identified five risk factors for all-cause mortality: advanced heart failure symptoms, atrial fibrillation, QRS duration greater than 120 milliseconds, age greater than 70 years, and blood urea nitrogen level between 27 and 50 mg/dL (Table 1). A small group of patients who had more advanced renal disease was separately classified as "very high risk." Patients who had no risk factors had no improvement in survival with ICD therapy. Patients who had three or more risk factors and the very high risk group also had no improvement in survival with an ICD. These findings resulted in what the investigators described as a U-shaped curve for ICD efficacy.

As cardiologists and electrophysiologists deal with increasingly elderly patients who have

Table 1
Risk factors for all-cause mortality in the Multicenter Defibrillator Implantation Trial II

Risk factor	HR (95% CI)	P
NYHA functional class > II	1.87 (1.23–2.86)	.004
Atrial fibrillation at baseline	1.87 (1.05–3.22)	.034
QRS > 120 ms	1.65 (1.08–2.51)	.020
Age > 70 y	1.57 (1.02–2.41)	.042
BUN 26–50 mg/dL	1.56 (1.00–2.42)	.048

Abbreviations: BUN, blood urea nitrogen; CI, confidence interval; HR, hazard ratio; NYHA, New York Heart Association.
From Goldenberg I, Vyas AK, Hall WJ, et al for the MADIT-II Investigators. Risk stratification for primary implantation of a cardioverter-defibrillator in patients with ischemic left ventricular dysfunction. J Am Coll Cardiol 2008;51:292; with permission.

multiple concomitant diseases, they will need to realize that guidelines based on clinical trials should not be employed without first carefully considering all the factors that might influence the treatment decision in that individual patient. In many cases, comorbid conditions will limit any potential benefit from an ICD implant, and the risks and costs of the procedure may be avoided. This principle should also apply to decisions regarding elective ICD generator replacements for battery depletion because changes in the patients' condition may now make them unsuitable candidates for continued ICD therapy. As recently reported by Hauptman and colleagues [21], however, few physicians discuss these issues with their patients, even if they agree with the general principle.

Cardiac resynchronization therapy with or without an implantable defibrillator

Prior the release of large cardiac resynchronization therapy (CRT) trials, defibrillator therapy was contraindicated in patients who had class IV heart failure except as a bridge to transplant. This group of patients has such high morbidity and mortality from heart failure–related complications that defibrillators have not been shown to improve survival. In addition, these patients are prone to excess complications from defibrillator therapy, including inappropriate shocks and device infections [22].

The COMPANION trial compared treatment strategies for patients who had severe heart failure [23]. Patients were randomly assigned to receive medical therapy, a CRT device, or a CRT device with a defibrillator (CRT-D). The primary combined end point of time to hospitalization and mortality from any cause was substantially improved in the group receiving CRT-D. This end point was also statistically improved in patients receiving CRT alone. The secondary end point of time to death from any cause was not statistically different between the CRT group and the medication group, but there was a trend toward the CRT group having decreased time to death, and the CRT-D group had a clear decreased time to death. The patients in the CRT and CRT-D groups experienced improved quality of life over those on medication alone.

In a subgroup of patients who had ambulatory class IV symptoms, the CRT-D group had a significant reduction in time to sudden death [24]; however, the CRT and CRT-D groups experienced similar reduction in time to death or hospitalization for any cause. Both groups also experienced similar reduction in time to death from any cause and heart failure hospitalization.

The Cardiac Resynchronization–Heart Failure (CARE-HF) study had even more dramatic findings [25]. This study evaluated patients who had class III or IV heart failure and either a QRS greater than 150 milliseconds or, if the QRS was between 120 and 149 milliseconds, echocardiographic evidence of dyssynchrony. The patients were randomized to receive medical therapy or CRT using a pacemaker with defibrillation capacity. There was a substantial decrease in total mortality in the patients who received CRT. The mortality was 55% in the medication group versus 39% for the CRT group over a mean of 29.4 months of follow-up. This benefit continued to be seen over long-term follow-up [26].

These findings altered the indications for defibrillator therapy. Patients who have end-stage heart failure have high mortality from causes other than ventricular arrhythmias, and these patients derive questionable benefit from defibrillators; however, if CRT can improve the morbidity and possibly the mortality in class IV congestive heart failure, then defibrillator therapy seems to be more reasonable. Current guidelines still define class IV heart failure as a contraindication for defibrillator therapy unless the patient is receiving a CRT device. Essentially, by guidelines, virtually any patient who is receiving a CRT device also qualifies for a defibrillator. But does that mean that every patient who receives a CRT device should get a defibrillator?

Although guidelines suggest that every patient who gets a CRT device also qualifies for a defibrillator, these studies raise several important issues. CRT alone may have antiarrhythmic properties. Defibrillators are substantially larger than biventricular pacemakers, and patients who have class IV heart failure are often elderly, thin, and relatively immune incompetent. They have higher risk for erosion and infection of the device. Patients who have defibrillators are also at risk for inappropriate shocks. In contrast, implantation of coronary sinus left ventricular leads in the CARE-HF study had a low risk for complications [27]. It is possible that the added complication rate of defibrillators offsets any incremental benefit over CRT alone.

The cost differential between CRT and CRT-D is also substantial. One study of the long-term cost-effectiveness of CRT versus CRT-D found that both were cost effective [28]; however, CRT-D was only moderately cost-effective compared with CRT plus medication and only in patients who had a life expectancy of at least several years.

At this point, it seems best to evaluate patients who have end-stage heart failure for CRT versus CRT-D devices on a case-by-case basis, taking into account clinical history and patient preferences. There are still not enough data to determine which groups of patients benefit the most from CRT and the incremental benefit incurred by the addition of a defibrillator. Until further data become available, these decisions will need to be made on an individual basis.

Device malfunctions

The number of patients who have ICDs has dramatically increased over the last several years. Concomitantly, the number of patients having a device that is recalled or that malfunctions has increased. The numbers of ICD recalls and malfunctions have proportionally increased more than would be expected compared with pacemaker malfunctions. One recent meta-analysis of device registries demonstrated a 20-fold higher incidence of ICD failure compared with pacemakers [29].

There are multiple reasons for this finding. ICD technology is much newer than pacemaker technology and far more complex. The expanding competitive market has also led to a "short product life cycle" in which new innovations are being developed and implemented at a rapid pace. Finally, there may be a lower threshold for ICD recalls than pacemaker recalls because an acute ICD malfunction has a greater potential to cause death.

Most device malfunctions are not due to recall-related failures. Most malfunctions are due to random component failures. Currently, there is no ICD ever marketed that has a malfunction rate lower than 0.1%. Recent data suggest that 2% of all implanted defibrillators are removed due to malfunction [30]. ICD leads have an even more striking failure rate. A long-term study of ICD leads showed a 20% failure rate at 10 years of follow-up [31]. This observation should be particularly concerning for younger patients who might have the potential for multiple lead failures during their lifetime.

Most devices that are recalled by the manufacturer never malfunction, but large numbers of patients are affected in a recall. In 2000, there were only two ICD advisories, but over 20,000 patients were affected [32]. Recalls present unique issues for physicians and patients. Due to widespread media coverage of the more recent device recalls, patients are more aware of the potential for device recalls but often do not have a sophisticated understanding of what a recall means. Most recalls do not require the device to be explanted because the risk of malfunction may be small or substantially mitigated by programming changes or closer device follow-up; however, it is unsettling to many patients to have a "defective" device, and many of them will want a new one. The difficulty with this is that explanting and replacing a device has a significant complication rate. One study of patients who had device explants for recall-related issues showed a major complication rate of 6%, with a postoperative mortality rate of 0.4%. The control subjects, who did not have their recalled devices explanted, had an advisory-related complication rate of 0.1% [33].

Review of device registries over the last several years suggests that the numbers of ICD malfunctions and recalls is stabilizing somewhat after a marked increase in prior years [29]. Nonetheless, with the substantial increase in device implants, a single recall affects a large number of patients, and even if the number of malfunctions decline, it is still significant. It is important for implanting centers to have the resources available to evaluate patients who have recalled devices and to address their concerns appropriately.

Summary

ICD therapy is a powerful intervention with a clear ability to prolong life. Few other therapies are able to reduce mortality by 20% to 30% when added to standard treatment in well-managed patients. As discussed, however, the answers to questions regarding the optimal use of ICD are not contained in results of clinical trials. Careful clinical judgment is still required to use this powerful tool wisely.

References

[1] Al-Khatib SM, Sanders GD, Mark DB, et al. Expert panel participating in a Duke Clinical Research Institute-sponsored conference. Implantable cardioverter defibrillators and cardiac resynchronization therapy in patients with left ventricular dysfunction: randomized trial evidence through 2004. Am Heart J 2005;149:1020–34.

[2] Ezekowitz JA, Rowe BH, Dryden DM, et al. Systematic review: implantable cardioverter defibrillators for adults with left ventricular systolic dysfunction. Ann Intern Med 2007;147:251–62.

[3] CMS Manual System. Pub. 100–03 Medicare National Coverage Determinations. Department of Health & Human Services (DHHS). Centers for Medical & Medicaid Services (CMS). Implantable Automatic Defibrillators. Transmittal 29. March 4, 2005.

[4] Center for Disease Control and Prevention. State-specific mortality from sudden cardiac death—United States, 1999. MMWR Morb Mortal Wkly Rep 2002;51(6):123–6.

[5] Rosamond W, Flegal K, Friday G, et al. American Heart Association Statistics Committee and Stroke Statistics Subcommittee. Heart disease and stroke statistics—2007 update: a report from the American Heart Association Statistics Committee and Stroke Statistics Subcommittee. Circulation 2007;115: e69–171.

[6] Cobb LA, Fahrenbruch CE, Olsufka M, et al. Changing incidence of out-of-hospital ventricular fibrillation, 1980–2000. JAMA 2002;288:3008–13.

[7] Bardy GH, Lee KL, Mark DB, et al. Sudden Cardiac Death in Heart Failure Trial (SCD-HeFT) Investigators. Amiodarone or an implantable cardioverter-defibrillator for congestive heart failure. N Engl J Med 2005;352:225–37.

[8] Kadish A, Dyer A, Daubert JP, et al. Defibrillators in Non-Ischemic Cardiomyopathy Treatment Evaluation (DEFINITE) Investigators. Prophylactic defibrillator implantation in patients with nonischemic dilated cardiomyopathy. N Engl J Med 2004;350: 2151–8.

[9] Moss AJ, Zareba W, Hall WJ, et al. Multicenter Automatic Defibrillator Implantation Trial II investigators. Prophylactic implantation of a defibrillator in patients with myocardial infarction and reduced ejection fraction. N Engl J Med 2002;346: 877–83.

[10] Hohnloser SH, Dorian P, Roberts R, et al. Effect of amiodarone and sotalol on ventricular defibrillation threshold: the Optimal Pharmacological Therapy In Cardioverter Defibrillator Patients (OPTIC) trial. Circulation 2006;114:104–9.

[11] Pacifico A, Hohnloser SH, Williams JH, et al. Prevention of implantable-defibrillator shocks by treatment with sotalol. d, l-Sotalol Implantable Cardioverter-Defibrillator Study Group. N Engl J Med 1999;340:1855–62.

[12] Dorian P, Borggrefe M, Al-Khalidi HR, et al, SHock Inhibition Evaluation with azimiLiDe (SHIELD) Investigators. Placebo-controlled, randomized clinical trial of azimilide for prevention of ventricular tachyarrhythmias in patients with an implantable cardioverter defibrillator. Circulation 2004;110:3646–54.

[13] Dhruva SS, Redberg RF. Variations between clinical trial participants and Medicare beneficiaries in evidence used for Medicare national coverage decisions. Arch Intern Med 2008;168:136–40.

[14] Zipes DP, Camm AJ, Smith SC, et al. ACC/AHA/ESC practice guidelines—executive summary. ACC/AHA/ESC 2006 guidelines for management of patients with ventricular arrhythmias and the prevention of sudden cardiac death – executive summary. A report of the American College of Cardiology/American Heart Association Task Force and the European Society of Cardiology Committee for Practice Guidelines (writing committee to develop guidelines for management of patients with ventricular arrhythmias and the prevention of sudden cardiac death) developed in collaboration with the European Heart Rhythm Association and the Heart Rhythm Society. J Am Coll Cardiol 2006;48:1064–108.

[15] Hammill SC, Stevenson LW, Kadish AH, et al. Review of the registry's first year, data collected, and future plans. Heart Rhythm 2007;4:1260–3.

[16] Krahn AD, Connolly SJ, Roberts RS, et al. Diminishing proportional risk of sudden death with advancing age: implications for prevention of sudden death. Am Heart J 2004;147:837–40.

[17] Stecker EC, Vickers C, Waltz J, et al. Population-based analysis of sudden cardiac death with and without left ventricular systolic dysfunction: two-year findings from the Oregon Sudden Unexpected Death Study. J Am Coll Cardiol 2006;47:1161–6.

[18] Parkash R, Stevenson WG, Epstein LM, et al. Predicting early mortality after implantable defibrillator implantation: a clinical risk score for optimal patient selection. Am Heart J 2006;151:397–403.

[19] Lee DS, Tu JV, Austin PC, et al. Effect of cardiac and noncardiac conditions on survival after defibrillator implantation. J Am Coll Cardiol 2007;49:2408–15.

[20] Goldenberg I, Vyas AK, Hall WJ, et al. Risk stratification for primary implantation of a cardioverter-defibrillator in patients with ischemic left ventricular dysfunction. J Am Coll Cardiol 2008;51:288–96.

[21] Hauptman PJ, Swindle J, Hussain Z, et al. Physician attitudes toward end-stage heart failure: a national Survey. Am J Med 2008;121:127–35.

[22] Tsai V, Chen H, Hsia H, et al. Cardiac device infections complicated by erosion. J Interv Card Electrophysiol 2007;19:133–7.

[23] Bristow MR, Saxon LA, Boehmer J, et al. Cardiac-resynchronization therapy with or without an implantable defibrillator in advanced chronic heart failure. N Engl J Med 2004;350:2140–50.

[24] Lindenfeld J, Feldman AM, Saxon L, et al. Effects of cardiac resynchronization therapy with or without a defibrillator on survival and hospitalizations in patients with New York Heart Association class IV heart failure. Circulation 2007;115:204–12.

[25] Cleland JG, Daubert J-C, Erdmann E, et al. The effect of cardiac resynchronization on morbidity and mortality in heart failure. N Engl J Med 2005;352:1539–49.

[26] Cleland JG, Daubert J-C, Erdmann E, et al. Longer-term effects of cardiac resynchronization therapy on mortality in heart failure [the Cardiac Resynchronization–Heart Failure (CARE-HF) trial extension phase]. Eur Heart J 2006;27:1928–32.

[27] Gras D, Docker D, Lunati M, et al. Implantation of cardiac resynchronization therapy systems in the CARE-HF trial: procedural success rate and safety. Europace 2007;9:516–22.

[28] Yao G, Freemantle N, Calvert MJ, et al. The long-term cost-effectiveness of cardiac resynchronization therapy with or without an implantable cardioverter-defibrillator. Euro H J 2007;28:42–51.

[29] Maisel WH. Pacemaker and ICD generator reliability. JAMA 2006;295:1929–34.

[30] Maisel WH, Moynahan M, Zuckerman BD, et al. Pacemaker and ICD generator malfunctions: analysis of Food and Drug Administration annual reports. JAMA 2006;295:1901 6.

[31] Kleemann T, Becker T, Doenges K, et al. Annual rate of transvenous defibrillation lead defects in implantable cardioverter-defibrillators over a period of >10 years. Circulation 2007;115:2474–80.

[32] Maisel WH, Sweeney MO, Stevenson WG, et al. Recalls and safety alerts involving pacemakers and implantable cardioverter-defibrillator generators. JAMA 2001;286:793–9.

[33] Gould PA, Krahn AD, Canadian Heart Rhythm Society Working Group on Device Advisories. Complications associated with implantable cardioverter-defibrillator replacement in response to device advisories. JAMA 2006;26:1907–11.

Problems with Implantable Cardiac Device Therapy

Marcin Kowalski, MD[a], Jose F. Huizar, MD[a,b], Karoly Kaszala, MD, PhD[a,b], Mark A. Wood, MD[a,*]

[a]Department of Cardiac Electrophysiology Service, Virginia Commonwealth University Medical Center, PO Box 980053, Richmond, VA 23298-0053, USA
[b]Department of Cardiac Electrophysiology Service, Hunter Holmes McGuire VA Medical Center, 1201 Broad Rock Boulevard, Richmond, VA 23249, USA

Implantable cardioverter-defibrillators (ICDs) are known to improve survival in patients who have left ventricular dysfunction. Nevertheless, ICD implantation is associated with numerous problems at implant and during follow-up. At implant, acute surgical complications, including pneumothorax, vascular perforation, hematoma, and acute lead dislodgement, occur in approximately 2% to 4% of patients. The diagnosis and management of these problems is usually straightforward. More difficult problems at implant include the management of patients who have elevated energy requirements to terminate ventricular fibrillation (VF) or of those who have postoperative device infections. Long-term issues in ICD patients include the occurrence of inappropriate or frequent appropriate shocks. Finally, ICD generators and leads are more prone to failures than are pacing systems alone. The management of patients potentially dependent on "recalled" devices to deliver life-saving therapy is a particularly complex issue involving competing risks. The purpose of this article is to review the diagnosis and management of these more troublesome ICD problems.

Defibrillation threshold

Due to the need for ICD reliability to terminate life-threatening arrhythmias, it is common practice to induce VF to ensure appropriate sensing, detection, and defibrillation during ICD

implantation. The success of defibrillation depends on the relationship between the spatial and temporal characteristics of the electrical field of the ICD shock (distribution of potential gradients) and the VF (critical regions or wave fronts). After an ICD shock, according to the critical mass hypothesis, the entire myocardium must be depolarized to establish a critical spatial electrical gradient to terminate VF. Thus, failure of an ICD to defibrillate maybe due failure to achieve this gradient due to inadequate shock waveform, shock vector, or delivered energy [1].

Successful defibrillation is probabilistic in nature, likely due to the spatial and temporal heterogeneities of ventricular myocardium during VF. Defibrillation threshold (DFT) is commonly defined as the minimum shock energy required to terminate VF. Although the term *threshold* is used, clinically, there is no single energy level above which defibrillation is always successful or an energy level below which it always fails. Instead, any given level of energy has a probability of defibrillating the heart [1]. DFT testing is commonly performed with a step-down protocol, which consists of reducing in a step-down fashion the delivered energy with each VF induction until a shock fails to defibrillate. The lowest delivered energy shock that successfully defibrillated VF is termed the DFT. This energy will, on average, achieve a 70% success rate of defibrillation (DFT_{70}), whereas twice the DFT energy will obtain a 98% successful defibrillation [2]. Due to the complexity of DFT protocols, a common practice is to perform two VF inductions with defibrillation energy 10 J below the maximum

* Corresponding author.
E-mail address: mwoodmd@pol.net (M.A. Wood).

device delivery output, thereby establishing at least a 10-J defibrillation safety margin. Thus, successful defibrillation is achieved in 96% when ICD is programmed at maximum delivery output [2].

A practical alternative to potentially avoid VF induction during DFT testing is to use the upper limit of vulnerability (ULV) test. The ULV is defined as the lowest energy shock that does not induce VF when delivered during the vulnerable phase of ventricular repolarization. The ULV hypothesis of defibrillation links the ULV to the minimum shock strength that defibrillates VF reliably. The ULV has been shown to be a surrogate for DFT. A shock delivered at the ULV plus 5 J has been shown to consistently defibrillate VF [3], reaching a near DFT_{100}. Thus, a 5-J vulnerability safety margin between the ULV and the maximum device delivery shock has been suggested as an acceptable end point during ICD testing [4]. Some clinicians have not accepted inductionless ICD testing because the ULV lacks the confirmation of appropriate VF sensing by the device and occasional large discrepancies exist between the ULV and DFT in individual patients.

DFT testing is considered overall safe and rarely associated with serious complications such as myocardial stunning, cerebral hypoperfusion, intractable VF, pulseless electrical activity, and death. Predictors of high morbidity and mortality during DFT testing include multiple VF inductions, advanced heart failure, and severe left ventricular dysfunction [5–7]. Although no clinical data are published, the authors believe that patients who have severe pulmonary hypertension may carry a high morbidity and mortality during DFT testing.

Successful defibrillation requirements for VF can vary on a daily basis. Several conditions are known to affect DFT, such as electrolyte and acid-base disturbances, hypoxemia, heart failure, sympathetic tone, and drugs (Box 1) [5,7]. Therefore, DFT testing should be performed in stable and ideal conditions. Reversible causes and predictors of high DFT (see Box 1), if present, should be addressed before testing. The intraoperative mortality and morbidity rates during a transvenous ICD implantation have been estimated to be 0.1% and 1.2%, respectively [6,8]. DFT testing is overall contraindicated in the setting of high-risk features such as hemodynamic instability and left atrial or ventricular thrombus (Box 2) [5,7].

High DFT refers to the clinical scenario in which the ICD is unable to consistently defibrillate with an adequate safety margin. The medical literature usually refers to high DFT when the

---

Box 1. Causes and predictors of high defibrillation threshold

Causes of high defibrillation threshold
Intrinsic myocardial process
  Electrolyte or acid-base disturbance
  Hypoxemia
  Heart failure
Inadequate vector of shock
  Poor shock lead placement
  Shunting current between coils
High shock voltage impedance
  Pneumothorax/chronic obstructive
    pulmonary disease[a]
  Defective connection or loose setscrew
Suboptimal shock waveform
  Excessively long pulse duration
    reinitiates VF
  Excessively short duration truncates
    energy delivery
  Inadequate second phase reinitiates
    VF
  Waveform mismatch with time
    constant of membrane electrical
    response
Drugs
  Antiarrhythmics: amiodarone,
    mexiletine
  Cocaine or illicit drug use
  Other: fentanyl, isoflurane, halothane,
    sildenafil[a], venlafaxine
Other
  Inactive epicardial patches[a]

Predictors of high defibrillation threshold
Amiodarone use
Heart failure class III/IV
Severe left ventricular dysfunction
  and dilatation
Body size
Prolonged DFT testing
History of cocaine use

---

[a] Controversial or limited data.

---

defibrillation safety margin is less than 10 J. The reported prevalence of high DFT has ranged from 5% to 10% [5,7]. One prospective study [7], however, did not find a higher mortality at 6-month follow-up in patients who had high DFT (>18 J).

Several causes of high DFT (see Box 1) are considered reversible and should be treated before

Box 2. Contraindications for defibrillation threshold testing

Left atrial or ventricular thrombus
Severe coronary artery stenosis
Absence of anesthesia
Recent stroke or transient ischemic event
Atrial fibrillation without adequate
    anticoagulation[a]
Hemodynamic instability
Critical aortic stenosis[a]
Severe pulmonary hypertension[a]

––––––––––
[a] Relative contraindication.

testing. Known predictors of high DFT include (1) amiodarone therapy, (2) New York Heart Association class III/IV heart failure, (3) severe left ventricular systolic dysfunction or dilatation, (4) nonischemic cardiomyopathy or no previous history of bypass surgery, (5) device upgrade or replacement, (6) older age, (7) body size, and (8) prolonged device implantation time [6,7,9]. Right-sided and abdominal implants have not been shown to be independent predictors of high DFT; however, they have a higher average DFT compared with left-sided implants [9]. The Optimal Pharmacological Therapy in Cardioverter Defibrillator Patients trial [10], a randomized controlled study, corroborated that amiodarone significantly increased the DFT ($+1.29 \pm 4.39$ J) compared with small a decrease of the DFT with β-blocker agents (-1.64 ± 3.54 J on β-blockers and -0.87 ± 3.78 J on sotalol). All patients on amiodarone, however, achieved an appropriate defibrillation safety margin and experienced no effect on outcome. In addition, this trial clarified that carvedilol and other β-blockers do not increase DFT as previously reported [5].

Current ICDs with proper lead implantation can reliably defibrillate most patients successfully. Due to advances in lead technology and defibrillators, appropriate defibrillation safety margins are usually obtained without the need to modify the ICD system. In addition, no difference in long-term mortality has been demonstrated in patients who have high DFT (<10-J safety margin) and who require ICD modification [9]. Moreover, some devices may still result in effective defibrillation despite an inadequate safety margin at implant due to the probabilistic nature of DFT

[2]. Therefore, recent debate has arisen questioning the true need for ICD testing [8,9].

The authors strongly believe that it is important to perform ICD testing during implantation or generator replacement, particularly in patients who have clear predictors of high DFT (see Box 1). Besides, the medicolegal implications of failure to defibrillate or unexplained death in patients who have ICD is important. Patients who have high DFTs could be identified with minimal ICD testing involving one or two VF inductions. Advances in technology and the understanding of VF and defibrillation have led to different interventions that can address the problem of high DFTs (see Box 2). The potential advantages of lowering DFT are (1) a further decrease in size of devices, (2) an increase of device longevity, and (3) shorter charge and shock delivery times.

Approach to high defibrillation thresholds

Invasive and noninvasive interventions can be made to improve defibrillation energy requirements. All interventions are intended to optimize shock configuration or vector, with subsequent improvement in defibrillation outcome. Invasive interventions are performed during ICD implantation and obviously carry a higher morbidity, whereas the noninvasive interventions can be performed in patients at implantation or during follow-up. Fig. 1 describes a suggested algorithm to approach high DFTs based on current clinical evidence for new ICD implants and chronic devices.

When high DFT and high shock impedance are noted during implantation, it is important that pneumothorax and a defective connection or a loose setscrew of the shocking coil always be excluded [5]. Invasive interventions include (1) the repositioning of right ventricular lead in an apical-septal location; (2) the use of a high-output device; (3) the addition of coils (superior vena cava [SVC], subclavian, axillary, azygous vein, and coronary sinus) and subcutaneous (SQ) arrays; and (4) alternative right ventricular coil locations such as right ventricular outflow tract.

One of the best initial interventions to lower DFTs is to reposition the right ventricular lead to a more apical-septal position, particularly if a basal position was achieved initially [5]. The most easy and straightforward approach to high DFTs is to replace the standard energy output device with a high-output energy device (maximum energy stored of 35–40 J). Even though

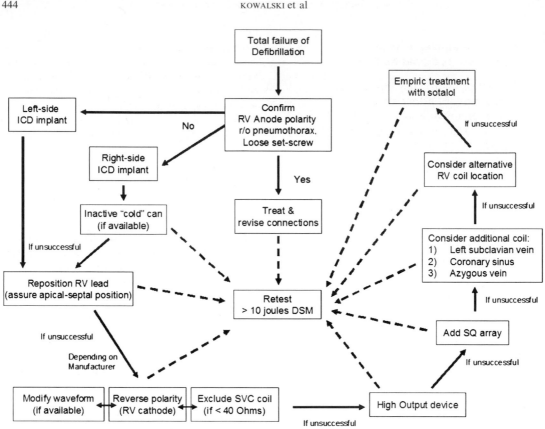

Fig. 1. Approach to high defibrillation threshold. DSM, defibrillation safety margin; RV, right ventricle; SQ, subcutaneous array; SVC, superior vena cava. (*Adapted from* Mainigi SK, Callans DJ. How to manage the patient with a high defibrillation threshold. Heart Rhythm 2006;3:45; with permission.)

a high-output device as a first option is not unreasonable, the use of a high-output device alone does not achieve an adequate safety margin in 48% of cases [9]. In addition, these devices are more expensive. Thus, the authors believe that this should not be the first option unless there is a circumstance that forces the surgeon to finish the case in a prompt manner.

The addition of coils is intended to improve the defibrillation vector, with subsequent reduction in DFTs. The SVC coils and SQ arrays have proved to lower DFTs, with few complications [11,12]. The SVC coil appears to significantly reduce defibrillation requirements, lower the percentage of high DFTs, lower shock impedance, and increase peak current, regardless of position of the SVC coil [11]. Moreover, the SQ arrays further decrease mean DFT by 4 J compared with SVC coils [12]. Other coils have limited data, such as inferior vena cava, left subclavian, brachiocephalic and azygous vein, and coronary sinus [5]. Epicardial patches appear to have lower DFTs than

transvenous systems; however, these are frequently associated with lead failure, constrictive pericarditis, and patch crinkling [13].

Noninvasive interventions include (1) reverse shock polarity, (2) waveform tilt and pulse width optimization, (3) electronic exclusion of SVC, (4) "cold can" or exclusion of can, and (5) drugs known to decrease DFTs. It is unfortunate that some approaches are manufacturer specific and not always available.

Anodal right ventricular polarity decreases DFT by 15% and up to 31% in patients who have a DFT greater than 15 J [1,5]. Over the past few years, most ICD manufacturers have changed and adopted right ventricular coil anode polarity based on clinical data. Even though anodal right ventricular polarity has better defibrillation outcome, occasionally reverse polarity (cathode right ventricular polarity) may help to lower DFT and reach an acceptable safety margin. This recommendation, however, is based solely on sporadic cases.

The presence of an SVC coil (right ventricular dual-coil leads) or an SQ array makes it possible to exclude the can as part of the cathode to limit the delivered shock between anodal right ventricular coil and cathodal SVC coil, or so-called "cold can." This methodology can improve DFTs, particularly in patients who have right-sided implants. This feature, however, is only available from specific ICD manufacturers.

Occasionally, electronic exclusion of SVC may be helpful to reach an appropriate defibrillation safety margin, especially when shock impedance is below 40 Ω [5]. Exclusion of the SVC can be performed by some manufacturers by way of software.

Shock optimization is performed by modifying the percentage-voltage delivered (tilt-based waveform) or the pulse width (fixed-duration waveform) in each phase of the biphasic shock. This feature is limited to a few ICD manufacturers. Most studies concur that shorter 42/42% and 50/50% tilt waveforms decrease DFTs by 15% to 25% compared with 65/65% tilt waveforms; however, other studies have not found similar results. Fixed-duration waveforms based on high-voltage impedance appear to reduce DFT by 20% to 30% versus tilt-based waveforms [1].

Finally, an important step to improve DFTs is the discontinuation of medications known to increase DFTs (see Box 1) or the addition of drugs such as sotalol that may improve DFT [10], or both. Sotalol may have a modest effect, decreasing DFT by 1 to 1.5 J in the overall ICD population. It is surprising that even though class III antiarrhythmics (except amiodarone) have been used to decrease DFTs, there have been no randomized controlled trials to assess their effectiveness in achieving appropriate safety margins in patients who have high DFTs.

The understanding of VF and the new ICD technology has decreased the energy requirements and improved the outcome of defibrillation during VF. A few patients, however, still require high-energy shocks to restore normal cardiac rhythm. By combining all these interventions, most centers can achieve an acceptable safety margin in most patients (85%) who have high DFTs [5].

Appropriate implantable cardioverter-defibrillator shocks and electrical storm

The incidence of appropriate ICD shocks is approximately 5% per year for primary prevention devices [14] and approximately 20% to 60% per year for secondary prevention devices [15,16]. ICD therapies are frequent in patients who have advanced heart failure, reaching a 20% to 40% incidence at 6 months after implant [17]. The incidence of appropriate shocks in secondary prevention patients is reduced post implant by prophylactic use of amiodarone combined with a β-blocker, with a trend toward reduction by sotalol [15]. Each ICD shock measurably reduces patient quality of life, with the cumulative effect becoming clinically significant after five or more shocks received [18]. When the frequency of ICD therapies becomes problematic, aggressive antitachycardia pacing, antiarrhythmic drug therapy (typically amiodarone or sotalol), or radiofrequency ablation are therapeutic options.

The long-term temporal patterns of ventricular arrhythmias in ICD patients are nonrandom and clustered in more than 80% of patients who have recurrent arrhythmias. The recurrence pattern can be described by a Weibull distribution [19]. The time between consecutive arrhythmic episodes is less than 1 hour for 78% of events and less than 91 hours for 94% of events [19]. After ICD therapies, patients may experience long periods of quiescence, making decisions about the necessity and efficacy of new therapies difficult. The statistical methodology in clinical trials should take into consideration the nonrandom pattern of arrhythmia recurrences [16].

Electrical storm is arbitrarily defined as two or more or three or more appropriate ICD therapies (shock or antitachycardia pacing) delivered within a 24-hour period. This pattern occurs in 10% to 20% of ICD patients. The recurrent arrhythmia is usually monomorphic ventricular tachycardia (VT), and hundreds of shocks can be delivered during a "storm." The causes of electrical storm are numerous (Box 3), but in approximately two thirds of cases, no clear etiology can be identified [20,21]. Approximately one third of cases are attributed to acute ischemia, decompensated heart failure, or metabolic disturbances [20,21]. Predictors of electrical storm include monomorphic VT as the indication for ICD implant, left ventricular ejection fraction less than 25%, chronic renal failure, QRS greater than 120 milliseconds, digoxin use, coronary artery disease, and absence of β-blocker therapy [20–23].

Electrical storm with multiple ICD shocks should be considered a medical emergency. The first goal is to suppress the arrhythmia to prevent further shock deliveries. Treatment should percentage of patients, perhaps reflecting the sporadic and self-limiting clustering of events [20,21]. Other common therapies include treatment of heart failure, revascularization, ICD reprogramming, and correction of metabolic derangements. Refractory cases occasionally require emergent radiofrequency ablation to eliminate the responsible arrhythmia.

Although death during an episode of electrical storm is rare, some studies have demonstrated increased mortality in the months following the storm. In the Antiarrhythmics Versus Implantable Defibrillators trial, electrical storm was an independent predictor of mortality, with a relative risk of death of 5.4 in the first 3 months after the storm [22]. Fifty percent of deaths were nonsudden cardiac deaths. Thus, electrical storm may be an indicator of a mechanically failing heart. Because of the increased mortality, the care of the patient after electrical storm should include aggressive revascularization and optimal treatment of heart failure. In addition, the repeated painful shocks can result in a ''posttraumatic'' type of syndrome with anxiety and depression [18].

commence simultaneously with a search for the etiology of the electrical storm. ICD therapies can be inhibited by application of a magnet to the device in the case of nonsustained arrhythmias triggering shocks or for recurrent hemodynamically tolerated arrhythmias. Drug therapy with intravenous β-blockers is the best management for electrical storm occurring in the setting of acute ischemia or in the days following myocardial infarction [24]. Otherwise, intravenous antiarrhythmic therapy (typically amiodarone) is the most frequently applied treatment (Box 4) [20,21]. No new therapy is required in a significant

Inappropriate implantable cardioverter-defibrillator therapy

The term *inappropriate ICD therapy* is used when ICD therapy is delivered in the absence of ventricular tachyarrhythmia. The incidence remains high even with modern devices, affecting 10% to 20% of ICD recipients [14]. Inappropriately delivered therapy may cause severe psychologic distress, decrease quality of life, impede on the cost-effectiveness, and may be proarrhythmic [25]. Although mechanisms are diverse, the two main causes for inappropriate ICD therapy are oversensing and inappropriate classification of rapid supraventricular tachycardia (SVT) (Box 5). In broader terms, inappropriate ICD therapy may also include withholding ICD therapy in the presence of ventricular arrhythmia.

Implantable cardioverter-defibrillator sensing

Heart rate has proved to be a sensitive parameter to detect VT or VF and it remains the primary parameter of rhythm classification even in modern devices. Appropriate rate sensing is therefore a key feature and one of the main pillars of normal ICD function. Recorded signals undergo filtering and augmentation (gain) to minimize signals that fall into nonphysiologic range

Box 5. Causes of inappropriate therapy

Oversensing
QRS
T wave
P wave
Myopotential
Electromagnetic interference

Algorithm-specific events
Frequent nonsustained VT
Frequent ventricular premature complex
Ventricular premature complex/
    oversensing during confirmation
    before ICD shock
Combined counter use in VT/VF zone

Mechanical complication
Lead fracture
Loose setscrew
Chatter between leads
Header problem

Supraventricular tachycardia
Atrial fibrillation
Sinus tachycardia
Atrial flutter

and to enhance signals of interest. Increasing the use of true bipolar leads instead of integrated bipolar leads allows more specific sampling of the myocardial signals. Further complexity and difficulty of sensing in ICDs results from the fact that ICDs have to recognize and treat brady- and tachyarrhythmias. For example, differentiation between asystole and VF requires special sensing algorithm that allows beat-to-beat adjustment of gain or sensitivity to appropriately sense R waves during fine VF but without sensing other parts of the EKG, such as the P wave or T wave. The drawback of increased sensitivity or gain is that signals from noncardiac or nonarrhythmic sources may be augmented and inappropriately sensed as if they were cardiac signals. A particularly vulnerable period is during bradycardia or following a pacing stimulus, when sensitivity of the ICD is maximized (Fig. 2). Programming options for the correction of oversensing in general are limited to decreasing sensitivity, but at a price of possible undersensing during VF. Defibrillation testing is therefore prudent following any modification of sensing parameters.

Oversensing of intracardiac signals

P waves, R waves, and T waves may be spuriously sensed and cause double counting of each cardiac cycle, which may lead to acceleration of the counter to a tachycardia zone. Recorded electrograms show ventricular-sensed events that correspond to the timing of the oversensed signal, such as a second R-wave component, P wave, or T wave. The timing of the sensed ventricular events shows beat-to-beat alternating cycle length (see Fig. 2). P-wave oversensing is commonly a result of ICD lead dislodgement to the tricuspid annulus as seen in twiddler's syndrome. R-wave oversensing is uncommon in modern devices and requires an alteration of ventricular blanking period or lead repositioning. Oversensing of T waves is more frequently seen in hypertrophic cardiomyopathy, short and long QT syndrome, and Brugada syndrome (see Fig. 2) [26–28]. Another common cause is a temporary or permanent decline in R-wave amplitude (<5 mV) that triggers autoadjustment in sensitivity. Increased sensitivity in turn may be sufficient to sense the T wave. Device-specific filtering may also contribute to differences in T-wave sensing. Initial management of T-wave oversensing is often noninvasive. Decreasing ventricular sensitivity may be sufficient, but lead repositioning is required in select cases. In some devices, a programmable option allows modification of the timing and slopes of sensitivity adjustment after sensed events and may be sufficient to allow noninvasive correction.

Oversensing of extracardiac signals

Myopotential oversensing is a result of sensing skeletal muscle signals, commonly from the diaphragm. Skeletal muscle activity is characterized by a continuous high frequency signal that usually overlaps several cardiac cycles. The high-frequency signals are sensed as rapid ventricular events and therefore inhibit pacing and may induce ICD therapy (see Fig. 2). Diaphragmatic oversensing is more commonly seen in the ventricular sensing channel in integrated bipolar leads in the right ventricular apex and in devices that use automatic gain adjustment for sensing. Clinical evaluation shows unchanged lead parameters, and noise may be reproduced with special maneuvers. Diaphragmatic oversensing might be corrected by manually adjusting sensitivity without impairing the detection of VF. In some extreme cases, it may be required to reposition the lead higher on the right ventricular septum or to insert

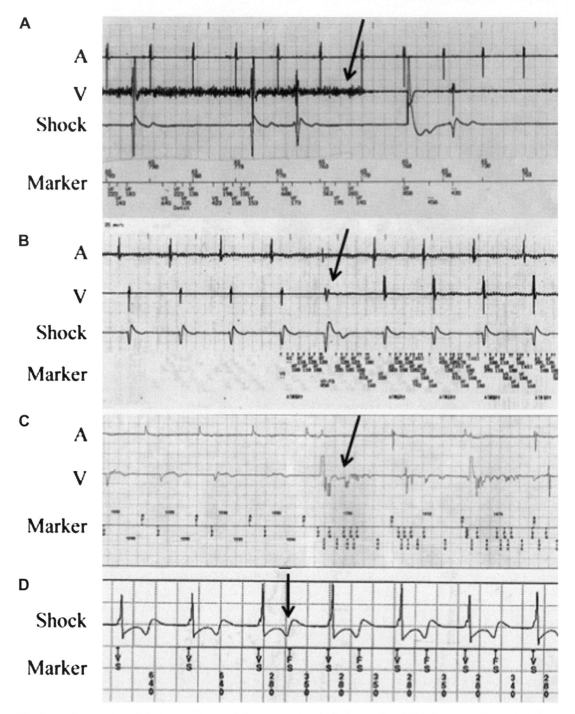

Fig. 2. (*A*) Oversensing of diaphragmatic signals in a pacemaker-dependent patient. High-frequency signals (noise) are noted on V that disappear when the patient stops straining (*arrow*). VF is detected and there is inhibition of ventricular pacing. (*B*) Electromagnetic interference during transcutaneous electrical nerve stimulation. Initially, noise is only present on the atrial lead. Atrial oversensing results in spurious detection of atrial fibrillation. Ventricular pacing at fall-back rate is initiated. There is postpacing automatic gain adjustment, which results in ventricular oversensing (*arrow*). Inappropriate ICD shock was delivered later (not shown). (*C*) Noise on ventricular lead due to lead fracture. Patient presented with ICD storm due to oversensing as a result of ventricular lead fracture. High frequency, nonphysiologic signals are pointed out (*arrow*). (*D*) T-wave oversensing. Arrow points to a sensed event that falls into VT zone and corresponds to oversensing T wave. A, atrial sensing channel; Shock, far-field electrogram from the ICD coil; V, ventricular sensing channel.

a separate dedicated sensing lead to prevent oversensing.

Increasing the use of electronics that emit electromagnetic signals pose challenges in ICD detection. Environmental electromagnetic interference (EMI) may be detected by ICDs and trigger therapy. EMI is a high frequency signal present in all leads, often with highest amplitude in far-field electrograms. Careful clinical correlation is required to identify the exact sources. In general, properly grounded common household appliances carry no substantial risk for EMI. Commonly encountered nonmedical and medical sources include electrocautery, MRI, lithotripsy, transcutaneous nerve stimulation, radiofrequency ablation, gasoline combustion engines, welding equipment, electronic article surveillance systems, and cellular phones. The general approach is avoidance and shielding from the source. If EMI cannot be avoided, especially during hospital care, inhibition of tachycardia detection with magnet application or temporary programming is required to avoid inappropriate ICD shocks. Special attention should be paid to pacemaker-dependent patients to assure appropriate pacing and monitoring because magnet application does not affect pacing mode in ICDs.

Mechanical complications of the ICD system may compromise the integrity of the sensing circuit. Thus, lead fracture and header or setscrew problems may present as intermittent noise. There usually are fluctuations in the lead impedance, and special maneuvers may reproduce the clinical findings. The solution is revision of the failed component.

Inappropriate classification of supraventricular tachycardia

Overlap between the rate of VT detection and supraventricular arrhythmia results in inappropriate therapy unless discriminators are applied to withhold therapy during SVT. Differentiation between SVT and VT remains a challenging task. Special algorithms are used in an attempt to distinguish typical features of arrhythmias and are applied to withhold inappropriate therapy without significantly compromising identification of VT.

In single-chamber ICDs, sudden onset, interval stability, and electrogram morphology are common primary discriminators. Applications and limitations of these discriminators are summarized in Table 1. In general, the combined use of discriminators is needed to improve specificity (ie, reject therapy for SVT) [29,30] but may impede on the sensitivity to detect VT (ie, VT may be misclassified as SVT). An arrhythmia duration timer may be used as a safety feature, which mandates ICD therapy regardless of the classification of the arrhythmia after the timer is expired, but it erodes on specificity [30].

Dual-chamber algorithms use atrial sensing information to assess atrioventricular relationship and are used in combination with single-chamber discriminators. Adequate atrial sensing is of key importance. Atrial undersensing, for example, may accelerate therapy delivery by producing V>A count. Despite the increasingly sophisticated detection algorithms, specificity of dual-chamber detection remains suboptimal [31,32]. For example, a recent multicenter study compared

Table 1
Single-chamber detection enhancement parameters

Detection enhancement parameter	General use of parameter	Common reasons for incorrect arrhythmia classification
Sudden onset	Reject gradual-onset tachycardia (SR)	Nonsudden onset of ST due to VPC VT may appear "sudden onset" if starts during ST
Stability	Reject irregular tachycardia (AF) as opposed to regular monomorphic VT	Regularized conduction in AF Frequent VPC
ECG morphology	Reject tachycardia if morphology is unchanged from SR	Aberrant conduction/BBB during SVT Minimal change in morphology during VT Processing errors of the signals

Abbreviations: AF, atrial fibrillation; BBB, bundle branch block; SR, sinus rhythm; ST, sinus tachycardia; VPC, ventricular premature complex.

single- and dual-chamber detection algorithms. SVT occurred commonly (in 34% of all patients) within 6 months after ICD implantation. Using single-chamber discriminators, 40% of the SVT episodes were classified inappropriately. Dual-chamber discriminators, on the other hand, significantly reduced the rate of inappropriate detection to 31% and reduced ICD shocks by half [33]. Other studies, including a meta-analysis, also confirmed a small but significant difference in favor of dual-chamber detection to reduce inappropriate ICD shocks [34].

Significant differences exist in detection algorithms between different models, and it is imperative to understand device-specific properties in detection algorithms to maximize specificity and maintain high sensitivity for VT therapy [30,33,35]. Additional strategies to reduce inappropriate shocks include increasing VT/VF detection time, increasing VT/VF detection rate, and the liberal use of antitachycardia pacings (ATPs), even for rapid VT [35]. Application of full energy shocks may terminate SVT and may help to minimize the number of shocks.

Undersensing

Suboptimal sensing may occur with a decline in R wave, such as following lead dislodgement, fracture, development of new bundle branch block, or ICD shock; with progression of heart disease; or because of electrolyte disturbances. Defibrillation testing should be considered when there is significant change in R-wave amplitude, when sensing parameters are modified, or when there is clinical suspicion for undersensing. Tachycardia detection may also fail when the tachycardia rate is less than the programmed detection rate or when the device therapy is inadvertently programmed off.

The identification and treatment of device infections

Currently, over 100,000 new ICDs are implanted in the United States per year [36]. In light of the expanded recommendations for ICD implantation, this number has significantly increased, as has the complication rate [37]. The files collected by the National Hospital Discharge Survey revealed that between 1996 and 2003, the rates of hospitalization for infections of implantable antiarrhythmic systems increased faster than the rates of system implants [38]. The estimated rate

of infection after implantation of permanent endocardial leads is between 1% and 2%, although the variability described in the literature is 0.13% to 12.6% [39,40]. Device infection carries significant public health consequences and is responsible for significant increases in morbidity, mortality, and financial cost. Reported mortality can range from 31% to 66% when the device is not removed and is 18% when the combined approach of device removal and antibiotic therapy is employed [41,42]. The combined average cost of medical and surgical treatment of an infected defibrillator may reach $57,000 [39].

Diagnosis

Correct diagnosis of device infection may prove difficult, even to an experienced clinician. An ICD infection is manifest by pocket cellulitis, erosion or fistula, wound dehiscence, abscess, persistent bacteremia, or endocarditis. The infection may involve the skin, the generator, the defibrillator pocket, or the leads as they track the tissue and enter the venous system. The most common signs and symptoms of device infection are shown in Table 2 [43]. Fever is an unreliable symptom and is reported in less than half of patients who have device infections. Most symptoms are nonspecific. Erythema, pain, and swelling at the device site are the most common signs. Leukocytosis and positive blood cultures occur in a minority of patients [43].

One must recognize less serious but common signs of infection such as local irritation around the incision site and superficial stitch abscess that are not considered device infections and that respond to local measures alone [44]. The average time to device infection from implant is approximately 1 year but may be manifest at almost any time after device surgery [43].

Blood cultures have the highest yield when the patient is febrile or directly after lead extraction and should be obtained before administration of antibiotics. Swab culture of the pocket or purulent exudate expressed from the fistula may facilitate identification of the organism; however, it has been shown that pocket tissue cultures are more effective than pocket swab cultures for the isolation of the pathogens in cardiac device infections [37,45]. Incubation and culture of explanted leads and devices appears to provide the highest yield of all [46]. Despite the need for a high index of suspicion for ICD infections, routine pocket cultures of asymptomatic patients should be

Table 2
Clinical presentation of patients who have permanent pacemaker or implantable cardioverter-defibrillator infection

Clinical presentation	n (%)
Systemic symptoms	
Fever (>38°C)	82 (43)
Chills	73 (39)
Malaise	79 (42)
Anorexia	32 (17)
Nausea	16 (8)
Sweating	34 (18)
Hypotension (systolic blood pressure <90 mm Hg)	18 (10)
Murmur on examination	66 (35)
Symptomatic heart failure	52 (28)
Local findings at generator site	
Erythema	128 (68)
Pain	93 (49)
Swelling	127 (67)
Warmth	71 (38)
Tenderness	86 (46)
Drainage	95 (50)
Purulent drainage	65 (34)
Skin ulceration	59 (31)
Generator/lead erosion	48 (25)
Intraoperative purulence at generator pocket	151 (80)
Laboratory abnormalities	
Leukocytosis (WBC >10 × 10^9/L),	82 (43)
Anemia (HCT <38% in men; <35% in women)	94 (50)
High ERS (>22 mm/h in men; >29 mm/h in women)	47 (25)
Positive blood culture	76 (40)

Abbreviations: ESR, erythrocyte sedimentation rate; HCT, hematocrit; WBC, white blood cell count.

From Sohail MR, Uslan DZ, Khan AH, et al. Management and outcome of permanent pacemaker and implantable cardioverter-defibrillator infections. J Am Coll Cardiol 2007;49:1853; with permission.

discouraged [45]. Positive cultures by pocket swab or tissue cultures are not uncommon in the absence of clinical signs and symptoms of infection, due to contamination or chronic innocuous colonization. This situation does not appear to require therapy [45]. Patients who have positive blood cultures or negative blood cultures after antibiotics should have a transesophageal echocardiogram to assess for device-related endocarditis [43].

Approximately two thirds of device infections are caused by *Staphylococcus* species (Fig. 3). Methicillin-resistant *Staphylococcus aureus* occurs in 4% of infections, gram-negative organisms

occur in 9%, and fungal infections are rare (2%) [43]. The most common source of the infection appears to be local contamination from the skin at the time of implant or generator change [47].

Risk factors

A number of studies examined and found multiple risk factors associated with development of ICD or permanent pacemaker infection (Table 3). In a retrospective multicenter study that evaluated 6319 patients who had permanent pacemaker and ICD implant, early repeat intervention for hematoma or lead dislodgement was the leading risk factor for infection, associated with an odds ratio of 15.0 [48]. Although repeated intervention for lead dislodgment or hematoma might seem essential in some cases, the risk of infection must be weighted against the absolute necessity of the revision procedure. Secondary procedures such as pulse generator replacements are well established to be a risk factor for infection. The rate of infectious complications is increased in patients who undergo multiple implantations of devices in their lifetime. In a retrospective analysis, the infection rate in young patients who had undergone a median of two pacemaker implantations was 5.5% [49].

The absence of antibiotic prophylaxis at the time of procedure is another risk factor for developing device infection. A meta-analysis showed a possible benefit conferred by systemic antibiotic administered before the procedures [50]. The antibiotics used in these trials included penicillin or cephalosporins. Classen and colleagues [51] showed that the risk of infection is best reduced when antibiotics are administered 2 hours before the initial incision.

Patients in whom a temporary pacing system is present at the time of implantation of the permanent antiarrhythmic systems are more than twice as likely to develop device-related infections [48]. Fever within 24 hours before implantation of the permanent system also increases the risk of postprocedure infection [48]. Renal insufficiency impairs cellular and humoral immunity and is a contributing factor in device infection. Patients who have renal insufficiency are nearly five times more likely to develop device infection than those who have preserved renal function [52].

Treatment

The management of ICD infection can be a challenge for the electrophysiologist and the infection disease specialist. Extraction of the

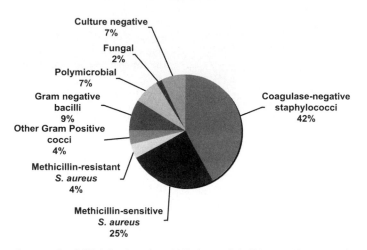

Fig. 3. Microbiology of pacemaker/ICD infections (n = 189). (*From* Sohail MR, Uslan DZ, Khan AH, et al. Management and outcome of permanent pacemaker and implantable cardioverter-defibrillator infections. J Am Coll Cardiol 2007;49:1853; with permission.)

generator and leads is mandatory in cases of sepsis or endocarditis involving any intravascular part of the pacing system (class I indication) [53]. In the case of localized pocket infection, erosion, or chronic draining sinus, multiple studies have shown high rates of relapsing infection (even after prolonged medical therapy) when the entire system is not removed. In a case series of 123 patients who had an infected device, only 1 of 117 (0.86%) patients who underwent removal of the entire system had infection relapse. In contrast, 3 of 6 (50%) patients who did not have complete hardware removal suffered relapse [37]. Complete device extraction is therefore recommended when infection of any part of the system is diagnosed; however, if the diagnosis is not certain, one can wait and reassess the pocket until the infection becomes more apparent and then proceed with lead extraction.

Based on a retrospective analysis and review of the published literature, Sohail and colleagues [43]

Table 3
Predictors of device infections

Risk factor	Odds ratio
Fever within 24 h before system implantation [48]	4.8
Early reintervention [48]	55.3
Antibiotic prophylaxis [48]	0.4
Renal insufficiency (creatinine ≥ 1.5) [52]	4.6
Generator change [52]	2.2

proposed guidelines for the management of cardiac device infections (Fig. 4). These guidelines include complete extraction of all hardware after infection is identified regardless of the clinical presentation and complete debridement of the infected scar tissue. Blood cultures should be repeated in all patients after device extraction. Patients who have positive blood cultures and patients who have complicated infection should be treated for at least 4 weeks with antibiotics even if transesophageal echocardiography is negative for vegetations or other evidence of infection. Adequate debridement and control of infection should be achieved at all sites before reimplantation of a new device at a remote anatomic location. Implanting devices submuscularly does not appear to prevent infection. It is extremely important before initiation of treatment to plan the course of the treatment. For example, if the patient is pacer dependent, provision for extended temporary pacing may be needed. Also, an alternative location for new implant must be identified [44]. Every implanter needs to keep in mind that the best method to treat device infection is to prevent it.

Lead extraction

Progressive growth of fibrous tissue around the electrode tip and the defibrillator coils and along the entire length of the lead body create a major barrier to the removal of leads [53]. Guidelines for lead extraction have been previously published [53,54]. In experienced hands, lead extraction

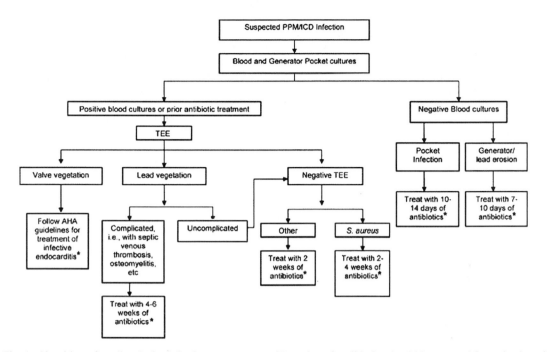

Fig. 4. Algorithm of cardiac device infection management. *Duration of antibiotics should be counted from the day of device explantation. AHA, American Heart Association; PPM, permanent pacemaker; TEE, transesophageal echocardiography. (*From* Sohail MR, Uslan DZ, Khan AH, et al. Management and outcome of permanent pacemaker and implantable cardioverter-defibrillator infections. J Am Coll Cardiol 2007;49:1857; with permission.)

can be a very successful procedure, with a success rate between 90% and 94% [55,56]. Nevertheless, the procedure can carry a significant rate of major complications (1%–5%) [55,56]. Potential lethal complications requiring extensive surgical procedures include tearing of the SVC/subclavian vein or the heart wall leading to tamponade, arterial tears causing arteriovenous fistula or dissecting hematoma, and tearing into the thoracic cavity causing a hemothorax. The mortality rate associated with laser lead extractions has been reported as high as 0.8% [55,56].

Prevention

Useful methods to prevent device infection are listed in Box 6. The infection rate for each implanting laboratory should be monitored, annually evaluated, and held under 0.5% [44]. Adherence to surgical conditions such as careful skin preparation and sterile operating room conditions is crucial in prevention of infections. The highest risk of infection is associated with generator changes and reimplants; therefore, some practitioners prefer to debride the device capsule to

facilitate increased blood flow and migration of inflammatory cells.

Implantable cardioverter-defibrillator generator and lead failure

Over their 20 years of evolution, ICD generators have undergone a fourfold to fivefold reduction in size along with incredible increases in function and complexity. Implanted ICDs and leads must endure a hostile physiologic environment and are subject to physical stresses imposed by the body. ICD generators and leads may fail due to design flaws, manufacturing problems, implant techniques, mechanical stress, or aging and fatigue of materials [36,57,58].

Implantable cardioverter-defibrillator generator failure

A recent study suggests that the reliability of ICD generators has decreased over recent years concomitant with an exponential rise in device implants [36]. As with any manufactured device, all ICD generators are subject to a random failure rate, but when failures are systematic due to

---

**Box 6. Useful methods to prevent
device infection**

Perform chlorhexidine skin scrubs up to
    24 hours pre procedure
Administer antibiotics 2 hours before the
    first incision
Observe strict sterile techniques and
    sterile operating room conditions
Perform careful chlorhexidine skin
    preparation
Limit duration of pocket exposure
Perform antibiotic flush of pocket
Redose antibiotics for long procedure

---

design or manufacturing problems, the device
may be subject to a safety advisory issued by the
manufacturer or imposed by the Food and Drug
Administration (FDA). Between 1990 and 2000,
18 safety alerts involving more than 114,000
ICDs were issued by the FDA [36,58]. In 2005,
four major ICD manufacturers issued alerts involving more than 200,000 devices. There were
several deaths directly attributed to ICD failures.
With expanded indications for ICD implants,
the absolute number of ICD and lead failures is
certain to grow.

*Recognizing implantable cardioverter-defibrillator
generator failure*

ICD failure modes that result in loss of pacing
may produce symptoms of bradycardia or syncope. Sudden death may occur from loss of pacing
in pacemaker-dependent patients or from failure
to treat ventricular tachyarrhythmias. Current
ICD generators have patient alert capabilities
(audible tone or vibratory alert) that may be
activated by failure modes resulting from battery
depletion, abnormal lead impedances, or prolonged capacitor charge times. A unique symptom
of one manufacturer's failure mode is warmth at
the device site due to heat generated by a sudden
battery short-circuit. Most device failures are
detected by device interrogation at follow-up.
Remote monitoring capabilities of some devices
allow for daily device follow-up, enabling rapid
recognition of some failure modes. Nevertheless,
some failure modes result in loss of critical
functions only at the time of their activation and
cannot be recognized in advance.

Management of device failure and safety alerts

Management of a failed device is straightforward: replace the device. A critical but overlooked
part of device replacement is the reporting of
a device failure (known or suspected) to the manufacturer and the FDA (www.fda.gov/medwatch).
The FDA compiles, analyzes, and posts these
reports in the Manufacturer and User Device
Experience database, which is accessible to the
public (www.fda.gov/cdrh/maude.html). Because
the reporting of device failures is voluntary at the
provider level, it is essential that health care profes-
sionals report all malfunctions to form the most
complete picture of device behavior.

The more difficult problem is the management
of a patient who has a device under safety alert
but who has not experienced problems. Safety
advisories are issued to physicians who are
following such patients. It then falls to the
physician to inform each patient regarding the
advisory. The authors' policy is to notify each
patient in writing and to have the patient come to
the clinic for device follow-up, to answer questions, and to make management decisions in-
dividually. The patient who has an ICD under
advisory faces the competing risks of harm from
device failure and the risks of surgical replacement
(primarily infection from lead extraction leading
to complications or death). The decision to replace a device or to continue monitoring the
patient is complex, and physician practice is
nonuniform [59–61]. Guidelines from scientific
agencies are based on expert opinion alone [62].
These guidelines suggest that device replacement
should be considered when failure could result in
serious harm and when the patient is pacemaker
dependent, has a secondary prevention ICD indication, or has received an appropriate therapy
from the device. Clinical data suggest, however,
that widespread categorical replacement of devices under advisory may be misguided [59,60].
Gould and Krahn [60] found that major complications including death were more common in
patients undergoing elective "recalled" device
replacement (43/533 replacements [8.1%]) compared with no adverse events directly attributable
to device failures in 2382 patients.

In the absence of controlled clinical data to
direct decisions regarding replacement of devices
under advisory, a decision analysis model has
been developed [61]. This form of analysis simu-
lates a two-armed clinical trial. Using a hypothetic
cohort of patients who have ICDs under advisory

for failure, half of the patients have device replacement and the other half continue to be monitored. The primary outcome variable is average survival for each strategy. According to the model, the most important considerations for device replacement are (1) estimated advisory failure rate, (2) procedural mortality rate for device replacement, (3) degree of pacemaker dependency, and (4) remaining generator life (Fig. 5). Patient age, indication for ICD (primary or secondary prevention), and frequency of follow-up had much less influence on the decision-making process. According to this model, to favor routine device replacement for highly pacemaker-dependent patients, the device failure rate should exceed 3 in 10,000 for the lowest procedural mortality rates (0.1% death per procedure) and more than 3 in 100 for the highest procedural mortality rates (1.0% death per procedure). For non–pacemaker-dependent patients, ICD failure rates should exceed 1 to 3 in 100 to favor routine replacement over the range of procedural mortality rates. Of interest, remaining device life favors replacement only when less than 10% of service life remains. These findings suggest that ongoing monitoring of "recalled" devices is likely to be the preferred strategy in most cases.

Implantable cardioverter-defibrillator lead failure

ICD leads have always been the "weakest link" in the ICD system, with failure rates far exceeding those of ICD generators. The failure rate for ICD leads may be 15% at 5 years and 40% at 8 years [57]. The reasons for the high failure rates are many, including the complex physical stresses placed on the leads by cardiac motion, subclavian "crush" due to implant technique, the complex construction compared with pacemaker leads, the high voltage stresses (up to 800 V) imposed on the leads, chemical reactions between insulation materials and metallic components, and attempts to downsize the lead diameters. Most lead problems result from insulation failure [57]. Lead failure appears to be more likely in women, younger patients, coaxial lead designs, multiple lead implants, and with the subclavian implant technique [57]. Despite the high failure rate for ICD leads in general, only one lead model has been subjected to an FDA safety alert, perhaps acknowledging the low expectations for the performance of these devices. Like ICD generators, ICD leads should be considered to have a finite service life.

Recognizing implantable cardioverter-defibrillator lead failures

One third of ICD lead failures are recognized by electrical noise producing inappropriate therapies from the device [57]. Syncope or presyncope may result from inhibition of pacing or loss of ventricular capture. Activation of patient alerts due to abnormal lead impedances may occur.

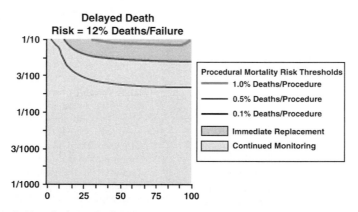

Fig. 5. Three-way threshold analysis graph identifying combinations of values for which device replacement or continued observation is the preferred strategy. This graph represents the case of a primary prevention ICD generator under safety advisory. The estimated risk of patient death is 12%/y if the device fails. The three lines in the graph represent different procedural mortality rates for device replacement of 0.1%, 0.5%, and 1.0% per procedure. By finding the position on the graph using coordinates of device failure rate and remaining generator life, the decision to replace the device is favored for a given procedural mortality rate when the point falls above the procedural mortality rate line; monitoring is favored when the point falls below the line. (*From* Amin MS, Matchar DB, Wood MA, et al. Management of recalled pacemakers and implantable cardioverter-defibrillators: a decision analysis model. JAMA 2006;296:417; with permission.)

Most failures (65%), however, are diagnosed at follow-up from the review of stored electrograms, the recording of nonphysiologically short R–R intervals, or abnormal lead impedance trends [57]. Noise on the ICD lead must be differentiated from intermittent exposure to EMI. Occasionally, the electrical noise may be reproduced by motion of the ipsilateral arm, body movement, or palpation of the lead.

Management of implantable cardioverter-defibrillator lead failure

Management of a known ICD lead failure is simple in theory (ie, provide a new lead) but often difficult in practice. Difficulties attend the decision to extract the failed lead or, more simply, to add a new lead. A small retrospective study suggests that both strategies carry equal risks, but the high likelihood of future lead malfunction favors extraction in younger patients [63]. Thrombosis of the venous system may complicate lead replacement by requiring lead extraction to restore vascular access or by requiring movement of the ICD system to the contralateral side. Extraction of ICD leads carries a major complication rate (including death) of 1% to 3% [56]. There are no randomized studies for these treatment strategies, and the decisions must be individualized for each patient.

As with ICD generator advisories, there is no consensus on the optimal management strategy. Although the incidence of ICD lead failures may greatly exceed that of generator failure, the risks of lead replacement or extraction are significant. For ICD leads under advisory, it is likely that continued monitoring will be favored in most cases. In these cases, increased surveillance including the use of home monitoring is warranted.

Summary

ICD technology has advanced greatly since its initial development a quarter of a century ago. Although improvements in technology have solved many problems associated with ICD therapy, others problems remain. Some new clinical syndromes have even resulted from these technical advances, such as inappropriate shocks. Despite their unquestioned benefits, with the increasing use of ICDs, especially in primary prevention patients who have an anticipation of long life spans spent with an ICD, we can expect continued

problems with ICD systems and must remain vigilant.

References

[1] Kroll MW, Swerdlow CD. Optimizing defibrillation waveforms for ICDs. J Interv Card Electrophysiol 2007;18:247–63.

[2] Strickberger SA, Daoud EG, Davidson T, et al. Probability of successful defibrillation at multiples of the defibrillation energy requirement in patients with an implantable defibrillator. Circulation 1997; 96:1217–23.

[3] Swerdlow CD. Implantation of cardioverter defibrillators without induction of ventricular fibrillation. Circulation 2001;103:2159–64.

[4] Day JD, Doshi RN, Belott P, et al. Inductionless or limited shock testing is possible in most patients with implantable cardioverter-defibrillators/cardiac resynchronization therapy defibrillators: results of the multicenter ASSURE Study (Arrhythmia Single Shock Defibrillation Threshold Testing Versus Upper Limit of Vulnerability: Risk Reduction Evaluation with Implantable Cardioverter-Defibrillator Implantations). Circulation 2007;115:2382–9.

[5] Mainigi SK, Callans DJ. How to manage the patient with a high defibrillation threshold. Heart Rhythm 2006;3:492–5.

[6] Schuger C, Ellenbogen KA, Faddis M, et al. Defibrillation energy requirements in an ICD population receiving cardiac resynchronization therapy. J Cardiovasc Electrophysiol 2006;17:247–50.

[7] Shukla HH, Flaker GC, Jayam V, et al. High defibrillation thresholds in transvenous biphasic implantable defibrillators: clinical predictors and prognostic implications. Pacing Clin Electrophysiol 2003;26:44–8.

[8] Strickberger SA, Klein GJ. Is defibrillation testing required for defibrillator implantation? J Am Coll Cardiol 2004;44:88 91.

[9] Russo AM, Sauer W, Gerstenfeld EP, et al. Defibrillation threshold testing: is it really necessary at the time of implantable cardioverter-defibrillator insertion? Heart Rhythm 2005;2:456–61.

[10] Hohnloser SH, Dorian P, Roberts R, et al. Effect of amiodarone and sotalol on ventricular defibrillation threshold: the Optimal Pharmacological Therapy in Cardioverter Defibrillator Patients (OPTIC) trial. Circulation 2006;114:104–9.

[11] Gold MR, Olsovsky MR, Degroot PJ, et al. Optimization of transvenous coil position for active can defibrillation thresholds. J Cardiovasc Electrophysiol 2000;11:25–9.

[12] Kuhlkamp V, Dornberger V, Khalighi K, et al. Effect of a single element subcutaneous array electrode added to a transvenous electrode configuration on the defibrillation field and the defibrillation threshold. Pacing Clin Electrophysiol 1998;21:2596–605.

[13] Brady PA, Friedman PA, Trusty JM, et al. High failure rate for an epicardial implantable cardioverter-defibrillator lead: implications for long-term follow-up of patients with an implantable cardioverter-defibrillator. J Am Coll Cardiol 1998;31:616–22.

[14] Bardy GH, Lee KL, Mark DB, et al. Amiodarone or an implantable cardioverter-defibrillator for congestive heart failure. N Engl J Med 2005;352:225–37.

[15] Connolly SJ, Dorian P, Roberts RS, et al. Comparison of beta-blockers, amiodarone plus beta-blockers, or sotalol for prevention of shocks from implantable cardioverter defibrillators: the OPTIC Study: a randomized trial. JAMA 2006;295:165–71.

[16] Dorian P, Borggrefe M, Al-Khalidi HR, et al. Placebo-controlled, randomized clinical trial of azimilide for prevention of ventricular tachyarrhythmias in patients with an implantable cardioverter defibrillator. Circulation 2004;110:3646–54.

[17] Desai AD, Burke MC, Hong TE, et al. Predictors of appropriate defibrillator therapy among patients with an implantable defibrillator that delivers cardiac resynchronization therapy. J Cardiovasc Electrophysiol 2006;17:486–90.

[18] Passman R, Subacius H, Ruo B, et al. Implantable cardioverter defibrillators and quality of life: results from the defibrillators in nonischemic cardiomyopathy treatment evaluation study. Arch Intern Med 2007;167:2226–32.

[19] Wood MA, Gunderson B, Xia A, et al. Temporal patterns of ventricular tachyarrhythmia recurrences follow a Weibull distribution. J Cardiovasc Electrophysiol 2005;16:181–5.

[20] Brigadeau F, Kouakam C, Klug D, et al. Clinical predictors and prognostic significance of electrical storm in patients with implantable cardioverter defibrillators. Eur Heart J 2006;27:700–7.

[21] Verma A, Kilicaslan F, Marrouche NF, et al. Prevalence, predictors, and mortality significance of the causative arrhythmia in patients with electrical storm. J Cardiovasc Electrophysiol 2004;15: 1265–70.

[22] Exner DV, Pinski SL, Wyse DG, et al. Electrical storm presages nonsudden death: the Antiarrhythmics Versus Implantable Defibrillators (AVID) trial. Circulation 2001;103:2066–71.

[23] Arya A, Haghjoo M, Dehghani MR, et al. Prevalence and predictors of electrical storm in patients with implantable cardioverter-defibrillator. Am J Cardiol 2006;97:389–92.

[24] Nademanee K, Taylor R, Bailey WE, et al. Treating electrical storm: sympathetic blockade versus advanced cardiac life support-guided therapy. Circulation 2000;102:742–7.

[25] Kamphuis HC, de Leeuw JR, Derksen R, et al. Implantable cardioverter defibrillator recipients: quality of life in recipients with and without ICD shock delivery: a prospective study. Europace 2003;5:381–9.

[26] Perry GY, Kosar EM. Problems in managing patients with long QT syndrome and implantable cardioverter defibrillators: a report of two cases. Pacing Clin Electrophysiol 1996;19:863–7.

[27] Schimpf R, Wolpert C, Bianchi F, et al. Congenital short QT syndrome and implantable cardioverter defibrillator treatment: inherent risk for inappropriate shock delivery. J Cardiovasc Electrophysiol 2003;14:1273–7.

[28] Porres JM, Brugada J, Marco P, et al. T wave oversensing by a cardioverter defibrillator implanted in a patient with the Brugada syndrome. Pacing Clin Electrophysiol 2004;27:1563–5.

[29] Kettering K, Dornberger V, Lang R, et al. Enhanced detection criteria in implantable cardioverter defibrillators: sensitivity and specificity of the stability algorithm at different heart rates. Pacing Clin Electrophysiol 2001;24:1325–33.

[30] Brugada J, Mont L, Figueiredo M, et al. Enhanced detection criteria in implantable defibrillators. J Cardiovasc Electrophysiol 1998;9:261–8.

[31] Kuhlkamp V, Wilkoff BL, Brown AB, et al. Experience with a dual chamber implantable defibrillator. Pacing Clin Electrophysiol 2002;25:1041–8.

[32] Kouakam C, Kacet S, Hazard JR, et al. Performance of a dual-chamber implantable defibrillator algorithm for discrimination of ventricular from supraventricular tachycardia. Europace 2004;6: 32–42.

[33] Friedman PA, McClelland RL, Bamlet WR, et al. Dual-chamber versus single-chamber detection enhancements for implantable defibrillator rhythm diagnosis: the Detect Supraventricular Tachycardia study. Circulation 2006;113:2871–9.

[34] Theuns DA, Rivero-Ayerza M, Boersma E, et al. Prevention of inappropriate therapy in implantable defibrillators: a meta-analysis of clinical trials comparing single-chamber and dual-chamber arrhythmia discrimination algorithms. Int J Cardiol 2007;(125):352–7.

[35] Sweeney MO, Wathen MS, Volosin K, et al. Appropriate and inappropriate ventricular therapies, quality of life, and mortality among primary and secondary prevention implantable cardioverter defibrillator patients: results from the Pacing Fast VT REduces Shock ThErapies (PainFREE Rx II) trial. Circulation 2005;111:2898–905.

[36] Maisel WH, Moynahan M, Zuckerman BD, et al. Pacemaker and ICD generator malfunctions: analysis of Food and Drug Administration annual reports. JAMA 2006;295:1901–6.

[37] Chua JD, Wilkoff BL, Lee I, et al. Diagnosis and management of infections involving implantable electrophysiologic cardiac devices. Ann Intern Med 2000;133:604–8.

[38] Voigt A, Shalaby A, Saba S. Rising rates of cardiac rhythm management device infections in the United States: 1996 through 2003. J Am Coll Cardiol 2006; 48:590–1.

[39] Ferguson TB Jr, Ferguson CL, Crites K, et al. The additional hospital costs generated in the

management of complications of pacemaker and defibrillator implantations. J Thorac Cardiovasc Surg 1996;111:742–51.

[40] Bluhm G. Pacemaker infections. A clinical study with special reference to prophylactic use of some isoxazolyl penicillins. Acta Med Scand Suppl 1985; 699:1–62.

[41] Cacoub P, Leprince P, Nataf P, et al. Pacemaker infective endocarditis. Am J Cardiol 1998;82:480–4.

[42] Klug D, Lacroix D, Savoye C, et al. Systemic infection related to endocarditis on pacemaker leads: clinical presentation and management. Circulation 1997;95:2098–107.

[43] Sohail MR, Uslan DZ, Khan AH, et al. Management and outcome of permanent pacemaker and implantable cardioverter-defibrillator infections. J Am Coll Cardiol 2007;49:1851–9.

[44] Wilkoff BL. How to treat and identify device infections. Heart Rhythm 2007;4:1467–70.

[45] Dy CJ, Abdul-Karim A, Mawhorter S, et al. The role of swab and tissue culture in the diagnosis of implantable cardiac device infection. Pacing Clin Electrophysiol 2005;28:1276–81.

[46] Klug D, Wallet F, Lacroix D, et al. Local symptoms at the site of pacemaker implantation indicate latent systemic infection. Heart 2004;90:882–6.

[47] Da Costa A, Lelievre H, Kirkorian G, et al. Role of the preaxillary flora in pacemaker infections: a prospective study. Circulation 1998;97:1791–5.

[48] Klug D, Balde M, Pavin D, et al. Risk factors related to infections of implanted pacemakers and cardioverter-defibrillators: results of a large prospective study. Circulation 2007;116:1349–55.

[49] Klug D, Vaksmann G, Jarwe M, et al. Pacemaker lead infection in young patients. Pacing Clin Electrophysiol 2003;26:1489–93.

[50] Da Costa A, Kirkorian G, Cucherat M, et al. Antibiotic prophylaxis for permanent pacemaker implantation: a meta-analysis. Circulation 1998;97:1796–801.

[51] Classen DC, Evans RS, Pestotnik SL, et al. The timing of prophylactic administration of antibiotics and the risk of surgical-wound infection. N Engl J Med 1992;326:281–6.

[52] Bloom H, Heeke B, Leon A, et al. Renal insufficiency and the risk of infection from pacemaker or defibrillator surgery. Pacing Clin Electrophysiol 2006;29:142–5.

[53] Love CJ, Wilkoff BL, Byrd CL, et al. Recommendations for extraction of chronically implanted transvenous pacing and defibrillator leads: indications, facilities, training. North American Society of Pacing and Electrophysiology Lead Extraction Conference Faculty. Pacing Clin Electrophysiol 2000;23:544–51.

[54] Byrd CL, Schwartz SJ, Hedin N. Lead extraction. Indications and techniques. Cardiol Clin 1992;10: 735–48.

[55] Kennergren C, Bucknall CA, Butter C, et al. Laser-assisted lead extraction: the European experience. Europace 2007;9:651–6.

[56] Epstein LM, Byrd CL, Wilkoff BL, et al. Initial experience with larger laser sheaths for the removal of transvenous pacemaker and implantable defibrillator leads. Circulation 1999;100:516–25.

[57] Kleemann T, Becker T, Doenges K, et al. Annual rate of transvenous defibrillation lead defects in implantable cardioverter-defibrillators over a period of > 10 years. Circulation 2007;115:2474–80.

[58] Maisel WH, Sweeney MO, Stevenson WG, et al. Recalls and safety alerts involving pacemakers and implantable cardioverter-defibrillator generators. JAMA 2001;286:793–9.

[59] Costea A, Rardon DP, Padanilam BJ, et al. Complications associated with generator replacement in response to device advisories. J Cardiovasc Electrophysiol 2007;19:266–9.

[60] Gould PA, Krahn AD. Complications associated with implantable cardioverter-defibrillator replacement in response to device advisories. JAMA 2006; 295:1907–11.

[61] Amin MS, Matchar DB, Wood MA, et al. Management of recalled pacemakers and implantable cardioverter-defibrillators: a decision analysis model. JAMA 2006;296:412–20.

[62] Carlson MD, Wilkoff BL, Maisel WH, et al. Recommendations from the heart rhythm society task force on device performance policies and guidelines endorsed by the American College of Cardiology Foundation (ACCF) and the American Heart Association (AHA) and the International Coalition of Pacing and Electrophysiology Organizations (COPE). Heart Rhythm 2006;3:1250–73.

[63] Wollmann CG, Bocker D, Loher A, et al. Two different therapeutic strategies in ICD lead defects: additional combined lead versus replacement of the lead. J Cardiovasc Electrophysiol 2007;18: 1172–7.

Role of Ablation Therapy in Ventricular Arrhythmias

Mithilesh K. Das, MD, MRCP, FACC*, Gopi Dandamudi, MD, Hillel Steiner, MD

Krannert Institute of Cardiology, 1800 North Capitol Avenue, Indianapolis, IN 46202, USA

Sustained ventricular tachycardia (VT) and ventricular fibrillation (VF) are associated with a poor prognosis because of an increased risk for sudden cardiac death (SCD), particularly in patients who have structural heart disease (SHD) [1]. In addition, frequent nonsustained VT (NSVT), premature ventricular complexes (PVCs), or ventricular couplets may cause tachycardia-induced cardiomyopathy, a rare consequence of these arrhythmias. In the present era, the implantable cardioverter defibrillator (ICD) is the mainstay therapy for primary and secondary prevention of SCD. Recurrent VT develops in 20% and 40% to 60% in patients who receive an ICD for primary and secondary prophylaxis for SCD, respectively [2]. ICDs terminate most ventricular arrhythmia (VA) episodes. ICDs do not prevent recurrence of VAs or change the underlying substrate of VA, however. In fact, there is evidence that ICDs may increase the incidence of VA. Repeated ICD shocks reduce quality of life and increase mortality. Recurrent VAs in these patients often are treated with antiarrhythmic agents with only moderate success. Furthermore, these drugs are associated with an increased risk of proarrhythmia, systemic toxicity, and increased defibrillation threshold (especially amiodarone). Catheter ablation is the treatment of choice to cure or reduce the recurrences of VA in patients who have an ICD [3]. Catheter ablation can be life-saving for electrical storms (ES), defined as three separate episodes of VT or VF within a 24-hour period, each separated by 5 minutes.

ES is an independent predictor of short-term mortality and occurs in 3.5% and 20% of patients who have an ICD implanted for primary and secondary prophylaxis, respectively. Catheter ablation is also the treatment of choice for symptomatic idiopathic VT or PVCs. Polymorphic VT or VF initiated by a single monomorphic PVC also can be treated with catheter ablation. A recent randomized trial showed that ablation therapy in patients who have an ICD implanted for secondary prophylaxis reduces the risk for ICD therapy by 65% during a 2-year follow up as compared with the patients who do not receive ablation therapy.

Catheter ablation of VT or VF in the electrophysiology (EP) laboratory remains a challenging procedure. Patients who have SHD often have poor hemodynamic tolerance to the VA induced in the EP laboratory. Catheter ablation of VA requires a precise understanding of cardiac EP, the VA mechanism, and mapping techniques. Most VAs can be ablated endocardially. Epicardial ablation is needed for VTs with an epicardial circuit or focal source. The purpose of this article is to describe current mapping techniques and indications and to discuss the present status of catheter ablation for VA.

Mechanisms of ventricular arrhythmia

VA mechanism, like any arrhythmia, has either a focal source or a reentrant circuit. Sustained monomorphic VT (SMMVT) occurs predominantly because of reentry in patients who have SHD, whereas a focal VT or a PVC occurs because of enhanced automaticity or triggered activity in patients who have normal hearts and rarely, in patients who have SHD (Box 1, Table 1).

Dr. Steiner is a recipient of a Fellowship Grant from The American Physicians Fellowship for Medicine in Israel.

* Corresponding author.

E-mail address: midas@iupui.edu (M.K. Das).

0733-8651/08/$ - see front matter. Published by Elsevier Inc.
doi:10.1016/j.ccl.2008.03.010

Box 1. Classification of ventricular arrhythmia

Monomorphic VT
1. SHD
   a. CAD (Post-MI):
      - Scar related reentry
      - Focal VT
      - His-Purkinje related VT
   b. Cardiomyopathies and myocarditis:
      - DCM
      - Others
         - Myocarditis
         - Hypertrophic cardiomyopathy
         - ARVD/C
         - Infiltrative (Sarcoidosis)
         - Chagas disease
   c. Incisional (after cardiac surgery):
      - VSD or TOF repair
      - Aortic and mitral valve repair
      - LVAD
   d. Bundle branch reentry;
      - DCM
      - CAD
      - Myotonic dystrophy
      - Mitral and aortic valve-surgery
2. Structurally Normal Heart (Idiopathic VT):
   a. Idiopathic RVOT VT and its variants
   b. Verapamil-sensitive left ventricular fascicular VT
   c. Catecholamiergic monomorphic VT

Polymorphic VT/VF
1. SHD:
   a. CAD
      - Late post-MI
      - During acute myocardial ischemia
   b. DCM and other cardiomyopathies
2. Structurally Normal Heart (Idiopathic VT):
   a. Idiopathic RVOT VT (malignant variety)
   b. Idiopathic VF
3. Inherited arrhythmia sydromes
   a. Long QT syndrome
   b. Short QT syndrome
   c. Brugada syndrome
   d. Exercise induced catecholaminergic polymorphic VT
   e. Overlap syndrome (SCN5A mutation)

Abbreviations: ARVD/C, arrhythmogenic right ventricular dysplasia cardiomyopathy; CAD, coronary artery disease; DCM, dilated cardiomyopathy; LVAD, left ventricular assist device; RVOT, right ventricular outflow tract; SHD, structural heart disease; TOF, tetralogy of Fallot; VSD, ventricular septal defect; VT, ventricular tachycardia.

Ventricular arrhythmia in structural heart disease

The mechanism of VA in patients who have SHD is mostly scar-related reentry, but rarely can be focal in origin [4,5]. Reentry occurs at the border zone of myocardial infarction (MI) scar, around areas of scar in nonischemic dilated cardiomyopathy (DCM), and around surgical scars in patients who have congenital heart disease, valvular heart disease, or implanted hardware such as a left ventricular assist device (LVAD). SMMVT in patients who have an MI scar usually is caused by myocardial reentry in the infarct border zone. The reentrant circuit of scar-related VT can be modeled as having an isthmus or corridor bounded by two scars, or a scar and a line of anatomic barrier or physiologic conduction block. Most of these VT circuits have surviving strands of myocardium interlaced with interstitial fibrosis and diminished cell-to-cell coupling with slow conduction. Wave front conduction through these areas creates an excitation gap and promotes reentry. The conduction of wave fronts through these corridors is mapped as mid-diastolic or presystolic electrograms (Egms). These voltages, however, are too low to contribute to the surface ECG. The QRS complex is inscribed when the impulse exits the isthmus and spreads rapidly across the relatively healthier ventricular myocardium. The VT cycle length depends mainly upon the length of isthmus and conduction velocity of the impulse while passing through the isthmus (Fig. 1). During a slow VT, the isthmus can be mapped for a few centimeters with relatively slow conduction across the isthmus. Of note, a single area of the scar border zone may be a substrate for multiple channels giving rise to multiple VT morphologies of varying cycle lengths. Unlike coronary artery disease (CAD), DCM is associated with diffuse myocardial scar, which occurs mostly in the basal left ventricle, primarily in midmyocardial and epicardial layers [6]. In addition, His-Purkinje system-related reentrant arrhythmia such as bundle branch reentry and focal SMMVT preceded by Purkinje potentials are occasionally encountered in patients who have SHD [7,8].

Idiopathic and inherited ventricular arrhythmia

Focal SMMVT originating from right ventricular (or less commonly left ventricular [LV]) outflow tract (RVOT) is the most common type (approximately 90%) of VT in patients who have

Table 1

Comparisons between the electrophysiological characteristics of the focal and reentrant ventricular tachycardia

Characteristics	Focal ventricular tachycardia (VT)	Reentrant VT
Initiation	Spontaneous or during isoproterenol infusion	Spontaneous or programmed stimulation
Number of VT morphologies present	Single	Single or multiple
Electrogram voltage around site of successful ablation	Normal voltage in normal hearts or low voltage around the focal source in structural heart disease (SHD)	Low voltage area at the site and surrounding area usually has a protected corridor.
Electrogram (Egm) during VT	1. Shorter Egm to QRS interval 2. A lower ratio of Egm to QRS duration and diastolic interval	1. Isolated mid to early diastolic potential 2. Relatively higher ratio of Egm to QRS duration and diastolic interval
Pace map	Identical to nearly identical pace-map, short stimulus–QRS interval (approximates Egm–QRS interval in VT)	Identical to nearly identical pace map, long stimulus–QRS interval (approximates Egm–QRS interval in VT)
Entrainment	Cannot be entrained	Entrainment in most stable VT is possible.
Activation mapping (isochronal electroanatomical map)	Focal source with a centrifugal spread of activation	Reentrant excitation with a protected diastolic corridor

structurally normal hearts. The mechanism of these VTs is postulated to be cAMP-mediated delayed afterdepolarizations and triggered activity caused by an acquired somatic cell mutation in the inhibitory G protein. Idiopathic LV fascicular VT (ILVT), the second most common SMMVT, has a reentrant mechanism with a relatively small circuit in close proximity to the left posterior fascicle (10% in close proximity to the left anterior fascicle). Both these arrhythmias have a benign prognosis. Rarely, repetitive idiopathic PVCs from RVOT or originating from other sites in the ventricles can initiate polymorphic VT or VF (idiopathic VF), which is associated with a high risk for SCD. The mechanism of VA varies in inherited arrhythmia syndromes: early after depolarization-induced triggered activity (long QT syndrome), delayed afterdepolarization-induced triggered activity (exercise-induced catecholaminergic polymorphic VT), and phase 2 reentry (Brugada syndrome).

Indications for catheter ablation

Catheter ablation is indicated as a first-line therapy for symptomatic VT in patients who have normal hearts, and recurrent VT despite antiarrhythmic therapy in patients who have SHD (Table 2). Consideration of risks and benefits should be individualized. Procedural risks are likely to be increased in the elderly and in patients who have severe underlying heart disease. In many patients, VT recurrences are reduced acceptably by antiarrhythmic drug therapy, and ablation is not required. Recurrent PVCs or VT episodes can result in deterioration of LV systolic function (tachycardia-induced cardiomyopathy) and increase the risk for heart failure and SCD. Catheter ablation is indicated in these patients. Additionally, symptomatic frequent PVCs and monomorphic PVCs that repeatedly initiate polymorphic VT or VF (idiopathic VF and in rare cases of Brugada syndrome and long QT syndrome) can be treated with catheter ablation.

Preprocedural evaluation

Patients should be risk stratified according to their clinical status and the type of VA. Patients who have poor LV function or advanced heart failure may not tolerate VT induction necessary for precise mapping and ablation of VA. Therefore, active coronary ischemia and fluid as well as electrolyte status should be evaluated and treated appropriately before the procedure. Patients who present with polymorphic VT or VF and ischemic symptoms should be evaluated for active myocardial ischemia, whereas patients who have an SMMVT often have stable CAD and usually do not need ischemia evaluation. Therefore, evaluation for active coronary artery disease usually is not needed before catheter ablation of SMMVT.

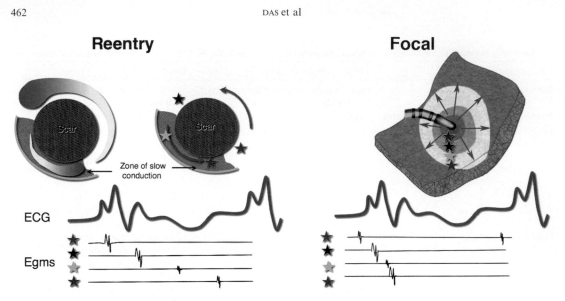

Fig. 1. Reentrant versus focal ventricular tachycardia (VT). The figure shows the timing of intracardiac recordings in relation to the surface ECG during mapping of a reentrant VT and a focal VT. Focal VT has a centrifugal activation.

Cardiac imaging before catheter ablation

Echocardiographic evaluation is required in patients who have SHD and poor systolic LV function to rule out any LV clot. It also may provide information regarding the location and extent of scar in the left ventricle. Traditional fluoroscopic mapping during EP study is a two-dimensional mapping system. Therefore, fine anatomic details such as papillary muscles and LV aneurysm are not visible. Recently, various mapping systems have been developed that create a three-dimensional map of the ventricles or the area of interest. These mapping systems recreate the geometry of the ventricles from point-by-point sampling while providing continuous display of the catheter position. Electrophysiological data such as the activation time, Egm amplitude, and impulse propagation are color-coded for display, which helps in localizing a focal source or a critical isthmus. This is possible only during a hemodynamically stable VT and allows mapping of multiple points during the VT. During a hemodynamically unstable VT, however, circuits cannot be localized well and therefore, ablation is performed in the scar border zones using substrate and pace mapping techniques. Scars in the left ventricle can be defined better by importing preacquired CT or cardiac magnetic resonance (CMR) images on mapping systems and using them as anatomic shells. These three-dimensional images can be incorporated into the three-dimensional map acquired during the EP study, which allows for a better understanding of the substrate and possible channels of VAs to be ablated.

Ventricular tachycardia morphology: an important guide to ablation

A careful analysis of ECGs of the clinical VT (mainly QRS morphology, QRS axis, and R wave transition in precordial leads) is prudent, because it is a major clue to the area of interest for mapping and ablation [9]. These serve only as a general guideline, however, because the QRS morphology in a reentrant VT also depends on several other factors such as the amount of scar, use of antiarrhythmic drugs, and orientation of the heart in the thorax (horizontal versus vertical) or on other pathology in the thoracic cavity (eg, pneumonectomy), causing alteration of the QRS vector.

Ventricular morphology in structural heart disease

As a general rule, in scar-based VT, all left bundle branch block (LBBB) morphology VTs arise from the LV septum (rarely from the right ventricle), whereas right bundle branch block (RBBB) morphology VTs can arise on the LV septum or the LV free wall. The QRS axis is the next major clue regarding the site of exit of a VT. A superior axis suggests an inferior wall exit site, whereas an inferior axis suggests an anterior wall exit site. The R wave amplitude in precordial leads is also a very important indication of the exit site

Table 2

Indications for catheter ablation of ventricular tachycardia and ventricular fibrillation according to current American College of Cardiology/American Heart Association guidelines [26]

	Indications	Level of evidence	Common scenario
Class 1	Patients who are otherwise at low risk for sudden cardiac death (SCD) and have sustained predominantly monomorphic ventricular tachycardia (VT) that is drug resistant, who are drug intolerant, or who do not wish long-term drug therapy	C	Idiopathic VT
	Patients with bundle-branch reentrant VT	C	Usually require an implantable cardioverter defibrillator (ICD) implant because of high recurrence of scar-related VT
	As adjunctive therapy in patients with an ICD who are receiving multiple shocks as a result of sustained VT that is not manageable by reprogramming or changing drug therapy or who do not wish long-term drug therapy	C	Patient with recurrent VT shocks or VT storm refractory to antiarrhythmic therapy
	Patients with WPW syndrome resuscitated from sudden cardiac arrest caused by atrial fibrillation and rapid conduction over the accessory pathway causing VF	B	High-risk patients with WPW syndrome
Class 2a	Patients who are otherwise at low risk for SCD and have symptomatic nonsustained monomorphic VT or monomorphic premature ventricular complex (PVC) that is drug-resistant, who are drug intolerant or who do not wish long-term drug therapy.	C	Idiopathic VT, tachycardia- induced cardiomyopathy
Class 2b	Ablation of Purkinje fiber potentials may be considered in patients who have ventricular arrhythmia storm consistently provoked by PVC of similar morphology	C	Idiopathic VF or VF in patients with structural heart disease (SHD) repeatedly initiated by a single monomorphic PVC
	Ablation of asymptomatic PVC may be considered when the PVCs are very frequent to avoid or treat tachycardia-induced cardiomyopathy.	C	Tachycardia- induced cardiomyopathy in patients with normal hearts and SHD
Class 3	Ablation of asymptomatic relatively infrequent PVC is not indicated	C	Asymptomatic PVC in patients with normal hearts or SHD

of a VT. Dominant R waves in precordial leads (V_1 to V_5) suggest a basal exit, and dominant R waves in the midprecordial leads (V_3 and V_4,) suggest an exit site between the base and apex. Apical VAs generate dominant S waves in all the precordial leads (similar to that encountered during right ventricular apical pacing).

Idiopathic ventricular tachycardia

Various algorithms have been described to localize idiopathic VTs also. VT originating from RVOT has an LBBB, inferior axis configuration with precordial transition to more positive QRS by V4, whereas the LV outflow tract (LVOT) VTs have RBBB inferior axis configuration [10]. A free wall origin is suggested by QRS duration greater than 140 milliseconds and notches in the inferior leads (II, III, AVF). Deeper S waves in aVL than in aVR suggest a leftward superior focus, and this ratio decreases with sites located more rightward and inferior in the RVOT. VT originating from the pulmonary artery and the aorta typically has large R waves in the inferior leads and greater R/S ratio in lead V2. The QRS axis depends on the location on the annulus.

Epicardial ventricular tachycardia

VTs that originate in the subepicardium generally have a slurred upstroke (pseudodelta wave). A pseudodelta wave of greater than or equal to 34 milliseconds (sensitivity: 83%, specificity: 95%), an intrinsicoid deflection time of greater than or equal to 85 milliseconds (sensitivity: 87%, specificity: 90%), and an RS complex duration of greater than or equal to 121 milliseconds (sensitivity: 76%, specificity: 85%) suggest an epicardial origin of a VT [11].

Ablation catheters and mapping techniques

Various mapping techniques are used to locate the circuit of a reentrant VT and the site of origin of a focal VT. VT that cannot be induced during EP study or be mapped because of hemodynamic compromise has a lower ablation success rate than the VTs in which the critical isthmus or the focal site can be localized. Several mapping techniques are used during catheter ablation of VT, including activation mapping, pace mapping, entrainment mapping, and substrate mapping (Table 3) [2,12]. Most commonly, a 4 mm or 5 mm tip mapping and ablation catheter is used for endocardial radiofrequency ablation (RFA). A 3.5 mm irrigated tip catheter is also used for VT ablation, especially for inflicting deeper tissue damage. Alternatively, an 8 mm catheter can be used for inducing a larger area of tissue damage; however, mapping is less precise because of a relatively larger antenna of these catheters. An irrigated tip catheter is preferred over the regular 4 mm tip RFA catheter for epicardial ablation. Cryoablation (4 mm to 6 mm tip) is another modality of catheter ablation, which inflicts tissue damage by decreasing the local temperature to −70° (usually applied for approximately 4 minutes at a single site). It has been used for VT ablation in the epicardium and the coronary sinus.

Activation mapping

Activation mapping is a very useful technique in patients who have hemodynamically stable VT. In focal VTs such as idiopathic RVOT VT, the earliest site of activation usually has a local intracardiac Egm 10 to 60 milliseconds earlier than the QRS onset. In reentrant VT in patients who have SHD, single or multiple presystolic or mid-diastolic Egms can be recoded in the isthmus or blind loop of the circuit (see Fig. 1).

Pace mapping

Pace mapping of VT and PVCs is performed by pacing from putative sites in the ventricles to entirely replicate the 12-lead QRS morphology of the VT induced in the EP laboratory or recorded on a standard ECG during the clinical arrhythmia, thereby to indicate the origin of a focal VT and critical isthmus of a reentrant VT. The QRS morphology obtained during pace mapping depends, not only on the location of the catheter in relation to the VT circuit or exit site, but also on several other factors. These include location of scar, catheter contact to the myocardial tissue, pacing output, unipolar versus bipolar pacing, and interelectrode distance during bipolar pacing. Pace mapping should be performed at a rate similar to the target VT using the minimum possible pacing output to ensure capture. Use of high pacing output may result in a relatively larger area of myocardial capture in the vicinity of the isthmus and may give rise to an erroneous QRS morphology, even when pacing is performed in the true isthmus. The 12-lead ECG during pace mapping should be matched carefully with the 12-lead ECG of the clinical VT or the target PVCs. An ideal pace map is considered perfect or exact if the QRS complexes in all 12 leads during pacing are identical to those of the targeted VT (ie, superimposable) (Fig. 2). A pace map is considered good if the QRS complexes during pacing and VT are identical in 10 or 11 of the 12 leads. An exact pace map (match) can be obtained in 49% to 81% of VTs [13]. Pace mapping at the site of fractionated Egms in the region of the suspected isthmus results in progressive prolongation of the S-QRS interval as the pacing site moves along the length of the isthmus, consistent with pacing progressively further from the exit site. Pace mapping is helpful in localizing the critical isthmus in up to 85% of VTs.

Entrainment mapping

Entrainment mapping is a very useful technique for mapping an SMMVT to determine the reentrant mechanism of the VT, and it can be performed from different sites in the ventricles. Usually, entrainment initially is performed from a site remote from the presumed isthmus by pacing at a cycle length marginally faster than that of the induced VT to demonstrate QRS fusion (manifest entrainment). Pacing also can be performed at progressively faster rates from the

Table 3
Comparison of mapping techniques and success rates of focal and reentrant ventricular tachycardia ablation

Hemodynamic status	Mechanism of VA	VT morphology	VA in structural heart disease (SHD)	Idiopathic VA	Mapping				Success rate
					Activation	Pace	Entrainment	Substrate	
Stable	Reentrant VT	SMMVT	Scar related	ILVT	+	±	+	+	High
	Focal	SMMVT or PVC	His-Purkinje disease	RVOT VT/PVC	+	+	−	−	High
Unstable	Reentrant VT	Sustained monomorphic VT	Scar-related reentry		−	±	−	+	Moderate to low
		Polymorphic VT/VF	Scar related reentry	Idiopathic VT/VF, BS, LQTS	−	−	−	−	Moderate to low
	Focal	Polymorphic	Monomorphic PVC-induced VT/VF		−	+	−	−	High

Abbreviations: BS, Brugada syndrome; ILVT, idiopathic left ventricular tachycardia; PVCs, premature ventricular complexes; SMMVT, sustained monomorphic ventricular tachycardia; VA, ventricular arrhythmia; VF, ventricular fibrillation; VT, ventricular tachycardia; +, useful; −, not useful; ±, sometimes useful.

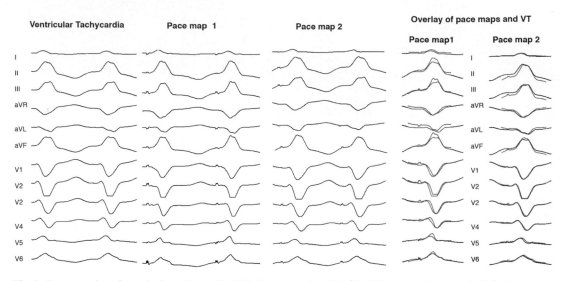

Fig. 2. Pace mapping of ventricular tachycardia (VT). Pace maps 1 and 2 of the VT are overlayed on the left. Pace map 1 is an example of a "not so good" pace map (9/12) of reentrant VT. At first look, the match appears to be close for QRS morphology in most of the leads but is obviously different in inferior leads (II, III and aVF), whereas pace map 2 is an excellent match (12/12) with the VT.

same site (or other sites remote from the presumed VT circuit) to demonstrate the progressive fusion of VT morphology on the 12-lead ECG, confirming its reentrant mechanism (entrainment with progressive fusion). Entrainment mapping then can be performed from additional sites, comparing the difference between the interval from the stimulus (S) artifact to the Egm at the pacing site on the first return complex of the VT (the postpacing interval, PPI) and the VT cycle length as a indicator of proximity of the pacing site to a critical isthmus. Finally, when entrainment is performed by pacing from the site of presumed critical isthmus, the 12-lead QRS morphology is identical to the VT, and the PPI at that site is equal or minimally longer (less than 30 milliseconds) than the VT cycle length (entrainment with concealed fusion) (see Fig. 2; Fig. 3).

Substrate mapping

Activation and entrainment mapping of rapid SMMVT, polymorphic VT, or VF is difficult because of a changing wavefront propagation, rapid heart rate, and hemodynamic instability. Careful analysis of clinical VT morphology helps to guide the regionalization of exit sites of VT. Because most of the VT circuits in CAD are located in the peri-infarct region (border zone),

pace mapping, along with substrate mapping, is helpful in localizing these areas. Single or multiple lines of ablation are performed perpendicular to the area of scar, which is extended from the scar tissue to the normal myocardium. Recently, a T-shaped line of ablation at the border zone has been used with reasonably good success [14]. Overall success rates of these types of ablation are less, because the precise circuit cannot be localized.

Therefore, these mapping techniques complement each other. All of these tools can be used to localize the critical isthmus of a hemodynamically stable sustained MMVT, whereas activation mapping and pace mapping are the only useful techniques available for localizing the exit sites of a focal VT or frequent symptomatic PVCs [15,16]. Mapping techniques for hemodynamically unstable MMVTs are limited to pace mapping and substrate mapping. Pace mapping complements the findings of activation and entrainment mapping [15]. Entrainment mapping is not helpful for focal VT mapping.

Ablation techniques

Most of the VT circuits are mapped and ablated endocardially. Epicardial ablation is needed for a minority of VTs associated with

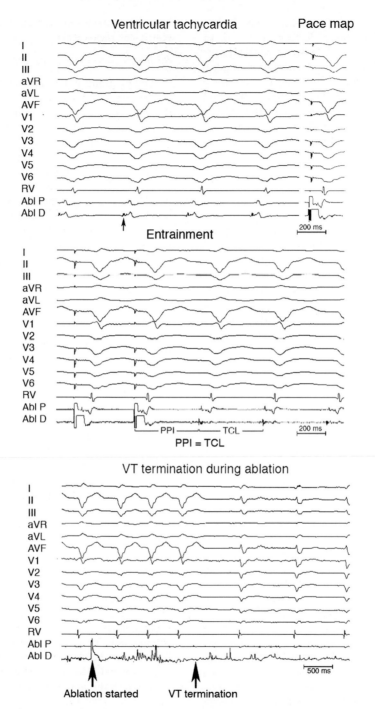

Fig. 3. Pace and entrainment mapping of a reentrant ventricular tachycardia (VT). A good pace map of VT (11/12) is displayed by pacing from the site where a presystolic potential (*small arrow*) was recorded by the ablation catheter (*upper panel*). Pacing during VT from the same site revealed concealed entrainment with a postpacing interval (PPI) equal to the tachycardia cycle length (TCL) (*middle panel*). Lower panel shows tachycardia termination during radiofrequency ablation. *Abbreviations:* Abl D: ablation distal, Abl P: ablation proximal, RV: right ventricle.

CAD, 30% to 40% of VTs associated with DCM, and a minority of idiopathic focal VTs [17]. In Chagas disease, 70% of VTs are epicardial in origin. Rarely, VT may arise from the pulmonary artery, the aortic sinus of Valsalva, the muscle bands in relation with the coronary sinus and the middle cardiac vein. Most idiopathic RVOT VTs and VTs associated with ARVD, congenital heart disease, or sarcoidosis arise from the right ventricle.

Endocardial ablation

LV mapping is performed retrogradely across the aortic valve or anterogradely across the mitral valve by means of a transseptal approach. The transseptal approach is the only method used for patients who have a mechanical aortic valve or severe peripheral vascular disease. LV mapping needs continuous anticoagulation during the procedure. The right ventricle is accessed by means of the femoral veins. The major risks of ablation include cardiac tamponade, thromboembolism including cerebral embolism (0% to 2.7%), coronary artery damage, incessant VT requiring multiple DC shocks, damage to the aortic valve, conduction system, or a coronary artery ostia, and rarely death. Significant vascular access complications, including bleeding, arterial dissection, and femoral arteriovenous fistulas can occur in about 2% of patients.

Epicardial ablation

Epicardial ablation is needed for VTs that originate in subepicardial or deep myocardial layers and cannot be ablated via the endocardium. The pericardial space is entered using an epidural needle under fluoroscopic guidance and contrast injection, followed by placement of a guidewire and introducer sheath for the mapping catheter [18]. Epicardial ablation is associated with a risk for epicardial coronary artery damage. Therefore, coronary angiography is recommended before the application of radiofrequency energy in all cases but infarct-related VT. Other risks include hepatic hemorrhage, phrenic nerve damage, pericardial effusion, and pericarditis. Pericarditis usually resolves in a few weeks, but patients may need aspirin or other anti-inflammatory drugs for that period.

Ablation strategies for sustained monomorphic ventricular tachycardia

Reentrant ventricular tachycardia

Mapping and ablation of a hemodynamically stable reentrant VT is very rewarding because of the high success rate of ablation. If a VT is inducible, then the QRS morphology guides toward the area of interest for mapping and ablation. Fig. 4 shows a reentrant circuit of an SMMVT with representation of different possible channels: critical isthmus, inner loop, outer loop, blind loop, and a bystander pathway. Careful manipulation of the mapping catheter locates the earliest mid-diastolic to late diastolic Egm during activation mapping (sites 1 and 3). Entrainment from these sites usually differentiates a blind loop (site 7) from the true isthmus (PPI–tachycardia cycle length is usually greater than 30 milliseconds at the blind loop). Additionally, pace mapping is performed within the isthmus. The stimulated wave front can proceed along certain paths, only which occur in at least two directions: the orthodromic and antidromic directions of propagation during the VT. Similar to the reentrant VT, the wave front during pace mapping only is detected on the surface ECG when it leaves this protected isthmus. Pacing from the exit site should give rise to a similar QRS morphology and a S-QRS interval that is relatively short and similar to the Egm to QRS (Egm–QRS) interval (sites 4 and 5). Pacing proximal to the exit sites should give similar results, except that the S-QRS and Egm-QRS intervals will be longer because of slow conduction of the impulse from those sites to the exit site [19]. Pace mapping from site 3 of the reentrant VT in Fig. 4 shows a long Egm-QRS (arrow) and similar S-QRS intervals with pacing, and a complete replication of each feature of each ECG lead. When the isthmus is short, or the catheter is positioned more proximally close to an entrance site of the critical isthmus (site 1), the stimulated antidromic wave front leaves the protected isthmus at the entrance and propagates to the surrounding myocardium producing a different QRS morphology. If the orthodromic wave front reaches the exit, a fused QRS complex is produced that includes depolarizations from both antidromic and orthodromic wave fronts. Therefore, the resultant QRS morphology depends upon the precise location of the pacing site relative to the reentrant circuit. As the mapping catheter is moved toward the

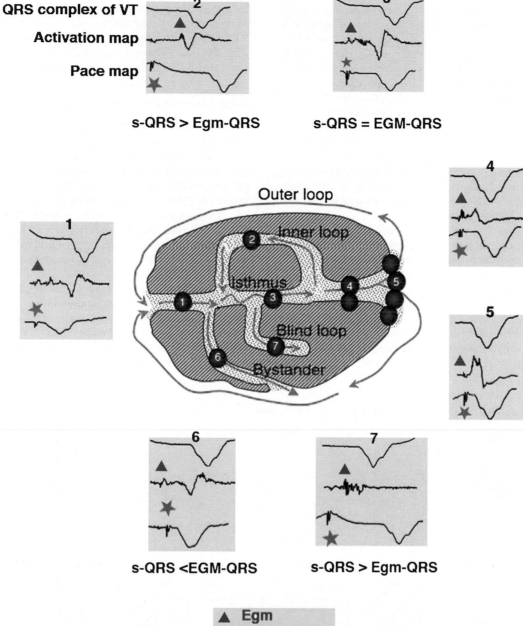

Fig. 4. Activation and pace mapping of a ventricular tachycardia (VT) from the presumed sites of VT circuits in a patient with structural heart disease. There is a long electrogram (Egm)–QRS interval (*arrow*) and similar stimulus (s)-QRS with pacing, and complete replication of each feature of each ECG lead when paced from the critical isthmus (*site 3*). Pacing during VT near entrance (proximal to slow conduction zone, (*site 1*) resulting in long S-QRS and QRS complexes identical to those of VT. Pacing at the same site, but during NSR, shows a completely different QRS, because the wave front can take a shorter path to normal myocardium than going through the diastolic corridor. Pacing near exit (*sites 4 and 5*) yields QRS match with a shorter S-QRS.

exit site (sites 4 and 5), pacing results in a QRS match of the VT but have a relatively shorter S-QRS interval. At the hypothetical bystander site (site 6), the activation map shows a relatively long Egm–QRS interval and a short S-QRS duration, whereas pace mapping shows a QRS morphology different from the clinical VT. In contrast to the entrance site of the critical isthmus (site 1), ablation at this site (site 6) will be unsuccessful. In the inner loop, the wavefront travels in the same direction as the outer loop. Therefore, the impulse reaches late during diastole at site 2, resulting in a relatively short Egm-QRS interval, whereas pacing from this site will show a relatively longer S-QRS interval, and ablation at this site also will be unsuccessful.

Fig. 5 shows various scar-related macroreentrant circuits encountered during mapping. Presystolic or mid- to late diastolic potentials (or Egms) are identified in approximately two thirds of patients during activation mapping of these VTs. A complete reentry circuit is defined in less than 20% of VTs with catheter mapping, whereas multielectrode and noncontact mapping systems identify endocardial exit regions of presystolic electric activity in greater than 90% of VTs. It is

not imperative to do this, however, because locating and ablating at the ideal site in the isthmus interrupts the particular circuit and terminate the VT. The participation of a particular isthmus with diastolic potential recorded during VT is confirmed by entrainment and pace mapping.

Focal ventricular arrhythmia

Focal MMVT (or PVC) generally is encountered in patients who have idiopathic VT, but it rarely may occur in patients who have MI scar. The bipolar Egm is used universally for this purpose, seeking a timing of 10 to 60 milliseconds before the QRS onset. The timing and morphology of unipolar recording from the catheter tip are also very helpful. At the suspected site of origin, this should have a sharp QS deflection that times with the bipolar recording and precedes the QRS onset by a similar amount.

As mentioned earlier, VTs in the setting of SHD have a reentrant mechanism in most patients, but a focal source of sustained MMVT has been reported also. A focal mechanism of VT has been found in 5% to 8% of VTs in patients who have CAD (Fig. 6). Similarly, a focal automatic

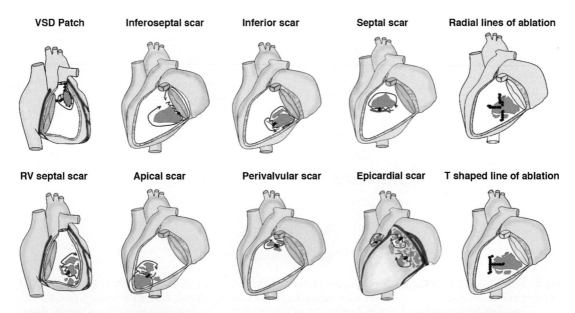

Fig. 5. Reentrant ventricular tachycardia (VT) circuits around myocardial scar in structural heart disease. The figure shows different endocardial and epicardial reentrant circuits with single loop or figure-of-eight wave fronts of VT, which can be ablated at critical isthmus sites. Reentry around a ventricular septal defect patch or right ventricular outflow tract (RVOT) patch can be ablated by connecting the ablation line from the patch to the pulmonary or the tricuspid valve. A single T-shaped line or multiple radial lines of ablation across the boarder zones often are drawn in patients in hemodynamically unstable VT. Blue lines denote potential circuits, red dots represent ablation points needed to interrupt the reentrant circuit.

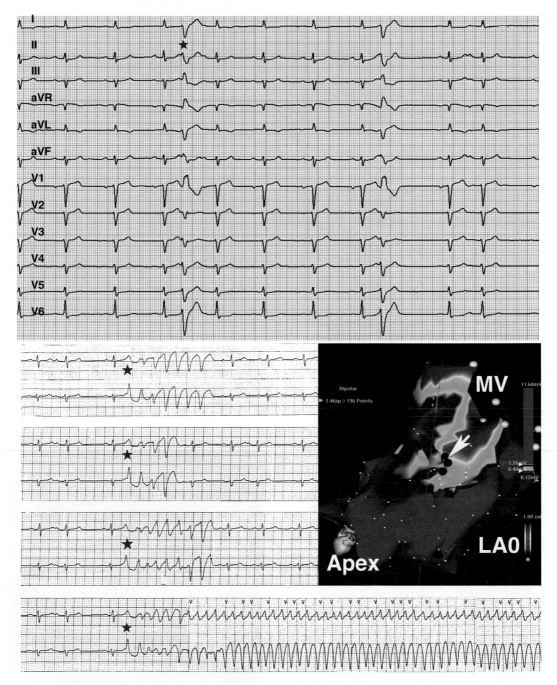

Fig. 6. Focal monomorphic premature ventricular complexes (PVCs) initiating nonsustained polymorphic ventricular tachycardia (VT) and ventricular fibrillation (VF). The telemetry recordings of a patient with history of myocardial infarction who presented with recurrent VF revealed frequent monomorphic PVCs and nonsustained VTs. Ablation of the PVC focus in the lateral left ventricle eliminated the ventricular arrhythmias.

mechanism was found to be responsible for VT in 27% of patients with DCM who underwent radiofrequency ablation for VT in one study [20].

Purkinje system ventricular tachycardia

His-Purkinje system-related SMMVT has been reported in patients who have SHD (8%) and in patients who have normal hearts [21].

Bundle branch reentrant ventricular tachycardia

Bundle branch reentrant VT occurs in 15% to 40% of patients who have DCM. It also can occur in ischemic cardiomyopathy (6%), after mitral or aortic valve surgery, myotonic dystrophy and rarely, in conduction system disease [22]. Typically, the VT has a LBBB pattern because of the wave fronts propagating retrogradely up the left bundle and anterogradely down the right bundle branch. Less frequently, the circuit revolves in the opposite direction, producing a RBBB configuration. Therefore, interruption of either of the bundles results in termination of the VT. Right bundle branch ablation, however, is preferred to avoid the hemodynamic consequences of chronic left bundle branch block (LV dyssynchrony). Usually, complete atrioventricular block does not occur. An ICD often is warranted, because of high risk of scar-related reentrant VT in these patients.

Ventricular tachycardias with participation of the left-sided His-Purkinje system

Interfascicular and fascicular VT occurs rarely in patients who have SHD. It can be cured by ablating the left posterior or left anterior fascicle depending upon the site of origin of the VT. It is associated with a considerable risk of complete heart block caused by preexisting conduction abnormalities. Similar VTs with a narrow QRS complex have been reported after acute or remote MI. During the VT, Purkinje potentials are captured orthodromically with decremental conduction properties, whereas presystolic Purkinje potentials are captured antidromically and appear between the His and QRS complex. In one study, catheter ablation at the site exhibiting a Purkinje–QRS interval of 58 plus or minus 26 milliseconds successfully eliminated VTs without provoking any conduction disturbances.

Idiopathic left ventricular tachycardia

ILVT involves the left posterior fascicle (less commonly, the anterior fascicle) and the posterior Purkinje network. The VT has a relatively narrow QRS (RBBB, superior axis), probably because of the conduction system being an integral part of the circuit. An abnormal diastolic potential within the posterior Purkinje network during sinus rhythm and VT can be used to guide successful catheter ablation of ILVT.

Ablation strategies for polymorphic ventricular tachycardia and ventricular fibrillation

Structural heart disease

For single or multiple unstable MMVTs and polymorphic VTs or VF, voltage maps are created from three-dimensional anatomic plots of low-voltage regions (less than 1.55 mV in bipolar recordings) to identify areas of scar and perinfarct zones. Pace mapping at the scar border zone usually is required for a SMMVT or PVC that triggers polymorphic VT/VF. Brief entrainment is tried and is often possible, even for unstable VTs, to confirm the location of a reentry circuit. Low-amplitude isolated potentials and late potentials inscribed after the end of the QRS complex during sinus rhythm also suggest potential isthmus sites. Connecting the two scar zones or scar and a line of conduction block/anatomic structure also is performed empirically (Fig. 7). A radial line or T-shaped line of ablation also is performed often at the scar border zones (see Fig. 5).

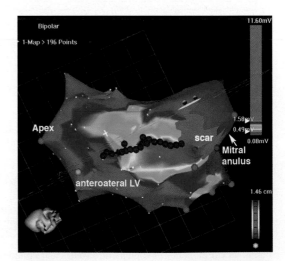

Fig. 7. Endocardial substrate mapping for ventricular tachycardia (VT). Endocardial substrate and pace mapping was performed for hemodynamically unstable reentrant VT with an exit site in the scar border zone of the anterolateral mid-left ventricle in a patients with history of myocardial infarction. Note a line of ablation was drawn across the border zone where good pace maps were achieved.

Polymorphic ventricular tachycardia and idiopathic ventricular fibrillation in normal hearts

Rare forms of polymorphic VT originate from the RVOT in structurally normal hearts and in the left ventricle in patients who have a history of MI. These VAs are triggered by monomorphic PVCs, which usually are preceded by a Purkinje-like potential. In idiopathic VF, activation and pace mapping of PVCs that initiate VF can be identified. Catheter ablation at these sites eliminates these trigger PVCs and prevents the recurrence of malignant polymorphic VT or VF episodes with a high success rate. Although this variety of life-threatening VA is initiated by repetitive monomorphic PVCs, the QRS morphology changes in the subsequent beats, and rapid pace mapping from the earliest site of activation also results in a change of QRS morphology similar to the clinical polymorphic VT. It is presumed that a shift in exit site during rapid pacing is responsible for the changing QRS morphology. Thus, PVCs that trigger polymorphic VT or VF in patients who have normal hearts, or SHD can be treated successfully with catheter ablation.

Ventricular tachycardia ablation in specific subpopulations

Coronary artery disease

Patients who have multiple VTs generally are tried on one or more antiarrhythmic drugs (most frequently, amiodarone) that have a limited response (19% to 50%). Most VTs can be ablated endocardially with a reasonably good long-term success rate of 77% to 95% for the clinical VT [2]. The epicardial approach for ablation is used for epicardial circuits or in presence of a LV thrombus (see Fig. 5).

Nonischemic dilated cardiomyopathy

SMMVT is uncommon in DCM. It occurs mostly (80%) because of scar-related reentry [20]. SMMVTs caused by reentry related to low-voltage regions (scars) often are located adjacent to a valve annulus that forms a border for the reentrant circuit. When a VT circuit cannot be defined during endocardial mapping, and significant low-voltage regions are not present on the endocardium, it often is present in the subepicardium (see Fig. 5). This likely contributes to the lower reported success rate of endocardial ablation. Some physicians start with epicardial ablation if

VT morphology suggests epicardial circuits. In Chagas disease, approximately 70% of VTs are epicardial in origin. Less commonly, it occurs because of bundle branch reentry [20]. Rarely, focal VTs are encountered. Of a series of 22 patients who had VT caused by reentry associated with DCM, endocardial ablation failed in 10 patients. Seven of these patients underwent epicardial mapping, with successful ablation in six patients. Fig. 8 demonstrates the endocardial and epicardial map of a patient with DCM in whom perivalvular and RV epicardial scar is demonstrated, whereas endocardial scar is minimal. His clinical VT was terminated by catheter ablation in the epicardial right ventricle medial to the proximal left anterior descending artery.

Other cardiomyopathies

Sustained VA is one of the major causes of SCD in cardiomyopathies such as hypertrophic cardiomyopathy, arrhythmogenic right ventricular dysplasia/cardiomyopathy (ARVD/C), various infiltrative cardiomyopathies such as sarcoidosis, and Chagas disease. ICD is indicated for most of these patients for secondary prophylaxis and for primary prophylaxis in high-risk patients.

Cardiac sarcoidosis

Cardiac manifestations of sarcoidosis include cardiomyopathy, AV block, and VA. Steroid treatment improves the heart block in 62% of patients, while the VT is unaffected. Many cases of VT related to sarcoidosis are misdiagnosed as idiopathic cardiomyopathy or ARVD. In a study of 98 patients who had nonischemic cardiomyopathy and VT, sarcoidosis was the cause in eight patients, and most were scar-related. Ablation abolished one or more VTs in six (75%) of eight patients, but other VTs remained inducible in all but one patient. After ablation, some form of sustained VT recurred in six of eight patients within 6 months. During a longer follow-up (range 6 months to 7 years), however, four of eight patients were free of VT with antiarrhythmic drugs and immunosuppression. Cardiac transplantation eventually was required in five of eight patients because of either recurrent VT (n = 4) or heart failure (n = 1). In another study, 68% of VTs were determined to be reentrant VTs.

Arrhythmogenic right ventricular dysplasia/cardiomyopathy

SMMVT occurs mostly because of reentry circuit in the vicinity of the tricuspid and

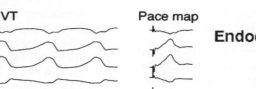

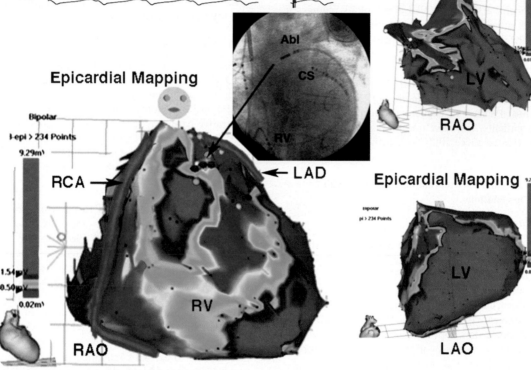

Fig. 8. Endocardial and epicardial bipolar voltage mapping to guide ablation. Endocardial and epicardial bipolar voltage mapping using an electroanatomical mapping system in a patient with dilated cardiomyopathy with sustained monomorphic ventricular tachycardia (VT). The endocardial mapping recorded minimal basal scar regions in the left ventricle (LV), whereas the epicardial mapping revealed extensive LV basal scars and right ventricular (RV) scar. The tachycardia was hemodynamically unstable. Pace mapping revealed an exit site medial to the proximal left anterior descending artery (LAD), which was ablated successfully. LAD and right coronary artery are drawn by mapping the coronary artery locations during coronary angiography. The fluoroscopic position of the catheter is shown in the left anterior oblique (LAO) view. *Abbreviations:* LL: left lateral view; RAO: right anterior oblique view.

pulmonary valve and the lateral right ventricle near the apex. The RV becomes paper-thin in scar regions; therefore, catheter ablation is associated with a 74% to 77% acute success rate. It also caries a higher risk for right ventricular perforation, and a high recurrence rate (11%–75%) due to the progressive nature of the disease [2].

Chagas disease. Cardiomyopathy caused by Chagas disease is associated with segmental scars, similar to ischemic cardiomyopathy. LV infero-lateral scar is often the source of VT (80%) and can be ablated successfully.

Congenital heart disease

Right ventriculotomy scar becomes a substrate for reentry in patients who have congenital heart disease such as repair of tetralogy of Fallot and ventricular septal defect. After repair of tetralogy of Fallot, the incidence of VT is 11.9%, with an 8.3% risk of SCD by 35 years of follow-up. Substrate mapping to evaluate congenital, surgical, and electrophysiological anatomy identifies the isthmus for successful VT ablation. Naturally occurring anatomic barriers in the right ventricle are limited, and the placement of a single ventriculotomy, outflow tract patch, or transannular patch, along with closure of the ventricular septal defect, would be expected to create only a limited number of possible tachycardia circuits (see Fig. 5). Unexcitable tissues from patch material or myocardial scar along with the tricuspid and pulmonary valve annuli form the channel. Common anatomic boundaries are isthmuses between the tricuspid or pulmonary annulus and septal scar or patch. These channels can be mapped with three-dimensional substrate mapping and connected by ablation lines during sinus rhythm. In one study, the acute success rate was 100%, and the long-term success rate was 91% (mean follow-up: 30.4 + 29.3 months).

Postvalve surgery

VTs after aortic or mitral valve surgery (without CAD) account for 4% of VTs. They have a bimodal presentation and occur either early after surgery (3 to 10 days) or years later (5 to 15 years) [23]. Most VTs are scar-related (70%). Nearly two thirds (64%) of patients have periannular scar in which an identifiable endocardial circuit isthmus (71%) and bundle branch reentry (10%) are present (see Fig. 5). The acute success rate of VT ablation is reported to be 98% [23].

Idiopathic monomorphic ventricular tachycardia in patients with normal hearts

Left ventricular outflow tract ventricular tachycardia and its variant

RVOT VT most commonly arises from RVOT (90%), and less commonly, it may originate from LV outflow tract, mitral annulus, pulmonary artery, aortic sinus of Valsalva, coronary sinus, and coronary veins. In fact, it may originate from any part of right ventricular or LV myocardium. These patients have frequent PVCs, nonsustained VT in salvos, or sustained VT. In a few patients, it is related to exercise [24]. These VTs or PVCs often are induced with burst pacing and with isoproterenol, adrenaline or aminophylline infusion, and terminated with intravenous injection of adenosine, β-blockers or calcium channel blockers. Success rates of ablation are higher in RVOT VTs and lower in septal VTs. The risks of ablation include RV perforation during RVOT or free wall ablation and complete heart block during septal ablation. The potential for acute occlusion of the left main or right coronary arteries is a major risk consideration, especially with VTs originating from the aortic sinuses of Valsalva. Coronary angiography and intracardiac ultrasound imaging have been used to define the proximity of the coronary ostia to the ablation site. Radiofrequency ablation has been performed safely at sites more than 8 mm away from the coronary artery ostia with careful continuous monitoring of catheter position during RF application. Standard RF ablation with tip temperature maintained at less than 55°C has been suggested to prevent aortic valve damage observed in animal studies. Epicardial origin of VT in close relation to coronary sinus can be ablated by means of the coronary sinus (Fig. 9).

Polymorphic ventricular tachycardia and ventricular fibrillation

The malignant variety of RVOT VT and idiopathic VF that is initiated by a single or two monomorphic PVCs can be ablated successfully with good long-term results (Fig. 10).

Inherited ventricular arrhythmia syndromes

Symptomatic and high-risk patients who have inherited arrhythmia syndromes are treated with an ICD. VT storm has been shown to have triggers (unifocal PVCs) from the Purkinje arborization or the RVOT. They play a crucial role in initiating VF in patients with long QT and Brugada syndromes. VT storm in Brugada syndrome is managed medically by infusion of isoproterenol. In one study, three patients who had long QT syndrome and four patients who had Brugada syndrome, episodes of polymorphic VT and VF, were associated with frequent isolated or repetitive PVCs, which could be ablated successfully without any recurrence during a follow-up of 17 + 17 months.

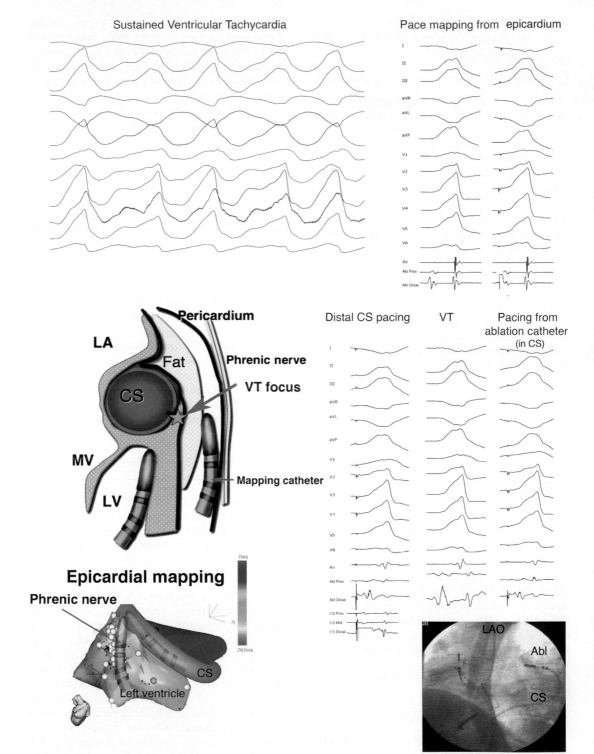

Sustained Ventricular Tachycardia

Pace mapping from epicardium

Pericardium

LA

Fat

CS

Phrenic nerve

VT focus

MV

LV

Mapping catheter

Epicardial mapping

Phrenic nerve

Left ventricle

CS

Distal CS pacing

VT

Pacing from ablation catheter (in CS)

LAO

Abl

CS

Electrical storms or ventricular tachycardia storm

Electrical storm (ES) is an important, independent marker for subsequent death among ICD recipients, particularly in the first 3 months after its occurrence. The development of VT/VF unrelated to ES, however, does not seem to be associated with an increased risk of subsequent death. Short- and long-term efficacy of catheter ablation for ES was studied in patients who had SHD (CAD, DCM and ARVD/C) [25]. After one to three procedures, induction of any clinical VT(s) by programmed electrical stimulation was prevented in 89% patients. VT storm was suppressed acutely in all patients; a minimum period of 7 days with stable rhythm was required before hospital discharge, and 92% patients were free of VT storm and 66% patients free of VT recurrence during a median follow-up of 22 months (range, 1 to 43 months). Eight of 10 patients who had persistent inducibility of clinical VT(s) had ES recurrence; four of them died suddenly despite ICD therapy.

Inducible ventricular tachycardias and ablation end points

Acute success

During EP study, in patients who have VT in the setting of SHD, an average of three different monomorphic VTs, including the clinical VT (VT requiring ablation) and nonclinical VTs, are induced. Of note, in many patients VT cycle length may be the only clue regarding the clinical VT, because the ICD promptly terminates VT. Ablation of incessant VTs and the inducible clinical VT is often an acceptable end point for success. Ablation of nonclinical VTs also is attempted because these VTs may recur subsequently. In one study, at least one VT was no longer inducible after ablation in 73% to 100% of patients, whereas all inducible VTs were abolished in 38% to 95% of patients [2].

Long-term results

VTs that are noninducible after ablation generally have low recurrence rates (less than 3% to 27%), whereas when the targeted VT remains inducible after ablation, the recurrence rate is greater than 60%. However, the frequency of episodes often is reduced in these patients. In a multicenter trial of 146 patients, the immediate effect on inducible VT did not predict outcomes; VT recurred in 44% of patients who had no inducible VT and 46% of those who had inducible VT. The frequency of spontaneous VT during short-term follow-up was reduced by more than 75% in most patients. Recurrence rate is higher after VT ablation in DCM [17].

The annual mortality after VT ablation ranges from 5% to greater than 20%, with death from progressive heart failure being the most common cause. The substantial mortality is consistent with the severity of heart disease and association of spontaneous VT with mortality and heart failure even when VT is treated effectively by an ICD. Older age, greater LV size, and LV dysfunction increase mortality. The potential for ablation to adversely affect LV function is a cause for concern, although assessment of LV ejection fraction after ablation has not shown any deterioration. Confining ablation lesions to regions of low-voltage scar and attention to appropriate medical therapy beneficial to patients who have LV dysfunction are prudent.

Future directions

VT ablation remains a relatively high-risk procedure with a success rate far from the desired because of several factors, including poor LV systolic function (in most patients who have SHD), inability to map the VT circuits with presently available mapping tools, hemodynamic instability, and changing activation patterns. Failure of ablation may be caused by organized thrombus preventing optimum energy delivery to the deeper myocardium, progression of disease, and multiple epicardial VT circuits that are not amenable to successful ablation due to epicardial fat and risk of coronary vessel and phrenic nerve injury. A high risk of recurrence after VT ablation occurs because of continued disease process,

Fig. 9. Mapping and ablation of epicardial ventricular tachycardia (VT). Initial mapping of the monomorphic premature ventricular complexes (PVCs) and VT with alternating QRS morphologies revealed a focal source originating from the epicardial surface of anterolateral mitral annulus. Because of the close proximity to the phrenic nerve (*white dots*), however, PVCs could not be ablated. Later, mapping of the same area was attempted by means of the coronary sinus, which revealed an early presystolic electrogram and an excellent pace map. The PVC was ablated successfully from this site. *Abbreviations:* CS: coronary sinus, LA: left atrium; LV: left ventrice; MV: mitral valve.

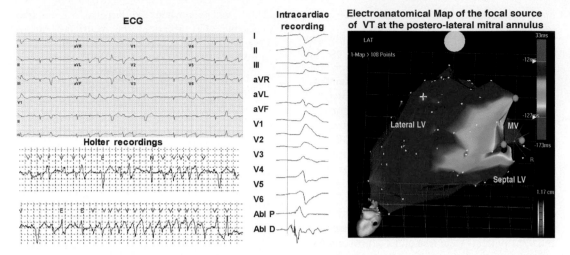

Fig. 10. Focal polymorphic ventricular tachycardia (VT) in a patient with normal heart. The 12-lead ECG shows a single monomorphic premature ventricular complex (PVC) that initiates frequent nonsustained polymorphic VT. The Holter recordings revealed multiple runs of symptomatic rapid nonsustained polymorphic VT. The intracardiac recording revealed a focal source originating from the lateral mitral annulus with a presytolic electrogram preceding the QRS during the premature ventricular complex by 30 milliseconds. Electroanatomical mapping shows a centrifugal activation pattern during the initiating premature complex that was ablated successfully (*red spot*). Follow-up Holter monitor did not show any polymorphic VT. Abl D and Abl P denote bipolar electrogram recordings form distal and proximal poles of ablation catheters, respectively.

electrolyte imbalance, ICD-induced proarrhythmia, and drug noncompliance. Development of better mapping tools (noninvasive and/or invasive modalities) with the capability to incorporate information regarding the substrate and pathophysiology of VT foci or reentrant circuits will reduce the procedure time and improve efficacy. The quest for alternative energy sources such as high intensity focused ultrasound, laser, and microwave are underway. VTs originating from deep within the ventricular myocardium may be treated by needle electrodes. Transcoronary ethanol ablation as an adjunctive therapy has been tried with limited success. Hemodynamic support with a percutaneous LV assist device may be used for ablation in patients with poor LV function. A recently published trial has opened the door for catheter ablation as a primary therapy in CAD patients who have VT.

Summary

Catheter ablation of VA may yield very satisfying palliation in most patients who have SHD and can be curative in those who have normal hearts. Catheter ablation, however, remains a challenging procedure for patients who have hemodynamically unstable VA. The success rate is less than desirable in patients who have unmappable VT and VT storm. Newer imaging modalities, mapping systems, and ablation techniques may improve the procedural success rate in the future.

References

[1] Zipes DP. Epidemiology and mechanisms of sudden cardiac death. Can J Cardiol 2005;21(Suppl A):37–40.

[2] Stevenson WG, Soejima K. Catheter ablation for ventricular tachycardia. Circulation 2007;115: 2750–60.

[3] Haissaguerre M, Shoda M, Jais P, et al. Mapping and ablation of idiopathic ventricular fibrillation. Circulation 2002;106:962–7.

[4] de Bakker JM, van Capelle FJ, Janse MJ, et al. Reentry as a cause of ventricular tachycardia in patients with chronic ischemic heart disease: electrophysiologic and anatomic correlation. Circulation 1988; 77:589–606.

[5] Pogwizd SM, Hoyt RH, Saffitz JE, et al. Reentrant and focal mechanisms underlying ventricular tachycardia in the human heart. Circulation 1992; 86:1872–87.

[6] Gottlieb I, Macedo R, Bluemke DA, et al. Magnetic resonance imaging in the evaluation of nonischemic cardiomyopathies: current applications and future perspectives. Heart Fail Rev 2006;11:313–23.

[7] Blanck Z, Dhala A, Deshpande S, et al. Bundle branch reentrant ventricular tachycardia: cumulative

experience in 48 patients. J Cardiovasc Electrophysiol 1993;4:253–62.

[8] Lopera G, Stevenson WG, Soejima K, et al. Identification and ablation of three types of ventricular tachycardia involving the his-Purkinje system in patients with heart disease. J Cardiovasc Electrophysiol 2004;15:52–8.

[9] Miller JM, Marchlinski FE, Buxton AE, et al. Relationship between the 12-lead electrocardiogram during ventricular tachycardia and endocardial site of origin in patients with coronary artery disease. Circulation 1988;77:759–66.

[10] Badhwar N, Scheinman MM. Idiopathic ventricular tachycardia: diagnosis and management. Curr Probl Cardiol 2007;32:7–43.

[11] Berruezo A, Mont L, Nava S, et al. Electrocardiographic recognition of the epicardial origin of ventricular tachycardias. Circulation 2004;109: 1842–7.

[12] Rothman SA, Hsia HH, Cossu SF, et al. Radiofrequency catheter ablation of postinfarction ventricular tachycardia: long-term success and the significance of inducible nonclinical arrhythmias. Circulation 1997;96:3499 508.

[13] Bogun F, Good E, Reich S, et al. Isolated potentials during sinus rhythm and pace-mapping within scars as guides for ablation of postinfarction ventricular tachycardia. J Am Coll Cardiol 2006;47:2013–9.

[14] Reddy VY, Reynolds MR, Neuzil P, et al. Prophylactic catheter ablation for the prevention of defibrillator therapy. N Engl J Med 2007;357(26):2657–65.

[15] Josephson ME, Waxman HL, Cain ME, et al. Ventricular activation during ventricular endocardial pacing. II. Role of pace mapping to localize origin of ventricular tachycardia. Am J Cardiol 1982;50: 11–22.

[16] Josephson ME, Horowitz LN, Spielman SR, et al. Role of catheter mapping in the preoperative evaluation of ventricular tachycardia. Am J Cardiol 1982; 49:207–20.

[17] Soejima K, Stevenson WG, Sapp JL, et al. Endocardial and epicardial radiofrequency ablation of ventricular tachycardia associated with dilated cardiomyopathy: the importance of low-voltage scars. J Am Coll Cardiol 2004;43:1834–42.

[18] Sosa E, Scanavacca M, d'Avila A, et al. Nonsurgical transthoracic epicardial catheter ablation to treat recurrent ventricular tachycardia occurring late after myocardial infarction. J Am Coll Cardiol 2000;35: 1442–9.

[19] Harada T, Tomita Y, Nakagawa T, et al. Pace mapping conduction delay at reentry circuit sites of ventricular tachycardia after myocardial infarction. Heart Vessels 1997;(Suppl 12):232–4.

[20] Delacretaz E, Stevenson WG, Ellison KE, et al. Mapping and radiofrequency catheter ablation of the three types of sustained monomorphic ventricular tachycardia in nonischemic heart disease. J Cardiovasc Electrophysiol 2000;11:11–7.

[21] Reithmann C, Hahnefeld A, Remp T, et al. Ventricular tachycardia with participation of the left bundle-Purkinje system in patients with structural heart disease: identification of slow conduction during sinus rhythm. J Cardiovasc Electrophysiol 2007;18:808–17.

[22] Mazur A, Kusniec J, Strasberg B. Bundle branch reentrant ventricular tachycardia. Indian Pacing Electrophysiol J 2005;5:86–95.

[23] Eckart RE, Hruczkowski TW, Tedrow UB, et al. Sustained ventricular tachycardia associated with corrective valve surgery. Circulation 2007;116: 2005–11.

[24] Morin DP, Lerman BB. Management of ventricular tachycardia in the absence of structural heart disease. Curr Treat Options Cardiovasc Med 2007;9: 356–63.

[25] Carbucicchio C, Santamaria M, Trevisi N, et al. Catheter ablation for the treatment of electrical storm in patients with implantable cardioverter defibrillators: short- and long-term outcomes in a prospective single-center study. Circulation 2008; 117:462–9.

[26] Zipes DP, Camm AJ, Borggrefe M, et al. ACC/ AHA/ESC 2006 guidelines for management of patients with ventricular arrhythmias and the prevention of sudden cardiac death: a report of the American College of Cardiology/American Heart Association Task Force and the European Society of Cardiology Committee for Practice Guidelines. Circulation 2006;114:e385–484.

ELSEVIER
SAUNDERS

CARDIOLOGY
CLINICS

Cardiol Clin 26 (2008) 481–496

A Comprehensive Approach to Management of Ventricular Arrhythmias

Fred Kusumoto, MD

*Electrophysiology and Pacing Service, Division of Cardiovascular Diseases, Department of Medicine,
Mayo Clinic School of Medicine, 4500 San Pablo Avenue, Jacksonville FL 32224, USA*

This review presents five cases that highlight the complexity of taking care of patients who have ventricular arrhythmias. Although there is a tendency to consider treatment of ventricular arrhythmias as a binary decision (ie, whether or not to implant a defibrillator), it is important to emphasize that treating ventricular arrhythmias and reducing the risk for sudden cardiac death in an individual patient requires a multifaceted approach. In addition, it should become apparent that extrapolating the results from clinical trials to management of individual patients can often be difficult because of the presence of comorbid conditions and the nuances of clinical trials that have small but important differences in design. Three of the cases discuss management of patients who have nonsustained ventricular tachycardia in the setting of structural heart disease: dilated cardiomyopathy, hypertrophic cardiomyopathy, and after myocardial infarction. A fourth case asks whether data from implantable cardioverter defibrillator (ICD) trials can be extrapolated to older patients, and the fifth case discusses management of recurrent ventricular arrhythmias in a patient who has an ICD.

Case 1: nonsustained ventricular tachycardia after a myocardial infarction with mildly reduced left ventricular function

A 64-year-old physician complains of 2 hours of substernal chest pain and is admitted with an acute inferior wall myocardial infarction. He undergoes primary angioplasty and stenting of an occluded right coronary artery. He has a residual ejection fraction (EF) of 45% with inferior hypokinesis, and on the third day of hospitalization, a six-beat run of nonsustained ventricular tachycardia is observed on telemetry. He was asymptomatic during the event.

Epidemiology and risk

Historically, frequent premature ventricular contractions (PVCs; generally considered > 10 per hour) or the presence of ventricular tachycardia after myocardial infarction has been considered important an independent prognostic marker for increased risk for overall mortality and sudden cardiac death [1]. In particular, the presence of nonsustained ventricular tachycardia (more than three beats) was found to be associated with a 2- to 3-fold increased risk for cardiac mortality [1,2]. In the prethrombolytic era, nonsustained ventricular tachycardia was observed in 12% to 25% of patients after myocardial infarction [1,2]. With the advent of early reperfusion strategies, the overall prevalence of nonsustained ventricular tachycardia after myocardial infarction has decreased substantially to 5% to 9% but continues to vary with the severity of left ventricular dysfunction [3]. In the Gruppo Italiano per lo Studio della Sporavvivenza nell' Infarto Miocardica (GISSI-2) trial, 8676 patients were followed for 6 months after thrombolytic therapy [3]. Nonsustained ventricular tachycardia was observed in 12% of patients with an EF less than 35% but in only 6% of patients with an EF greater than 35%. In addition to a lower prevalence with aggressive reperfusion strategies, the prognostic impact of nonsustained ventricular tachycardia

E-mail address: kusumoto.fred@mayo.edu

is less certain. For example, with multivariate analysis of the GISSI-2 data, the presence of non-sustained ventricular tachycardia was not associated with a worse prognosis (hazard ratio = 1.2, 95% confidence interval [CI]: 0.80–1.79) once other clinical factors, such as EF, were taken into account. Similarly, in a smaller study with longer follow-up (30 ± 22 months), the presence of nonsustained ventricular tachycardia was not associated with an increased risk for sudden death or significant ventricular arrhythmias [4]. In contrast, in a study of 700 patients followed for almost 4 years after myocardial infarction, the presence of nonsustained ventricular tachycardia was associated with a significant increased risk for sudden cardiac death (hazard ratio = 4.1, 95% CI: 1.3–13.0) [5]. In this patient cohort, the risk for sudden cardiac death began increasing approximately 2 years after the index event. To summarize, the presence of nonsustained ventricular tachycardia after myocardial infarction may identify a group of patients at higher risk for late sudden cardiac death, but all studies have found a low positive predictive value (5%–15%) that limits its use for guiding therapy.

Diagnostic testing

What additional tests can be considered to evaluate this patient's risk for sudden cardiac death? Left ventricular EF remains the most important prognostic factor for sudden cardiac death after myocardial infarction. In the Valsartan in Acute Myocardial Infarction Trial (VALIANT), 14,609 patients who had symptomatic heart failure after myocardial infarction were evaluated for risk for sudden cardiac death during a mean follow-up of 2 years [6]. Risk for sudden cardiac death was highest in patients with an EF less than 30% compared with patients with an EF greater than 30% (sudden death during the trial: EF <30%: 10%; EF 31%–40%: 6%; EF >40%: 5%). Regardless of EF, the risk for sudden cardiac death was highest in the first 30 days after myocardial infarction. In patients with an EF greater than 40%, the risk for sudden cardiac death was 0.88% per month during the first month, decreasing to 0.25% per month at 4 months. It is important to keep in mind that only patients who had symptomatic heart failure were enrolled in the VALIANT and that the sudden death risk for this patient is probably somewhat lower.

Impaired heart rate variability and reduced vagal tone have also been suggested as risk factors for sudden cardiac death after myocardial infarction. In the Autonomic Tone and Reflexes after Myocardial Infarction (ATRAMI) trial, heart rate variability and baroreceptor reflex sensitivity were evaluated after myocardial infarction in 1284 patients [7]. Reduced heart rate variability and a blunted baroreceptor reflex from a relative decrease in vagal tone were associated with increased mortality, particularly in those patients who had reduced left ventricular function. In a second cohort study of 244 patients who had myocardial infarction but relatively preserved left ventricular function (EF >35%, with 89% of patients with an EF >45%), the relative risk for overall mortality was 11.4 for patients with depressed baroreceptor receptor sensitivity [8]. Although reduced vagal tone seems to identify a group of patients who have a poorer overall prognosis, the specific effect of reduced vagal tone on sudden cardiac death remains unknown.

Instability of ventricular repolarization that can become manifest by the presence of microvolt T wave alternans during exercise testing has also been forwarded as another potential risk stratifier for sudden cardiac death after myocardial infarction. Ikeda and colleagues [9] evaluated the use of T wave alternans for predicting sudden cardiac death in patients with an EF of 40% or greater after myocardial infarction. They enrolled more than 1000 patients, almost all of whom had undergone revascularization (percutaneous coronary intervention in 94% and coronary artery bypass grafting in 5%) and performed microvolt T wave alternans testing 6 to 8 weeks after the myocardial infarction. Most patients (74%) had a negative microvolt T wave alternans test. Although a positive microvolt T wave alternans test was associated with a significant increase in the risk for sudden cardiac death (hazard ratio = 19.7), the positive predictive value was only 8%. In the same study, nonsustained ventricular tachycardia identified on 24-hour ambulatory electrocardiography and the presence of late potentials on signal-averaged electrocardiography were associated with lower but significant associated risk (nonsustained ventricular tachycardia: hazard ratio = 3.3 [range: 1.1–10.2]; late potentials: hazard ratio = 1.8 [range: 0.6–5.9]). Interestingly, lower EF (between 40% and 45%) did not confer additional risk for sudden cardiac death when compared with patients with an EF greater than 45%, suggesting that EF may be less useful as a marker for sudden cardiac death once the EF is greater than a threshold value of 40%.

Finally, there are provocative data from large epidemiologic studies that serum markers could be used to help evaluate the risk for sudden cardiac death. Several studies have found that elevated levels of free fatty acids are associated with an increased risk for sudden cardiac death (average relative risk = 1.7) [10,11]. Another analysis using serum samples from the Physicians' Health Study found that elevated levels of C-reactive protein were associated with an increased risk for sudden cardiac death [12].

To summarize, left ventricular function after myocardial infarction remains the most important prognostic tool for overall mortality and risk for sudden cardiac death. Specialized tests, such as heart rate variability, baroreflex sensitivity, and T wave alternans, and simple blood tests, such as C-reactive protein, may provide additional prognostic information, but low positive predictive values limit their clinical utility.

Treatment

Although not usually considered as management of sudden cardiac death risk, it is important to acknowledge the importance of modifiable risk factors in patients who have coronary artery disease. The Framingham Study found that cigarette smoking increased risk for sudden cardiac death by 2- to 3-fold [13]. Although not directly applicable to this case, in cardiac arrest survivors, cessation of cigarette smoking decreased the risk for recurrent sudden cardiac death by 33%, from 27% to 19% [14]. Obesity; psychosocial stressors, including economic and social problems; and a sudden increase in exercise in a previously sedentary individual have all been implicated as risk factors for sudden cardiac death [15–17] Finally, a large meta-analysis of randomized clinical trials of the utility of exercise rehabilitation programs after acute myocardial infarction reported a hazard ratio of 0.79 (95% CI: 0.57–1.09) for sudden cardiac death [18].

Several epidemiologic studies have evaluated the effects of ω-3 fatty acids on sudden cardiac death after myocardial infarction. In the Diet and Reinfarction Trial (DART), high fish oil intake was associated with a 29% reduction in total mortality in men after myocardial infarction [19]. Similarly, the GISSI Prevention Study demonstrated a 45% reduction in sudden cardiac death and a 20% reduction in all-cause mortality with ω-3 fatty acid intake [20]. Lipid-lowering agents may also reduce risk for sudden cardiac death.

In the Long-Term Intervention with Pravastatin in Ischemic Disease (LIPID) study, pravastatin was associated with a modest reduction in sudden cardiac death [21]. A meta-analysis of 10 trials with more than 20,000 patients found that statin therapy was associated with a 20% decrease in the risk for sudden cardiac death (hazard ratio = 0.81, 95% CI: 0.71–0.93) [22].

Beta-blockers are one of the cornerstones of therapy after myocardial infarction. In addition to their salutary effects on cardiac remodeling and reduced mortality, several trials have found that beta-blockers reduce the incidence of sudden cardiac death in patients after myocardial infarction. In the Norwegian Multicenter Study, timolol was associated with a 45% reduction in sudden cardiac death [23]. Similarly, in the Beta Blocker Heart Attack Trial (BHAT), a 28% reduction in sudden cardiac death was observed with propranolol therapy [24]. Angiotensin-converting enzyme inhibitors have been shown to reduce risk for sudden cardiac death in patients who have heart failure, although a beneficial effect in patients who have coronary artery disease and preserved left ventricular function has not been shown [25–27]. An integrated approach can reduce the risk for sudden cardiac death as illustrated by a cohort study of 2130 consecutive patients after myocardial infarction who were classified as receiving "optimal" therapy, defined as appropriate revascularization, beta-blockers, aspirin, statins, and angiotensin-converting enzyme inhibitors, or "nonoptimal" therapy (patients who did not receive these therapies if indicated by guidelines). After a mean follow-up of almost 3 years, the incidence of sudden cardiac death was 1.2% in the optimally treated group and 3.6% in the nonoptimal group [28].

Because patients who have coronary artery disease and ventricular arrhythmias have traditionally been considered to be at higher risk for sudden cardiac death, multiple older trials have evaluated the use of antiarrhythmic medications after myocardial infarction, unfortunately all with neutral or even harmful effects [29–32]. In the landmark Cardiac Arrhythmia Suppression Trial (CAST), patients who had ventricular ectopy after myocardial infarction were treated with encainide or flecainide, which was effective in suppressing the ventricular ectopy but was also more likely to cause sudden cardiac death because of proarrhythmia. [29]. This trial was the first to demonstrate that antiarrhythmic dugs can have harmful side effects and that surrogate end points (in this case, suppression of ventricular arrhythmias) are not adequate for evaluating the effectiveness of a medication. In the Canadian Amiodarone Myocardial Infarction Arrhythmia Trial (CAMIAT), 1202 patients who had ventricular ectopy observed after myocardial infarction were randomized to placebo or amiodarone [30]. After mean follow-up of 1.79 years, amiodarone was associated with a 38% reduction in sudden cardiac death but did not reduce total mortality. Similarly randomized trials of other antiarrhythmic medications, such as sotalol, dofetilide, or azimilide, after myocardial infarction have demonstrated no survival benefits [31–33].

Although ICDs can be effective for preventing sudden cardiac death, no trial has evaluated the use of an ICD for primary prevention of sudden cardiac death in the patient who has coronary artery disease and an EF greater than 40%. Because the incidence of sudden cardiac death in patients with preserved left ventricular function is low, ICDs in their present form are not likely to be used unless improved diagnostic tests become available that can select patients at higher risk. Given the temporal changes in risk for sudden cardiac death identified by analysis of the VALIANT, a large multicenter trial is currently being planned to evaluate the use of wearable external defibrillators during the initial period after myocardial infarction.

To summarize, the presence of ventricular arrhythmias has traditionally been considered a marker for higher risk, but this effect is attenuated by early reperfusion, the patient's preserved residual left ventricular function, and absence of clinical heart failure. Although diagnostic tests, such as T wave alternans and autonomic testing, may provide additional diagnostic information, their clinical utility is limited. Aggressive risk factor modification and treatment for smoking, hypertension, and diabetes should be initiated if applicable. A gradual exercise program coupled with diet and weight-loss counseling should be discussed. Standard post-myocardial infarction therapy with beta-blockade, antiplatelet drugs, and statins should be instituted, and ω-3 fatty acids can be considered as adjunctive therapy.

Case 2: elderly patient with a history of heart failure

An 80-year-old retired school teacher comes to your office for an annual evaluation. She has a known history of coronary artery disease and had an inferior wall myocardial infarction 4 years ago. Her most recent echocardiogram from several months ago reports an EF of 33%. She was hospitalized for heart failure 1 year ago but has done well since. She still complains of shortness of breath with mild to moderate exertion, but she is able to live independently. She is already being treated with optimal medical therapy, including beta-blockers and angiotensin-converting enzyme inhibitors. Her electrocardiogram shows inferior Q waves but with a normal QRS duration. Her family asks whether an ICD would be beneficial.

The most rapidly growing segment in the United States is the elderly (>65 years of age) with the "oldest old" (>80 years of age) comprising more than 7 million people [34]. The United States census bureau estimates that the worldwide population of people older than 80 years of age is going to increase from 75 million in 2002 to more than 400 million by 2050. It is estimated that almost 30% of the eligible population for ICDs in the United States is older than 79 years of age [35].

Several trials have evaluated the use of ICDs in patients who have heart failure after a myocardial infarction. The largest of these, the Sudden Cardiac Death in Heart Failure Trial (SCD-HeFT) could apply to this patient by clinical inclusion criteria [36]. This trial randomized 2521 patients who had ischemic and nonischemic cardiomyopathy, an EF less than 35%, and class II or III heart failure to placebo, amiodarone, or an implantable defibrillator implant. After mean follow-up of 45.5 months, ICD therapy was associated with a 23% reduction in overall mortality compared with amiodarone or placebo.

Currently published guidelines have subtle differences in recommendations for ICD implantation in patients who have heart failure. In the American Heart Association/American College of Cardiology (AHA/ACC) 2005 Heart Failure Guidelines, a patient who has class II/III heart failure and an EF less than or equal to 30% to 35% is considered to have a class IIa indication for implantation [37]. In the 2006 ACC/AHA Prevention of Sudden Cardiac Death Guidelines, indications for ICD implantation have been elevated to a class I recommendation for patients who have class II/III heart failure with a higher EF range of less than or equal to 30% to 40% and a new class IIa recommendation for patients who have class I heart failure symptoms and an

EF less than 35% has been added [38]. In both guidelines, an EF range acknowledges the vagaries of EF estimation and implicitly asks whether a patient with an EF reported as 36% truly has a lower risk for sudden cardiac death than a patient with an EF of 35%.

Although by both guidelines, this patient is a candidate for ICD implantation, can ICD implantation confer a survival benefit in our elderly but otherwise healthy patient and does the risk for ICD implantation increase with age? Unfortunately, limited data are available on whether the benefits of ICDs can be generalized to the older patient. In the SCD-HeFT, although no upper age limit criteria was specified, the median age was 60 years [36]. In a prespecified subgroup analysis, the survival benefit was greater in patients less than 65 years of age (hazard ratio = 0.68, 95% CI: 0.50–0.93) when compared with patients older than 65 years of age (hazard ratio = 0.86, 95% CI: 0.62–1.18). It is important to remember that the overall survival curves in the SCD-HeFT did not begin to separate until 2 years after ICD implantation. Indirect information on the potential utility of ICDs in the elderly is also available from the Multicenter Unsustained Tachycardia Trial (MUSTT) [39]. In the MUSTT, patients with an EF less than 40% and nonsustained ventricular tachycardia were randomized to electrophysiology-guided therapy (which could include ICD use) or no specific antiarrhythmic therapy. The 5-year rate of cardiac arrest or arrhythmic death was 33% for patients older than 70 years of age and 28% for patients younger than 70 years of age. Implantation of an ICD in the subgroup of patients older than 70 years of age was associated with a 57% decrease in the risk for sudden cardiac death, an effect that was actually greater than for the younger than 70-year-old age group.

Although no prospective randomized trial has specifically evaluated the effects of ICDs in the elderly patient, several cohort studies have attempted to evaluate the relation between age and ICD benefit [40–44]. In a single center study of 107 octogenarians who received ICDs, median survival depended on left ventricular function and renal function: 6.1 years if the EF was greater than 30% and the estimated glomerular filtration rate (eGFR) was greater than 60 mL/min, 4.7 years if the EF was 30% or less and the eGFR was 60 mL/min or less, and only 19 months if the EF was less than 30% and the eGFR was 60 mL/min or less [40]. Another study that compared

outcomes after ICD implant between 74 patients older than 75 years of age and 695 patients younger than 75 years of age found higher total mortality in the elderly patients but no sudden deaths during a mean follow-up of 29 months [41]. Taken together, the available data suggest that ICDs can be beneficial in selected elderly patients who are likely to have substantial survival (>2 years) because of the absence of comorbidities.

Several studies have evaluated the relation between age and operative risk for ICD implantation. Noseworthy and colleagues [42] found no difference in complication rates between octogenarians and septuagenarians undergoing ICD implantation, with no perioperative deaths in the study group. This low perioperative risk may not be generalizable to larger populations treated outside of studies, however. In a study of more than 23,000 Medicare beneficiaries with varying ages (65–74 years old: 39%; 75–84 years old: 40%; >84 years old: 6%) who underwent ICD implantation in 2003, an overall complication rate of 11% during the implant hospitalization was observed [43]. Another important issue is the development of complications during the lifetime of the device. In a long-term study of 500 patients with ICDs, 24% of patients observed at least one complication during a mean follow-up of 4 years [44]. The most common problem was inappropriate shocks, which can be associated with significant reductions in quality-of-life. The lingering effects of an ICD shock may be more important in the elderly patient.

After a discussion of the treatment options, our patient chose not to have an ICD implanted.

Case 3: ventricular arrhythmias in a patient who has recently identified idiopathic dilated cardiomyopathy

A 42-year-old attorney with no prior medical history came to your office 1 week ago complaining of a 2-week history of progressive shortness of breath. An echocardiogram revealed a reduced EF of 28%, and subsequent cardiac catheterization demonstrated normal coronary artery anatomy. A 24-hour ambulatory electrocardiogram revealed frequent PVCs (18,722 during the monitoring period) with several short runs of nonsustained ventricular tachycardia (three beats and seven beats). The patient is started on beta-blockers and afterload reduction. What therapies could be considered for treating his ventricular arrhythmias and his overall risk for sudden cardiac death?

Epidemiology and risk

Idiopathic dilated cardiomyopathy has multiple causes but is familial in 40% of cases, most frequently attributable to mutations in architectural or sarcomeric proteins [45]. The 5-year mortality rate is approximately 20%, with 30% of deaths occurring suddenly [45]. Unfortunately, risk stratification for prevention of sudden cardiac death is difficult in patients who have idiopathic dilated cardiomyopathy.

Similar to patients who have ischemic cardiomyopathy, it seems that left ventricular EF is an important predictor for sudden cardiac death. In the Marburg Cardiomyopathy Study, 343 patients who had idiopathic dilated cardiomyopathy were evaluated with multiple techniques, including echocardiography, ambulatory electrocardiography, signal-averaged electrocardiography, heart rate variability, baroreflex sensitivity, and microvolt T wave alternans, and they were followed for more than 4 years. On multivariate analysis, left ventricular EF was the only predictor for risk for sudden cardiac death, with a relative risk of 2.3 for each 10% reduction in left ventricular EF. Ventricular ectopy is common in patients who have idiopathic dilated cardiomyopathy, with nonsustained ventricular tachycardia observed in 25% to 30% of patients and frequent PVCs (>10 PVCs per hour) in 35% to 40% of patients [46–48]. Some but not all studies have suggested that the presence of nonsustained ventricular tachycardia is an independent risk factor for sudden cardiac death [46–48].

The ability of specialized tests for sudden death risk stratification has been evaluated in patients who have idiopathic dilated cardiomyopathy. Microvolt T wave alternans has been found to be a useful predictor for the development of ventricular arrhythmias in one study but not in another [46,49]. Recently, the relation between QT interval changes and heart rate (QT dynamicity) has been forwarded as a possible tool for predicting ventricular arrhythmias in patients who have idiopathic dilated cardiomyopathy [47]. Investigators found that a steeper slope of the ratio of the interval between QRS complexes and the QT interval (RR/QT slope) was associated with an increased risk for arrhythmic events. A steeper RR/QT slope could be attributable to excessive shortening of the QT interval with fast heart rates or to excessive prolongation of the QT interval with slow heart rates. Increased QT dynamicity could lead to ventricular arrhythmias by facilitating re-entry or by increasing the risk for after-depolarizations and triggered arrhythmias at slower heart rates. Similar to the situation with ischemic heart disease, these specialized tests, although promising, currently are not generally indicated for patients who have idiopathic dilated cardiomyopathy.

Treatment

Medical treatments, such as beta-blockade, angiotensin-converting enzyme inhibitors, and aldosterone antagonists, that have been associated with reduced overall mortality have also shown a reduced incidence of sudden cardiac death [50,51]. Amiodarone can be used in selected patients who have symptomatic ventricular arrhythmias and does reduce the incidence of sudden cardiac death but is not associated with improved survival [52].

Several prospective trials have evaluated the use of defibrillators in patients who have dilated cardiomyopathy. In the Cardiomyopathy Trial (CAT), 104 patients who had newly diagnosed dilated cardiomyopathy (≤ 9 months) were randomized to receive an ICD or not [53]. The trial was stopped after 1 year when no differences were detected between the two groups. There were no episodes of sudden cardiac death in either group during the trial. In the larger Defibrillators in Nonischemic Cardiomyopathy Treatment Evaluation (DEFINITE) trial, 458 patients who had idiopathic dilated cardiomyopathy (EF $\leq 35\%$) and frequent PVCs or nonsustained ventricular tachycardia were randomized to receive best medical therapy with or without an ICD [54]. ICD therapy was associated with a trend toward reduced mortality at 2 years (mortality: 8.1% with ICD versus 13.8% with no ICD) that did not reach statistical significance ($P = .06$). ICD implantation was associated with a significant reduction in the risk for sudden cardiac death, however, with the survival curves beginning to separate approximately 1 year after ICD implantation. The large SCD-HeFT (EF $\leq 35\%$, class II/III) enrolled more than 1200 patients who had idiopathic dilated cardiomyopathy and is the only trial to demonstrate improved survival associated with ICD implantation in this patient population [36].

The 2006 Guidelines for Prevention of Sudden Cardiac Death have placed the ICD as a class I indication for patients who have idiopathic dilated cardiomyopathy and an EF of 35% or less and class II or III symptoms [38]. In addition, they classify patients with an EF of 35% or less and class I symptoms as class IIb. Controversy exists over the timing of ICD implantation for newly identified dilated cardiomyopathy. Large trials have described recovery of left ventricular function in 20% to 30% of patients, and more than 50% of patients have a significant improvement in left ventricular function (absolute increase >10% in left ventricular EF) with aggressive pharmacologic therapy [55]. In a post-hoc analysis of the DEFINITE trial, however, a benefit from ICD implantation was identified even in those patients with a recent diagnosis of dilated cardiomyopathy (<3 months or <9 months); information on the impact of temporal changes in EF from the DEFINITE study are not available [56]. It may be that echocardiographic criteria, such as marked impairment of left ventricular function (<20%), enlarged spherical left ventricles, and the presence of pulmonary hypertension identify patients who are unlikely to respond to therapy [57,58]. The presence of significant fibrosis identified by late gadolinium enhancement with MRI has been thought to be associated with an increased risk for sudden cardiac death and reduced likelihood of reversibility [59]. In addition, patients with persistently elevated troponin, possibly attributable to ongoing myocyte degeneration, have been found by some investigators to have a worse prognosis [60].

In some circumstances, frequent PVCs (traditionally considered to be >20,000 over 24 hours) can be associated with cardiomyopathy [61]. It has been speculated by some investigators that the mechanism of cardiomyopathy in this condition is cardiac dyssynchrony [62]. Suppression of the ventricular ectopy with medications or ablation can be associated with improvement in left ventricular function [61–63]. In a selected group of 22 patients with frequent PVCs and accompanying cardiomyopathy, radiofrequency catheter ablation was associated with a significant improvement in left ventricular function in all 18 patients who could have their PVCs successfully ablated [63].

This patient underwent aggressive therapy with beta-blockade and angiotensin-converting enzyme inhibitors. The timing of whether to implant an ICD is much more difficult. The main problem in patients who have idiopathic dilated cardiomyopathy is our inability to predict natural history or the response to treatment. In this case, the patient underwent radiofrequency catheter ablation of a left ventricular outflow tract site with normalization of his EF after 1 month of follow-up (Fig. 1). It is not known whether left ventricular function would have spontaneously improved.

Case 4: multiple implantable cardioverter defibrillator discharges

A 47-year-old man with a history of idiopathic dilated cardiomyopathy had an ICD implanted for reduced EF (22%). He has come to the emergency room after receiving three shocks from his device. Interrogation of his device (Fig. 2) shows appropriate shocks for ventricular arrhythmias.

ICD shocks can be appropriate or inappropriate. Inappropriate ICD discharges can be attributable to multiple causes, including supraventricular arrhythmias or noise from lead fracture or outside interference. Unfortunately, inappropriate discharges are common and occur in 13% to 22% of cases [36,53,54]. In fact, in the DEFINITE study discussed previously, a patient was more likely to receive an inappropriate discharge (21%) than an appropriate discharge (18%) [54]. Evaluation of the stored electrograms from the event can provide important diagnostic clues on whether a shock was appropriate or inappropriate (Fig. 3).

In this case, the ICD delivered appropriate shocks for repetitive episodes of ventricular tachycardia. Frequent appropriate device discharges for repetitive bursts of sustained ventricular arrhythmias are often called electrical storm. Although there is no specific definition, two or three device shocks or therapies during a 24-hour period is used by most investigators [38]. Electrical storm is not uncommon, with a reported incidence of 10% to 20% [64–71]. One recent study found that although an appropriate shock in patients who have ischemic cardiomyopathy is often an isolated event (90%), patients who have dilated cardiomyopathy commonly have recurrent arrhythmias over the next 24-hour period after an appropriate shock [70]. Causes of electrical storm include ischemia, electrolyte disorders, and heart failure exacerbation; however, in most cases, a specific cause for electrical storm cannot be readily identified. In patients who have ischemic cardiomyopathy, the development of electrical storm is a poor prognostic sign and may be a sign of

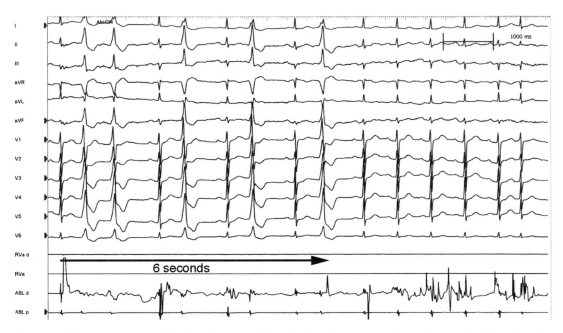

Fig. 1. Radiofrequency catheter ablation after 6 seconds. 12 lead ECG (I, II, III, aVR, aVL, aVF, V1-V6) and cardiac electrograms are shown. ABLd, ablation catheter, distal electrodes; ABLp, ablation catheter, proximal electrodes; RVA, right ventricular apex, proximal electrodes; RVAd, right ventricular apex, distal electrodes.

a failing heart. In an analysis of the Multicenter Automatic Defibrillator Implantation Trial-II (MADIT-II), there was a 3-fold increase in the risk for death after an appropriate device discharge and an 18-fold risk for death in the 3 months after electrical storm [69]. Patients who have dilated cardiomyopathy also have a grim prognosis after the development of electrical storm. In a cohort study of 106 patients, after 3 years of follow-up, 28% of patients had clusters of ventricular arrhythmias [70]. Once electrical storm developed, the subsequent 1-year survival rate was only 57%.

Acute treatment of electrical storm usually involves stabilizing patients with antiarrhythmic medications. Intravenous amiodarone is effective for acute treatment of electrical storm. In one of the few randomized trials available for treatment of electrical storm, 352 patients who had recurrent hemodynamically unstable ventricular arrhythmias that were refractory to lidocaine and procainamide were randomized to intravenous amiodarone or bretylium [72]. In this extremely ill patient group (14% 48-hour mortality rate), bretylium and amiodarone were effective in suppressing recurrent ventricular arrhythmias in approximately 50% of patients. Bretylium was associated with a significantly higher rate of

adverse effects, however, including hypotension, atrioventricular (AV) block, and heart failure. The class I drugs are less successful (30%) for treating electrical storm [71]. Although lidocaine has historically been the initial antiarrhythmic medication used for ventricular arrhythmias and may be effective in some circumstances, such as myocardial ischemia, it is now considered a second-tier medication [38,73]. Institution of antiadrenergic therapy is important in patients with electrical storm. In one noncontrolled study of 49 patients who had recurrent ventricular arrhythmias after a myocardial infarction, investigators found that sympathetic blockade was more effective than standard antiarrhythmic therapy [74]. As a corollary, anxiolytics are an important adjunctive therapy to reduce the sympathetic activity in electrical storm; there has been a case report of effective acute treatment of drug-refractory electrical storm with general anesthesia using propofol [75]. Patients who seem to have ventricular arrhythmias triggered by pauses or bradycardia can be treated with temporary pacing. In patients who have recurrent ventricular arrhythmias that become hemodynamically unstable, intra-aortic balloon pump (IABP) counterpulsation and ventricular assist devices (VADs) may be required.

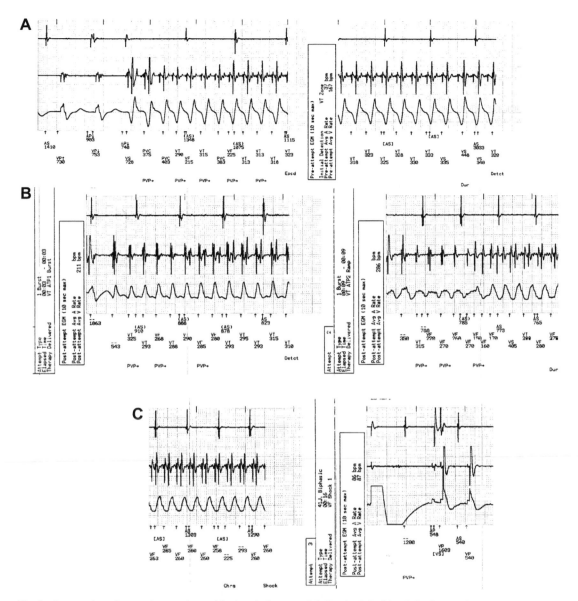

Fig. 2. Appropriate therapy in a patient with electrical storm. (*A*) On the left side of the figure, the patient is in sinus rhythm with sudden onset of ventricular tachycardia (note the atrioventricular dissociation of the atrial and ventricular electrograms). (*B*) The ICD first tries antitachycardia pacing that accelerates the ventricular tachycardia slightly and changes the QRS morphology. A second attempt with antitachycardia pacing causes transient polymorphic ventricular tachycardia that organizes to a different QRS morphology. (*C*) The patient receives a 41-J shock that terminates the ventricular tachycardia. AP, atrial pace event; AS, atrial sense event; Avg, average; bpm, beats per minute; Chrg, charge; Detct, detect; Epsd, episode; EGM, electrogram; max, maximum; PVC, premature ventricular contraction; PVP, post-shock ventricular protection period; VP, ventricular pace event; VS, ventricular sense event; VT, ventricular tachycardia.

Once the patient has been stabilized and optimal therapy for cardiac ischemia and heart failure is established, one of the first considerations for long-term management of electrical storm is assessing the programming of the ICD. Patients who have idiopathic cardiomyopathy tend to have longer episodes of self-terminating ventricular arrhythmias. It is important for the physician to program a sufficient interval to allow ventricular arrhythmias to self-terminate but not to delay delivery of necessary therapy. This can often be a delicate balance and may vary with

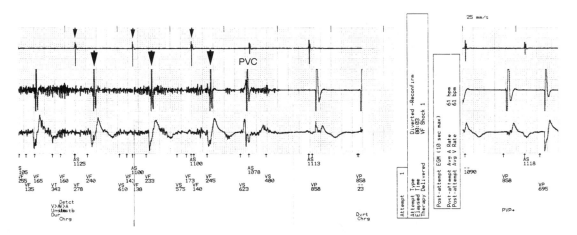

Fig. 3. Internal electrograms from a patient with an intermittent lead fracture. At baseline, the patient is in sinus rhythm (*small arrows*) and first-degree atrioventricular block (*large arrows* show intrinsic ventricular signal). The patient also has a single PVC. The intermittent fracture leads to high-frequency signals, which lead to the ICD inappropriately "diagnosing" ventricular fibrillation (VF). Fortunately, the problem is intermittent, and the ICD does not deliver a shock when it reconfirms for continued ventricular arrhythmia. AS, atrial sense event; bpm, beats per minute; Chrg, charge; Detct, detect; Dvrt, divert; EGM, electrogram; max, maximum; VS, ventricular sense event; VT, ventricular tachycardia.

changes in the patient's clinical condition. Antitachycardia pacing is an important therapy option available in all currently implanted ICDs. Antitachycardia pacing can be effective in patients who have ventricular arrhythmias in the setting of ischemic cardiomyopathy and prior myocardial infarction. One study composed mostly of patients who had coronary artery disease found that antitachycardia pacing was effective 72% of the time for terminating ventricular arrhythmias [76]. Patients with ICDs that were programmed for aggressive antitachycardia pacing had fewer shocks and higher quality-of-life indices than those patients with antitachycardia pacing programmed "off." Unfortunately, antitachycardia pacing is less effective in patients who have idiopathic dilated cardiomyopathy because ventricular arrhythmias are more likely to be attributable to a focal mechanism rather than to re-entry [77].

Long-term antiarrhythmic drug therapy for electrical storm can include sotalol, dofetilide, or amiodarone. Several studies have found that treatment with sotalol can decrease the likelihood of ventricular arrhythmias and ICD therapy [68,78]. Sotalol seems to be less effective in patients who have idiopathic dilated cardiomyopathy [68]. The Optimal Pharmacologic Therapy in Cardioverter Defibrillator Patients (OPTIC) trial found that amiodarone and beta-blockade were more effective than sotalol or beta-blockade alone for preventing shocks in patients with ICDs [78].

Amiodarone has several serious adverse side effects, however, including optic neuropathy or neuritis (1%–2%), hyperthyroidism (1%–2%), pulmonary toxicity (1%–17%), peripheral neuropathy (0.3% annually), blue skin discoloration (5%–9%), and photosensitivity (25%–75%) [79].

In some cases, medical therapy is not sufficient for treating patients with ICDs and recurrent electrical storm. In a study of 29 patients who had ischemic cardiomyopathy presenting with frequent ICD shocks attributable to recurrent ventricular fibrillation, 21 patients were controlled with antiarrhythmic drugs (16 patients: 15 with amiodarone and 1 with dofetilide) or with treatment of decompensated heart failure (5 patients). The remaining 8 patients underwent radiofrequency catheter ablation by targeting the PVCs that initiated the ventricular fibrillation [80]. After ablation and a mean follow-up of 10 months, none of the patients had recurrent storms of ventricular fibrillation. Similarly, in a single-center study of 95 patients who developed electrical storm despite medical therapy (maximal beta-blockade in 97% and long-term amiodarone use in 94%), radiofrequency catheter ablation was acutely successful in 70% to 90% of patients but required repeat procedures in 19% of patients [81]. After a median follow-up of 22 months, 66% of patients were free of recurrent ventricular tachycardia and 92% of patients did not have recurrent electrical storm. After ablation, patients were continued on antiarrhythmic medication, although the mean daily dose of amiodarone decreased from 350 to 225 mg/d, again emphasizing that hybrid therapy is often required for these extremely ill patients.

Finally, it is important for the physician to appreciate the significant psychologic effects of electrical storm [82,83]. In an analysis of the DEFINITE study, implantation of an ICD was not associated with a reduction in quality-of-life indices [82]. Although a single shock was associated with a slight decrease in the emotional and mental components of quality-of-life indices, more frequent shocks led to significant declines in quality of life. Most studies have described reduced quality of life with frequent shocks, particularly once a threshold of five shocks was reached [83–85]. Some preliminary data suggest that ICD shocks have a greater impact on women [83]. Reduced quality of life because of increased anxiety can persist for many months after an episode. Psychologic interventions and a social support network can be useful for treating the anxiety and depression associated with ICD shocks [83,86].

The patient was stabilized with intravenous amiodarone and beta-blockade. For long-term management, sotalol was tried initially, but the patient continued to have device discharges. Because of reluctance to use long-term amiodarone in this young patient, he underwent radiofrequency catheter ablation. He continued aggressive treatment with beta-blockade and afterload reduction. He also became an active member of a local ICD patient support group.

Case 5: hypertrophic cardiomyopathy and nonsustained ventricular arrhythmias

A 28-year-old police officer with the new diagnosis of hypertrophic cardiomyopathy undergoes extensive evaluation. He has complained of shortness of breath with high levels of exertion but has been able to pass the physical tests for his work. He denies any dizziness, syncope, or palpitations. He has undergone echocardiography that demonstrates left ventricular hypertrophy with a septal thickness of 2.5 cm with a minimal resting gradient (20 mm Hg) but a provocable gradient of 64 mm Hg. On exercise testing, he is able to exercise 14 minutes on a standard Bruce Protocol with a normal hemodynamic response during exercise, with his gradient increasing to only 25 mm Hg at peak exercise. He has undergone 24-hour ambulatory monitoring, which demonstrates a 6-beat run of nonsustained ventricular tachycardia at a rate of 130 beats per minute. An uncle died during an automobile accident several years ago. He has one brother and two children.

Hypertrophic cardiomyopathy is a genetic disease characterized by hypertrophy of the left ventricle. The prevalence is estimated to be 0.2%, with approximately 600,000 affected people in the United States [87]. Hypertrophic cardiomyopathy is usually caused by mutations of sarcomere myofilaments or their supporting proteins but can also be attributable to mutations in calcium handling (calcium ATPase, cardiac ryanodine receptor), mitochondria, and lysosomal proteins [88,89].

Two separate issues must be addressed when taking care of patients who have hypertrophic cardiomyopathy. First, the clinician must treat symptoms like shortness of breath or fatigue and determine whether or not symptoms are attributable to left ventricular outflow tract obstruction or diastolic dysfunction. Second, the clinician must estimate an individual patient's risk for sudden cardiac death. Hypertrophic cardiomyopathy is associated with myocyte disorder and development of localized fibrosis and scar tissue that can lead to life-threatening ventricular arrhythmias.

Risk stratification

Although initial data from tertiary medical centers gave the impression that hypertrophic cardiomyopathy is a rare disease with a poor prognosis and high risk for sudden cardiac death, recent population studies suggest that hypertrophic cardiomyopathy is a relatively common problem (prevalence of 1:500) with an annual mortality rate of approximately 1% and a sudden death rate of 0.5% to 0.7% [90–92]. In a single-center cohort study from the Minnesota region, investigators found that during a mean follow-up of 8 years, the diagnosis of hypertrophic cardiomyopathy did not significantly alter life expectancy [93]. Hypertrophic cardiomyopathy is one of the most common medical causes for sudden death in young athletes, however. Given the tragic consequences of sudden unexpected death, particularly in a young person, research has focused on identifying risk factors for sudden cardiac death (Table 1). Cardiac risk factors for sudden cardiac death include prior cardiac arrest or sustained ventricular tachycardia, syncope, a family history of sudden cardiac death

Table 1
Risk factors for sudden cardiac death in hypertrophic cardiomyopathy

Major risk factor	Possible risk factors in individual patients
Cardiac arrest (VF)	AF
Spontaneous sustained VT	Myocardial ischemia
Family history of premature sudden death	LV outflow obstruction
Unexplained syncope	High risk mutation
LV thickness ≥ 30 mm	Intense (competitive) physical exertion
Abnormal exercise BP	
Nonsustained spontaneous VT	

Abbreviations: AF, atrial fibrillation; BP, blood pressure; LV, left ventricular; VF, ventricular fibrillation; VT, ventricular tachycardia.
Data from Maron BJ, McKenna WJ. American College of Cardiology/European Society of Cardiology Clinical Expert Consensus document on hypertrophic cardiomyopathy. J Am Coll Cardiol 2003;42:1703.

(particularly in a first-degree relative), severe left ventricular hypertrophy (> 30 mm), nonsustained ventricular tachycardia on 24-hour ambulatory electrocardiographic monitoring, and a hypotensive response to exercise [92,94]. Several studies found that the presence of several risk factors increased the risk for sudden cardiac death, although a recent case report describes two young patients who had no traditional risk factors for sudden cardiac death but had subsequent appropriate use of their ICDs for treatment of malignant ventricular arrhythmias [90,92,94–96].

Treatment

Sudden cardiac death can be a devastating outcome in young patients who have hypertrophic cardiomyopathy. Although amiodarone and beta-blockade have been used, they are minimally effective for prevention of sudden cardiac death. In a retrospective study, similar sudden death rates were found between patients who had hypertrophic cardiomic cardiomyopathy taking cardiac medications (beta-blockers, calcium channel blockers, or antiarrhythmic medications) and those not on cardiac medications [97].

No prospective trial on the use of ICDs in patients who have hypertrophic cardiomyopathy has been performed, but recent data from a large multicenter registry provide important information. Outcomes in 506 patients who had

hypertrophic cardiomyopathy and ICDs were evaluated: 123 patients for secondary prevention and 383 patients for primary prevention. The annual rate of appropriate discharge was 10.6% per year for secondary prevention and 3.6% per year for primary prevention [96]. These investigators further stratified patients relative to risk factors. Traditional risk factors included a history of premature hypertrophic cardiomyopathy–related sudden death in one or more first-degree or other relatives younger than 50 years of age, massive left ventricular hypertrophy (septum > 30 mm), one or more runs of nonsustained ventricular tachycardia at heart rates of 120 beats per minute or greater on 24-hour ambulatory electrocardiographic monitoring, and prior unexplained syncope not thought to be attributable to neurocardiogenic causes. Interestingly, event rates were similar regardless of whether one, two, or three risk factors were present.

The 2006 sudden death guidelines suggest that ICD implantation is appropriate as a class IIa indication for patients with one or more risk factors for sudden cardiac death (see Table 1) [38]. The 2003 guidelines for management of hypertrophic cardiomyopathy place ICD as primary prevention in the class IIb category with no specific recommendations for the number of risk factors required and emphasize that the decision on whether to implant an ICD should be made after careful discussion between the physician and patient [94]. Major risk factors for sudden cardiac death and potential risk factors for sudden cardiac death in individual patients are listed in Table 1.

It is also important to acknowledge that certain professions may have different requirements for hypertrophic cardiomyopathy and ICD implantation. In Massachusetts, an ICD precludes employment as a police officer or fire fighter, whereas there is no specific discussion of hypertrophic cardiomyopathy other than left ventricular hypertrophy as a possible exclusionary criterion [98]. Similarly, the presence of a defibrillator precludes deployment with the United States Central Command (US CENTCOM), a force that is responsible for security for parts of Africa and Central Asia, with no specific mention of hypertrophic cardiomyopathy [99].

Finally, the role of genetic testing is a rapidly evolving field. Originally, it was hoped that knowledge of specific mutations would provide prognostic information and risk for sudden cardiac death. Unfortunately, because of variable penetrance and expression of the gene, this strategy has not been generally accepted. At this point, genetic testing can be useful for establishing a diagnosis of hypertrophic cardiomyopathy in patients with borderline criteria and for identifying family members at risk. It is important to emphasize the importance of counseling with genetic testing. Unlike most blood tests, results from genetic tests have an impact on family members and can have potentially beneficial (because of knowledge) and harmful (because of guilt and anxiety) effects on family dynamics.

The patient decided to undergo genetic testing that confirmed he had the mutation for hypertrophic cardiomyopathy. The rest of his family was tested, and his brother and son were found to be carriers of the gene but did not manifest any left ventricular hypertrophy on echocardiography. The patient was started on beta-blockade and chose to have a defibrillator implanted. In 1 year of follow-up, he has not had a defibrillator discharge. He was given a medical retirement from the police force and is currently working in sales.

References

[1] Bigger JT, Fleiss JL, Kleiger K, et al. The Multicenter Post-Infarction Research Group. The relationship between ventricular arrhythmias, left ventricular dysfunction, and mortality in the two years after myocardial infarction. Circulation 1984, 69:250–8.

[2] Kostis JB, Byington R, Friedman LM, et al. Prognostic significance of ventricular ectopic activity in survivors of acute myocardial infarction. J Am Coll Cardiol 1987;10:231–42.

[3] Maggioni AP, Zuanetti G, Franzosi MG, et al. Prevalence and prognostic significance of ventricular arrhythmias after acute myocardial infarction in the fibrinolytic era. Circulation 1993;87:312–22.

[4] Hohnloser SH, Klingenheben T, Zabel M, et al. Prevalence, characteristics and prognostic value during long-term follow-up of nonsustained ventricular tachycardia after myocardial infarction in the thrombolytic era. J Am Coll Cardio 1999;33:1895–902.

[5] Huikuri HV, Tapanainen JM, Lindgren K, et al. Prediction of sudden cardiac death after myocardial infarction in the beta-blocking era. J Am Coll Cardiol 2003;42:652–8.

[6] Solomon SD, Zelenkofske S, McMurray JJV, et al. Sudden death in patients with myocardial infarction and left ventricular dysfunction, heart failure, or both. N Engl J Med 2005;352:2581–8.

[7] La Rovere MT, Bigger JT Jr, Marcus FI, et al. Baroreflex sensitivity and heart rate variability in prediction of total cardiac mortality after myocardial infarction. ATRAMI (Autonomic Tone and Reflexes After Myocardial Infarction) Investigators. Lancet 1998;351:478–84.

[8] De Ferrari GM, Sanzo A, Bertoletti A, et al. Baroreflex sensitivity predicts long-term cardiovascular mortality after myocardial infarction even in patients with preserved left ventricular function. J Am Coll Cardiol 2007;50:2285–90.

[9] Ikeda T, Yoshino H, Sugi K, et al. Predictive value of microvolt T wave alternans for sudden cardiac death in patients with preserved cardiac function after acute myocardial infarction. J Am Coll Cardiol 2006;48:2268–74.

[10] Jouven X, Desnos M, Guerot C, et al. Predicting sudden death in the population: the Paris Prospective Study I. Circulation 1999;99:1978–83.

[11] Pilz S, Scharnagl H, Tiran B, et al. Elevated plasma free fatty acids predict sudden cardiac death: a 6.85-year follow-up of 3315 patients after coronary angiography. Eur Heart J 2007;28:2763–9.

[12] Albert CM, Ma J, Rafai N, et al. Prospective study of C-reactive protein, homocysteine, and plasma lipid levels as predictors of sudden cardiac death. Circulation 2002;105:2595–9.

[13] Kannel WB, Thomas HE Jr. Sudden coronary death. The Framingham Study. Ann N Y Acad Sci 1982;382:3–21.

[14] Hallstrom AP, Cobb LA, Ray R. Smoking as a risk factor for recurrence of sudden cardiac arrest. N Engl J Med 1986;314:271–5.

[15] Albert CM, Mittelman MA, Chae CU, et al. Triggering of sudden death from cardiac causes by vigorous exertion. N Engl J Med 2000;343:1355–61.

[16] Krantz DS, Sheps DS, Carney RM, et al. Effects of mental stress in patients with coronary artery disease: evidence and clinical implications. JAMA 2000;283:1800–2.

[17] Lampert R, Joska T, Burg MM, et al. Emotional and physical precipitants of ventricular arrhythmias. Circulation 2002;106:1800–5.

[18] Taylor RS, Brown A, Ebrahim S, et al. Exercise-based rehabilitation for patients with coronary heart disease: systematic review and meta-analysis of randomized controlled trials. Am J Med 2004;116: 682–92.

[19] Burr ML, Fehily AM, Gilbert JF, et al. Effects of changes in fat, fish, and fibre intakes on death and myocardial reinfarction: Diet and Reinfarction Trial (DART). Lancet 1989;2:757–61.

[20] Dietary supplementation with n-3 polyunsaturated fatty acids and vitamin E after myocardial infarction: results of the GISSI Prevenzione trial. Gruppo Italiano per lo Studio della Sopravvivenza nell'infarto Miocardico. Lancet 1999;354:447–55.

[21] The Long-Term Intervention with Pravastatin in Ischemic Disease (LIPID) Study Group. Prevention of cardiovascular events and death with pravastatin

in patients with coronary heart disease and a broad range of initial cholesterol levels. N Engl J Med 1998;339:1349–57.

[22] Levantesi G, Scarano M, Marfisi R, et al. Meta-analysis of effect of statin treatment on risk of sudden death. Am J Cardiol 2007;100:1644–50.

[23] The Norwegian Multicenter Study Group. Timolol induced reduction in mortality and reinfarction in patients surviving acute myocardial infarction. N Engl J Med 1981;304:801–7.

[24] Beta Blocker Heart Attack Trial Research Group. A randomized trial of propranolol in patients with acute myocardial infarction, I: mortality results. JAMA 1982;247:1707–14.

[25] Domanski M, Exner D, Borkowf C, et al. Effect of angiotensin converting enzyme inhibition on sudden cardiac death in patients following a myocardial infarction: a meta-analysis of randomized clinical trials. J Am Coll Cardiol 1999;33:598–604.

[26] Fox KM, European Trial on Reduction of Cardiac Events with Perindopril in Stable Coronary Artery Disease Investigators. Efficacy of perindopril in reduction of cardiovascular events among patients with stable coronary artery disease: randomised, double-blind, placebo-controlled, multicentre trial (the EUROPA study). Lancet 2003;362:782–8.

[27] Braunwald E, Domanski MJ, Fowler SE, et al, Peace Trial Investigators. Angiotensin-converting enzyme inhibition in stable coronary artery disease. N Engl J Med 2004;351:2058–68.

[28] Mäkikallio TH, Barthel P, Schneider R, et al. Frequency of sudden cardiac death among acute myocardial infarction survivors with optimized medical and revascularization therapy. Am J Cardiol 2006;97:480–4.

[29] Preliminary report: effect of flecainide and encainide on mortality in a randomized trial of arrhythmia suppression after myocardial infarction. The Cardiac Arrhythmia Suppression Trial (CAST) Investigators. N Engl J Med 1989;321:406–12.

[30] Cairns JA, Connolly SJ, Roberts R, et al. Randomised trial of outcome after myocardial infarction in patients with frequent or repetitive ventricular premature depolarisations: CAMIAT. Lancet 1997;349:675–82.

[31] Julian DG, Prescott RJ, Jackson FS, et al. Controlled trial of sotalol for one year after myocardial infarction. Lancet 1982;1:1142–7.

[32] Camm AJ, Pratt CM, Schwartz PJ, et al, Azimilide Post Infarct Survival Evaluation (ALIVE) Investigators. Mortality in patients after a recent myocardial infarction: a randomized placebo-controlled trial of azimilide using heart rate variability for risk stratification. Circulation 2004;109:990–6.

[33] Køber L, Bloch-Thomsen PE, Møller M, et al. Effect of dofetilide in patients with recent myocardial infarction and left-ventricular dysfunction: a randomised trial. Lancet 2000;356:2052–8.

[34] Available at: www.cdc.gov/MMWR/preview/mmwrhtml/mm5206a2.htm Accessed January 9, 2008.

[35] Ruskin JN. Implantable cardioverter defibrillator utilization based on discharge diagnoses from Medicare and managed care patients. J Cardiovasc Electrophysiol 2002;13:38–43.

[36] Bardy GH, Lee KL, Mark DB, et al. Amiodarone or an implantable cardioverter-defibrillator for congestive heart failure. N Engl J Med 2005;352:225–37.

[37] Hunt SA. ACC/AHA 2005 guideline update for the diagnosis and management of chronic heart failure in the adult: a report of the American College of Cardiology/American Heart Association Task Force on Practice Guidelines (Writing Committee to update the 2001 guidelines for the evaluation and management of heart failure). J Am Coll Cardiol 2005;46:E1–82.

[38] Zipes DP, Camm AJ, Borggrefe M, et al, American College of Cardiology/American Heart Association Task Force, European Society of Cardiology Committee for Practice Guidelines, European Heart Rhythm Association, Heart Rhythm Society. ACC/AHA/ESC 2006 guidelines for management of patients with ventricular arrhythmias and the prevention of sudden cardiac death: a report of the American College of Cardiology/American Heart Association Task Force and the European Society of Cardiology Committee for Practice Guidelines (Writing Committee to develop guidelines for management of patients with ventricular arrhythmias and the prevention of sudden cardiac death): developed in collaboration with the European Heart Rhythm Association and the Heart Rhythm Society. Circulation 2006;114:E385–484.

[39] Peterson MA, Hafley G, Lee KL, et al. Do the elderly benefit from defibrillator therapy as primary prevention in coronary artery disease and left ventricular dysfunction? Pacing Clin Electrophysiol 2003;26:973 [abstract].

[40] Koplen BA, Epstein LM, Albert CM, et al. Survival in octogenarians receiving implantable defibrillators. Am Heart J 2006;152:714–9.

[41] Pantopoulos PT, Axtell K, Snderson AJ, et al. Efficacy of the implantable cardioverter-defibrillator in the elderly. J Am Coll Cardiol 1997;29:556–60.

[42] Noseworthy PA, Lashevsky I, Dorian P, et al. Feasibility of implantable cardioverter defibrillator use in elderly patients: a case series of octogenarians. Pacing Clin Electrophysiol 2004;27:373–8.

[43] Reynolds MR, Cohen DJ, Kugelmass AD, et al. The frequency and incremental cost of major complications among Medicare beneficiaries receiving implantable cardioverter-defibrillators. J Am Coll Cardiol 2006;47:2493–7.

[44] Grimm W, Stula A, Sharkova J, et al. Outcomes of elderly recipients of implantable cardioverter defibrillators. Pacing Clin Electrophysiol 2007; 30(Suppl 1):34–8.

[45] Dec GW, Fuster V. Idiopathic dilated cardio-myopathy. N Engl J Med 1994;331:1564–75.

[46] Grimm W, Christ M, Bach J, et al. Noninvasive arrhythmia risk stratification in idiopathic dilated cardiomyopathy. Results of the Marburg Cardio-myopathy Study. Circulation 2003;108:2883–91.

[47] Iacoviello M, Forleo C, Guida P, et al. Ventricular repolarization dynamicity provides independent prognostic information toward major arrhythmic events in patients with dilated cardiomyopathy. J Am Coll Cardiol 2007;50:225–31.

[48] Baker RL, Koelling TM. Prognostic value of ambulatory electrocardiography monitoring in pa-tients with dilated cardiomyopathy. J Electrocardiol 2005;38:64–8.

[49] Hohnloser SH, Klingenheben T, Bloomfield D, et al. Usefulness of microvolt T-wave alternans for prediction of ventricular tachyarrhythmic events in patients with dilated cardiomyopathy: results from a prospective observational study. J Am Coll Cardiol 2003;41:2220–4.

[50] Effect of enalapril on survival in patients with reduced left ventricular ejection fractions and congestive heart failure. The SOLVD Investigators. N Engl J Med 1991;325:293–302.

[51] The Cardiac Insufficiency Bisoprolol Study II (CIBIS II): a randomized trial. Lancet 1999;353:9–13.

[52] Singh SN, Fletcher RD, Fischer SG, et al. Amiodar-one in patients with congestive heart failure and asymptomatic ventricular arrhythmia. Survival Trial of Antiarrhythmic Therapy in Congestive Heart Failure. N Engl J Med 1995;333:77–82.

[53] Bänsch D, Antz M, Boczor S, et al. Primary prevention of sudden cardiac death in idiopathic dilated cardiomyopathy: the Cardiomyopathy Trial (CAT). Circulation 2002;105(12):1453–8.

[54] Kadish A, Dyer A, Daubert JP, et al. Prophylactic de-fibrillator implantation in patients with nonischemic cardiomyopathy. N Engl J Med 2004;350:2151–8.

[55] Steimle AE, Stevenson LW, Foranow GC, et al. Prediction of improvement in recent onset cardio-myopathy after referral for heart transplantation. J Am Coll Cardiol 1994;23:553–9.

[56] Kadish A, Scaechter A, Subacius H, et al. Patients with recently diagnosed nonischemic cardio-myopathy benefit from implantable cardioverter defibrillators. J Am Coll Cardiol 2006;47:2477–82.

[57] Khanlou H, Paltoo B, Forbes W. Echocardio-graphic parameters in reversible idiopathic dilated cardiomyopathy. Am J Med Sci 2000;319:366–9.

[58] Cicoira M, Zanolla L, Latina L, et al. Frequency, prognosis and predictors of systolic left ventricular function in patients with 'classical' clinical diagnosis of idiopathic dilated cardiomyopathy. Eur J Heart Fail 2001;3:323–30.

[59] Assomull RG, Prasad SK, Lyne J, et al. Cardiovas-cular magnetic resonance, fibrosis, and prognosis in dilated cardiomyopathy. J Am Coll Cardiol 2006;48:1977–85.

[60] Sugiura T, Takase H, Toriyama T, et al. Circulating levels of myocardial proteins predict future deterio-ration of congestive heart failure. J Card Fail 2005;11:504–9.

[61] Duffee DF, Shen WK, Smith HC. Suppression of frequent premature ventricular contractions and im-provement of left ventricular function in patients with presumed idiopathic dilated cardiomyopathy. Mayo Clin Proc 1988;7:430–3.

[62] Takemoto M, Yoshimura H, Ohba Y, et al. Radio-frequency catheter ablation of premature ventricular complexes from the right ventricular outflow tract improves left ventricular dilation and clinical status in patients without structural heart disease. J Am Coll Cardiol 2005;45:1259–65.

[63] Bogun F, Crawford T, reich S, et al. Radiofrequency ablation of frequent, idiopathic premature ventricu-lar complexes: comparison with a control group without intervention. Heart Rhythm 2007;4:863–7.

[64] Verma A, Kilicaslan F, Marrouche NF, et al. Preva-lence, predictors, and mortality significance of the causative arrhythmia in patients with electrical storm. J Cardiovasc Electrophysiol 2004;15:1265–70.

[65] Villacastin J, Almendral J, Arenal A, et al. Incidence and clinical significance of multiple consecutive, ap-propriate, high energy discharges in patients with implanted cardioverter-defibrillators. Circulation 1996;93:753–62.

[66] Exner DV, Pinski SL, Wyse DG, et al. Electrical storm presages nonsudden death: the Antiarrhyth-mics Versus Implantable Defibrillators (AVID) Trial. Circulation 2001;103:2066–71.

[67] Arya A, Haghjoo M, Dehghani MR, et al. Preva-lence and predictors of electrical storm in patients with implantable cardioverter-defibrillator. Am J Cardiol 2006;97:389–92.

[68] Furushima H, Chinuhi M, Okamura K, et al. Effect of Dl sotalol on mortality and recurrence of ventricular tachyarrhythmias: ischemic compared to nonischemic cardiomyopathy. Pacing Clin Electrophysiol 2007;30:1136–41.

[69] Sesselberg HW, Moss AJ, McNitt S, et al. Ventricu-lar arrhythmia storms in postinfarction patients with implantable defibrillators for primary prevention indications: a MADIT-II substudy. Heart Rhythm 2007;4:1395–402.

[70] Bansch D, Bocker D, Brunn J, et al. Clusters of ventricular tachycardias signify impaired survival in patients with idiopathic dilated cardiomyopathy and implantable cardioverter defibrillators. J Am Coll Cardiol 2000;36:566–73.

[71] Credner SC, Klingenheben T, Mauss O, et al. Elec-trical storm in patients with transvenous implantable cardioverter-defibrillators. J Am Coll Cardiol 1998;32:1909–15.

[72] Kowey PR, Levine JH, Herre JM, et al. Random-ized, double-blind comparison of intravenous amiodarone and bretylium in the treatment of pa-tients with recurrent, hemodynamically destabilizing

ventricular tachycardia or fibrillation. The Intravenous Amiodarone Multicenter Investigators Group. Circulation 1995;92:3255–63.

[73] The International Guidelines 2000 for CPR and ECC. A comprehensive review of the current evidence and recommendation for antiarrhythmic usage in emergency cardiovascular care and cardiopulmonary resuscitation. Circulation 2000;102:I112–28.

[74] Nademanee K, Taylor R, Bailey WE, et al. Treating electrical storm: sympathetic blockade versus advanced cardiac life-support therapy. Circulation 2000;102:742–7.

[75] Burjorjee JE, Milne B. Propofol for electrical storm; a case report of cardioversion and suppression of ventricular tachycardia by propofol. Can J Anaesth 2002;49:973–7.

[76] Sweeney MO, Wathen MS, Volosin K, et al. Appropriate and inappropriate ventricular therapies, quality of life, and mortality among primary and secondary prevention implantable cardioverter defibrillator patients: results from the Pacing Fast VT REduces Shock ThErapies (PainFREE Rx II) trial. Circulation 2005;111:2898–905.

[77] Pogwizd SM, McKenzie JP, Cain ME. Mechanisms underlying spontaneous and induced ventricular arrhythmias in patients with idiopathic dilated cardiomyopathy. Circulation 1998;98:2404–14.

[78] Connolly SJ, Dorian P, Roberts RS, et al, Optimal Pharmacological Therapy in Cardioverter Defibrillator Patients (OPTIC) Investigators. Comparison of beta-blockers, amiodarone plus beta-blockers, or sotalol for prevention of shocks from implantable cardioverter defibrillators: the OPTIC Study: a randomized trial. JAMA 2006;295:165–71.

[79] Goldschlager N, Epstein AE, Naccarelli GV, et al, Practice Guidelines Sub-Committee, North American Society of Pacing and Electrophysiology (IIRS). A practical guide for clinicians who treat patients with amiodarone: 2007. Heart Rhythm 2007;4(9):1250–9.

[80] Marrouche NF, Verma A, Wazni O, et al. Mode of initiation and ablation of ventricular fibrillation storms in patients with ischemic cardiomyopathy. J Am Coll Cardiol 2004;43:1715–20.

[81] Carbucicchio C, Santamaria M, Trevisi N, et al. Catheter ablation for the treatment of electrical storm in patients with implantable cardioverter-defibrillators. Short- and long-term outcomes in a prospective single-center study. Circulation, 2008; 117(4):462–9..

[82] Passman R, Subacius H, Ruo B, et al. Implantable cardioverter defibrillators and quality of life: results from the defibrillators in nonischemic cardiomyopathy treatment evaluation study. Arch Intern Med 2007;167:2226–32.

[83] Bostwick JM, Sola CL. An updated review of implantable cardioverter/defibrillators, induced anxiety, and quality of life. Psychiatr Clin North Am 2007;30:677–88.

[84] Namerow PB, Firth BR, Heywood GM, et al. Quality-of-life six months after CABG surgery in patients randomized to ICD versus no ICD therapy: findings from the CABG Patch Trial. Pacing Clin Electrophysiol 1999;22:1305–13.

[85] Irvine J, Dorian P, Baker B, et al. Quality of life in the Canadian Implantable Defibrillator Study (CIDS). Am Heart J 2002;144:282–9.

[86] Pedersen SS, van den Broek KC, Sears SF Jr. Psychological intervention following implantation of an implantable defibrillator: a review and future recommendations. Pacing Clin Electrophysiol 2007;30:1546–54.

[87] Maron BJ, Gardin JM, Flack JM, et al. Prevalence of hypertrophic cardiomyopathy in a general population of young adults: echocardiographic analysis of 4,111 subjects in the CARDIA study: coronary artery risk development in (young) adults. Circulation 1995;92:785–9.

[88] Bos JM, Ommen SR, Ackerman MJ. Genetics of hypertrophic cardiomyopathy: one, two, or more diseases. Curr Opin Cardiol 2007;22:193–9.

[89] Arad M, Maron BJ, Gorham JM, et al. Glycogen storage diseases presenting as hypertrophic cardiomyopathy. N Engl J Med 2005;352:362–72.

[90] McKenna WJ, England D, Doi YL, et al. Arrhythmia in hypertrophic cardiomyopathy. I: influence on prognosis. Br Heart J 1981;46:168–72.

[91] Maron BJ, Casey SA, Poliac AC, et al. Clinical course of hypertrophic cardiomyopathy in a regional United States cohort. JAMA 1999;281:160–5.

[92] Ommen SR, Nishimura RA. Hypertrophic cardiomyopathy. Curr Probl Cardiol 2004;29:239–91.

[93] Maron BJ, Olivotto I, Spirito P, et al. Epidemiology of hypertrophic cardiomyopathy-related death: revisited in a large non-referral-based patient population. Circulation 2000;102:858–64.

[94] Maron BJ, McKenna WJ. American College of Cardiology/European Society of Cardiology Clinical Expert Consensus document on hypertrophic cardiomyopathy. J Am Coll Cardiol 2003;42:1687–713.

[95] Maron BJ, Maron MS, Lesser JR, et al. Sudden cardiac arrest in hypertrophic cardiomyopathy in the absence of conventional criteria for high risk status. Am J Cardiol 2008;101(4):544–7.

[96] Maron BJ, Spirito P, Shen WK, et al. Implantable cardioverter-defibrillators and prevention of sudden cardiac death in hypertrophic cardiomyopathy. JAMA 2007;298(4):405–12.

[97] Melacini P, Maron BJ, Bobbo F, et al. Evidence that pharmacological strategies lack efficacy for the prevention of sudden death in hypertrophic cardiomyopathy. Heart 2007;93(6):708–10.

[98] Available at: www.masschiefs.org/CIVIL%20 SERVICE%20INITIAL%20PUBLIC%20SAFETY %20MEDICAL%20STANDARDS.pdf. Accessed January 9, 2008.

[99] chppm. Available at: www.apgea.army.mil/ documents/FitnessforDeployment.pdf. Accessed January 9, 2008.

ELSEVIER
SAUNDERS

Cardiol Clin 26 (2008) 497–505

CARDIOLOGY
CLINICS

Index

Note: Page numbers of article titles are in **boldface** type.

A

Ablation, catheter, in ventricular arrhythmias, **459–479.** See also *Catheter ablation, in ventricular arrhythmias.*

Ablative therapy, in ventricular arrhythmia management in heart failure patients, 394–395

ACC/AHA Prevention of Sudden Cardiac Death Guidelines (2006), 484

Activation mapping, in catheter ablation in ventricular arrhythmias, 464

AHA/ACC 2005 Heart Failure Guidelines, 484

ALIVE trial. See *Azimilide Post-infarct Survival Evaluation (ALIVE) trial.*

Ambulatory ECG monitoring, in risk stratification, 359

American College of Cardiology/American Heart Association (ACC/AHA) Prevention of Sudden Cardiac Death Guidelines (2006), 484

American Heart Association, 433

American Heart Association Statistics Committee, 321

American Heart Association/American College of Cardiology (AHA/ACC) 2005 Heart Failure Guidelines, 484

Amiodarone, for VT/VF and sudden cardiac death, 408

Amiodarone Trials Meta-Analysis, 409

Amiodarone versus Implantable Cardioverter-Defibrillator Trial (AMIOVIRT), 425

AMIOVIRT. See *Amiodarone versus Implantable Cardioverter-Defibrillator Trial (AMIOVIRT).*

Antiarrhythmic drugs
for VT/VF and sudden death, 405–410

Class I, 405–406
Class II, 406
Class III, 407–408
Class IV, 410
digoxin, 413–414
statins, 410–411
unresolved issues related to, 434–435

Antiarrhythmics versus Implantable Defibrillators (AVID) trial, 419–422

Arrhythmia(s)
triggered, in heart failure patients, 382–384
ventricular. See also specific types and *Ventricular arrhythmias.*
antiarrhythmic drugs for, 405–410. See also *Ventricular arrhythmias, drug therapy for, antiarrhythmic drugs.*
management of, **481–496**

Arrhythmogenic cardiomyopathies, 346–350

Arrhythmogenic right ventricular dysplasia (ARVD), types of, 347–349

Arrhythmogenic right ventricular dysplasia/cardiomyopathy, VT ablation in, 473–474

Arrhythmogenic RV dysplasia/cardiomyopathy, in heart failure patients, 387–388

ARVD. See *Arrhythmogenic right ventricular dysplasia (ARVD),*

ATRAMI trial. See *Autonomic Tone and Reflexes after Myocardial Infarction (ATRAMI) trial.*

Automatic ventricular tachycardia, in normal hearts, 377

Autonomic Tone and Reflexes after Myocardial Infarction (ATRAMI) trial, 390, 482

Autosomal dominant inheritance, ventricular arrhythmias and, 335–336

Autosomal recessive inheritance, ventricular arrhythmias and, 336